D1739806

Novel Medical and General Hebrew Terminology from the 13th Century

Novel Medical and General Hebrew Terminology from the 13th Century

VOLUME 4

By

Gerrit Bos

BRILL

LEIDEN | BOSTON

The cover illustration hails from Biblioteca universitaria di Bologna Ms 2197, fol. 492r. It represents a scene in an open air pharmacy, featuring on the title page of Book five of Nathan ha-Me'ati's Hebrew translation of Ibn Sīnā's *Kitāb al-Qānūn*. The manuscript was copied c. 1440.

Library of Congress Cataloging-in-Publication Data

Names: Bos, Gerrit, 1948– author.
Title: Novel medical and general Hebrew terminology from the 13th century. Volume 4 / by Gerrit Bos.
Other titles: Hebrew terminology from the 13th century
Description: Leiden ; Boston : Brill, [2018] | Includes bibliographical references and indexes.
Identifiers: LCCN 2018040747 (print) | LCCN 2018044446 (ebook) | ISBN 9789004382626 (E-book) | ISBN 9789004382619 (hardback : alk. paper)
Subjects: LCSH: Medicine—Terminology. | Hebrew language, Medieval—Glossaries, vocabularies, etc. | Hebrew language—Technical Hebrew—History—13th century.
Classification: LCC R123 (ebook) | LCC R123 .B6682 2018 (print) | DDC 610.1/4—dc 3
LC record available at https://lccn.loc.gov/2018040747

Typeface for the Latin, Greek, and Cyrillic scripts: "Brill". See and download: brill.com/brill-typeface.

ISBN 978-90-04-38261-9 (hardback)
ISBN 978-90-04-38262-6 (e-book)

Copyright 2019 by Koninklijke Brill NV, Leiden, The Netherlands.
Koninklijke Brill NV incorporates the imprints Brill, Brill Hes & De Graaf, Brill Nijhoff, Brill Rodopi, Brill Sense, Hotei Publishing, mentis Verlag, Verlag Ferdinand Schöningh and Wilhelm Fink Verlag.
All rights reserved. No part of this publication may be reproduced, translated, stored in a retrieval system, or transmitted in any form or by any means, electronic, mechanical, photocopying, recording or otherwise, without prior written permission from the publisher.
Authorization to photocopy items for internal or personal use is granted by Koninklijke Brill NV provided that the appropriate fees are paid directly to The Copyright Clearance Center, 222 Rosewood Drive, Suite 910, Danvers, MA 01923, USA. Fees are subject to change.

This book is printed on acid-free paper and produced in a sustainable manner.

Printed by Printforce, United Kingdom

Contents

Abbreviations

a — Arabic text
Ms[1] — marginal note in the Ms
Ms[2] — supralinear note in the Ms

AB — A. Arberry, 'A Bagdad Cookery Book', in: *Medieval Arab Cookery: Essays and Translations*, ed. by M. Rodinson, A.J. Arberry, and C. Perry (Blackawton 2001), 37–89.

AEY — P. Auerbach and M. Ezrahi, 'Yalqut Ṣemahim', *Leshonenu* 1 (1929): 161–395.

BAN — W.S. van den Berg, *Eene middelnederlandsche vertaling van het 'Antidotarium Nicolaï' (Ms. 15624–15641, Kon. Bibl. Te Brussel) met den Latijnschen tekst der eerste gedrukte uitgave van het Antidotarium Nicolaï* (Leiden 1917).

BDB — F. Brown, S.R. Driver and C.A. Briggs, *A Hebrew and English Lexicon of the Old Testament*, with an Appendix containing the Biblical Aramaic, based on the Lexicon of William Gesenius as translated by Edward Robinson (Repr., Oxford 1978).

BK — Y. Brand, *Klei ha-Ḥeres be-Sifrut ha-Talmud* (*Ceramics in Talmudic Literature*) (Jerusalem 1953).

BM — E. Ben Yehuda, *Millon ha-Lashon ha-Ivrit: Thesaurus Totius Hebraitatis et Veteris et Recentioris*, 17 vols. (Repr., Tel Aviv 1948–59).

BMZ — G. Bos, G. Mensching and J. Zwink, *Medical Glossaries in the Hebrew Tradition: Shem Tov Ben Isaac, Sefer Almansur*, with a Supplement on the Romance and Latin Terminology (Leiden 2017).

CPD — D.N. MacKenzie, *A Concise Pahlavi Dictionary* (London 1971).

D — R.P.A. Dozy, *Supplément aux Dictionnaires arabes*, 2 vols. (Leiden 1927).

DAS — G. Dalman, *Arbeit und Sitte in Palästina*, 8 vols. (Repr., Hildesheim 1964–87).

DECLC — J. Coromines, *Diccionari etimològic i complementari de la llengua catalana*, Barcelona 1980–91.

DKT — P. De Koning, *Trois traités d'anatomie arabes*, ed. by F. Sezgin (Repr., Frankfurt 1986).

DT — *Dioscurides Triumphans: Ein anonymer arabischer Kommentar (Ende 12. Jahr. n. Chr.) zur Materia medica*, Arabischer Text nebst kommentierter deutscher Übersetzung, ed. by A Dietrich, 2 vols. = Abhandlungen der Akademie der Wissenschaften in Göttingen,

Philologisch-Historische Klasse, vol. 3.172 (Göttingen 1988).

EG J. N. Epstein, *Perush ha-Ge'onim le-Seder Tohorot: The Gaonic Commentary on the Order Tohorot attributed to Rav Hay Gaon*, ed. with Introduction and Notes (Jerusalem 1982).

EI^2 *The Encyclopaedia of Islam*, new ed., 12 vols. (Leiden 1960–2004).

EJ^2 *Encyclopaedia Judaica*, 2nd ed., 22 vols. (Detroit 2007).

EM A. Even-Shoshan, *Ha-Millon he- Ḥadash*, 7 vols. (Repr., Jerusalem 1983).

EP I. Efros, *Philosophical Terms in the Moreh Nebukim* (New York 1924).

FA S. Fraenkel, *Die aramäischen Fremdwörter im Arabischen* (Leiden 1886).

FAL A. Fonahn, *Arabic and Latin Anatomical Terminology, chiefly from the Middle Ages* (Kristiana 1922).

FAQ I. Fellmann, *Das Aqrābāḏīn al-Qalānisī: Quellenkritische und begriffsanalytische Untersuchung zur arabisch-pharmazeutischen Literatur* (Beirut 1986).

FEW W. von Wartburg, *Französisches Etymologisches Wörterbuch* (Bonn-Leipzig-Tübingen-Basilea 1922–87).

FZ U. Feldman, *Ṣimḥei ha-Mishnah* (Tel Aviv n.d.).

FL G. W. Freytag, *Lexicon Arabico-Latinum*, 4 vols. (Halis Saxonum 1830–37).

FM J. Feliks, *Mar'ot ha-Mishnah, Seder Zera'im* (Jerusalem 1967).

HA J. Hyrtl, *Das Arabische und Hebräische in der Anatomie* (Vienna 1879).

HM S. Heymans, *Ha-Millim ha-She'ulot mi-Yewanit u-mi-Latinit ba-Mishnah: Leksikon we-Torat Hegeh* (PhD diss., Tel Aviv 2013).

IBA *Ibn al-Bayṭār, al-Jāmiʿ li-mufradāt al-adwiya wa l-aghdhiya*, 4 pts. in 2 vols. (Beirut 1992).

IBF Ibn al-Bayṭār, *Traité des simples*, trans. by L. Leclerc, 3 vols. (Paris 1877–83).

IJ Ibn Janāḥ, *Abū l-Walīd Marwān, Kitāb al-uṣūl: The Book of Hebrew Roots*, ed. by A. Neubauer (Oxford 1875).

IJZ Ibn al-Jazzār, *Zād al-musāfir wa-qūt al-ḥāḍir, Provisions for the Traveller and Nourishment for the Sedentary, Book 7 (7–30)*. Critical ed. of the Arabic Text with English trans., and Critical ed. of Moses ibn Tibbon's Hebrew Translation (*Ṣedat ha-Derakhim*), ed. and trans. by G. Bos (Leiden 2015).

ISW Ibn Sayyār al-Warrāq, *Kitāb al-ṭabīkh*, ed. by K. Öhrnberg and S. Mroueh, = Studia Orientalia, vol. 60 (Helsinki 1987).

JAD Ad-Damīrī, *Ḥayāt al-Ḥayawān* (*A Zoological Lexicon*), trans.

by A. S. G. Jayakar, 2 vols. (London 1906–8).

JD M. Jastrow, *A Dictionary of the Targumim, the Talmud Bavli and Yerushalmi, and the Midrashic Literature*, 2 vols. (Repr., New York 1950).

JNK Judah Ben Solomon Natan, *Kelal Qaẓar mi ha-Sammim ha-Nifradim* (= Hebrew translation of Abū Ṣalt's *K. al-Adwiya al-mufrada* (*On Simple Medicines*), in: M. Steinschneider, 'Abu's-'Salt (gest. 1134) und seine Simplicia, ein Beitrag zur Heilmittellehre der Araber', *Archiv für pathologische Anatomie und Physiologie und für klinische Medicin* 94.9.4 (1883): 28–65.

KA A. Kohut, *Arukh shalem: Aruch Completum*, and S. Krauss, *Tosefet he-Arukh. Additamenta*, 9 vols. (Repr., Tel Aviv 1970).

KB L. Koehler and W. Baumgartner, *The Hebrew and Aramaic Lexicon of the Old Testament*, subsequently rev. by W. Baumgartner and J. J. Stamm, with assistance from B. Hartmann, Z. Ben-Hayyim, E. Y. Kutscher, P. Reymond., ed. and trans. under the supervision of M. E. J. Richardson, 2 vols. (Leiden 2001).

KDS D. Kaufmann, *Die Sinne: Beiträge zur Geschichte der Physiologie und Psychologie im Mittelalter aus hebräischen und arabischen Quellen* (Jahresbericht der Landes-Rabbinerschule in Budapest für das Schuljahr 1883–84), repr. in: idem., *Die Spuren al-Baṭaljûsi's* (*Budapest 1880*), *and Studien über Salomon Ibn Gabirol* (*Budapest 1899*), *and Die Sinne* (*Budapest 1884*), with an introduction by L. Jacobs (Farnborough 1972).

KL S. Krauss, *Griechische und Lateinische Lehnwörter im Talmud, Midrasch und Targum*, with comments by I. Löw, 2 vols. (Berlin 1898–9).

KM F. Käs, *Die Mineralien in der arabischen Pharmakognosie: Eine Konkordanz zur mineralischen Materia medica der klassischen arabischen Heilmittelkunde nebst überlieferungsgeschichtlichen Studien*, 2 vols. = Akademie der Wissenschaften und der Literatur Mainz. Veröffentlichungen der Orientalischen Kommission, vol. 54 (Wiesbaden 2010).

KT S. Krauss, *Talmudische Archäologie*, 3 vols. (Leipzig 1910–2).

KTD O. Kahl, *The Dispensatory of Ibn at-Tilmiḏ: Arabic Text, English trans., Study and Glossaries* (Leiden 2007).

KTM I. L. Katzenelsohn, *Ha-Talmud we-Hokmat ha-Refu'ah: Talmud und Medizin* (Berlin 1928).

KTP J. Klatzkin, *Thesaurus Philosophicus linguae hebraicae et veteris et recentioris*, 4 pts. in 2 vols. (Repr., New York 1968).

KZ H. Kroner, *Zur Terminologie der arabischen Medizin und zu ihrem zeitgenössischen hebräischen Ausdrucke: An der Hand dreier medizinischer Abhandlungen des Maimonides* (Berlin 1921).

L E. W. Lane, *Arabic-English Lexicon*, 8 vols. (London 1863–79).

LF I. Löw, *Die Flora der Juden*, 4 vols. (Repr., Hildesheim 1967).

LFA I. Löw, *Fauna und Mineralien der Juden*, with an introduction by A. Schreiber (Repr., Hildesheim 1969).

LOW A. Lowinger, 'Register of Hebrew and Aramaic Terms, translated and edited by S. Paley': in: J. Preuss, *Biblisch-talmudische Medizin. Beiträge zur Geschichte der Heilkunde und der Kultur überhaupt* (Repr., New York 1971).

LR F. J. Raynouard, *Lexique roman: Ou dictionnaire de la langue des troubadours comparée avec les autres langues de l'Europe latine* (Heidelberg 1970).

LRM R. E.Latham, *Revised Medieval Latin Word-list from British and Irish Sources*, with Supplement (Repr., London 2008).

LS C. Lewis and C. Short, *A Latin Dictionary Founded on Andrews' Latin Dictionary*, rev., enl., and in great part rewritten (Oxford 1966).

LSG H. G. Liddell and R. Scott, *A Greek English Lexicon*, rev. and augmented throughout by H. S. Jones, a.o., with a supplement (Repr., Oxford 1989).

LW J. Levy, *Wörterbuch über die Talmudim und Midraschim*, nebst Beiträgen von H. Leberecht Fleischer. 2nd ed., mit Nachträgen und Berichtigungen von L. Goldschmidt, 4 vols. (Berlin 1924).

LZ L. Lewysohn, *Zoologie des Talmuds* (Frankfurt 1858).

MA A. Melzer, *Asaph the Physician—The Man and his Book: A Historical-Philological Study of the Medical Treatise, The Book of Drugs* (ספר רפואות). (PhD diss., Wisconsin 1927).

MB M. Marin, 'Beyond Taste: The Complements of Colour and Smell in the Medieval Arab Culinary Tradition,' in: *Culinary Cultures of the Middle East*, ed. by R. Tapper and S. Zubaida (London 1994).

MIG Marwan Ibn Ǧanāḥ, *Kitāb al-Talḫīṣ*, ed. and trans. By G. Bos, F. Käs, G. Mensching and M. Lübke (forthcoming).

MK Maimonides, *Mishnah ʿim Perush Rabbeinu Mosheh Ben Maimon. Maqor we-Targum*, ed. by J. Kafiḥ, 6 pts. in 7 vols.

(Jerusalem 1963–1969): MK 1 = *Zeraʿim*; MK 2 = *Moʿed*; MK 3 = *Nashim*; MK 4 = *Nezikin*; MK 5 = *Kodashin*; MK 6 = *Toharot*.

MM S. Muntner, *Mavo-le-Sefer Asaph ha-Rofe* (Jerusalem 1957).

MMS Maimonides, *Sharḥ asmāʾ al-ʿuqqār, un glossaire de matière médicale composé par Maïmonide*, ed. by M. Meyerhof (Cairo 1940), repr. in: *Islamic Medicine*, vol. 63, ed. by F. Sezgin (Frankfurt 1996).

MMT M. Meyerhof (ed.), *The Book of the Ten Treatises on the Eye Asribed to Ḥunain ibn Isḥāq (809.877 AD)* (Cairo 1928), and: *Al-morchid fi'l kohhl ou le guide d'oculiste: Ouvrage inédit de l'oculiste arabe-espagnol Mohammad ibn Qassoûm ibn Aslam al-Ghâfiqî* (Barcelona 1933); repr. in: *Augenheilkunde im Islam: Texte, Studien und Übersetzungen*, vol. 2: *Werke von Ḥunain b. Ishaq und Muḥammad al-Ġāfiqī*, ed. by F. Sezgin. = Veröffentlichungen des Institutes für Geschichte der Arabisch-Islamischen Wissenschaften, Reihe B: Nachdrucke, Abteilung Medizin, vol. 3.2 (Frankfurt 1986).

MWK M. Marín and D. Waines (eds.), *Kanz al-fawāʾid fī tanwīʿ al-mawāʾid* (*Medieval Arab/Islamic Culinary Art*) (Stuttgart 1993).

NA N. Nasrallah, *Annals from the Kaliphs' Kitchens: Ibn Sayyār al-Warrāq's Tenth-Century Baghdadi Cookbook*, English trans. with Introduction and Glossary, = Islamic History and Civilization, vol. 70 (Leiden 2007).

NM 1 G. Bos, *Novel Medical and General Hebrew Terminology from the 13th Century: Translations by Hillel Ben Samuel of Verona, Moses Ben Samuel Ibn Tibbon, Shem Tov Ben Isaac of Tortosa, and Zeraḥyah Ben Isaac Ben She'altiel Ḥen*, = *Journal of Semitic Studies*, Suppl. 27 (Oxford 2011).

NM 2 G. Bos, *Novel Medical and General Hebrew Terminology from the 13th Century, Volume Two*, = *Journal of Semitic Studies*, Suppl. 30 (Oxford 2013).

NM 3 G. Bos, *Novel Medical and General Hebrew Terminology: Hippocrates' Aphorisms in the Hebrew Tradition*, = *Journal of Semitic Studies*, Suppl. 37 (Oxford 2016).

PD C. Perry (trans.), 'The Description of Familiar Foods. *Kitāb waṣf al-aṭʿima al-muʿtāda*', in: *Medieval Arab Cookery: Essays and Translations*, ed. by M. Rodinson, A. J. Arberry, and C. Perry (Blackawton 2001), 275–465.

PDA *Pedanius Dioscorides of Anabarzus: De materia medica*, trans. by L. Y. Beck, 2nd rev. and enl. ed. (Hildesheim 2011).

PI C. Perry, '*Isfīdhabāj*, Blancmanger and no Almonds', in: *Medieval Arab Cookery: Essays and Translations*, ed. by M. Rodinson, A.J. Arberry, and C. Perry (Blackawton 2001), 263–6.

PK C. Perry (trans.), '*Kitāb al-Ṭibākha*: A Fifteenth-Century Cookbook', in: *Medieval Arab Cookery: Essays and Translations*, ed. by M. Rodinson, A.J. Arberry, and C. Perry (Blackawton 2001), 467–75.

QA al-Qalānisī, *Aqrābādīn*, ed. by Z. al-Bābā (Aleppo 1983).

RMA R. Mielck, *Terminologie und Technologie der Müller und Bäcker im islamischen Mittelalter* (Ing. diss., Glückstadt 1914).

ROT al-Rāzī, *On the Treatment of Small Children* (*De curis puerorum*)*: The Latin and Hebrew Translations*, ed. and trans. by G. Bos and M. McVaugh (Leiden 2015).

RR M. Rodinson, 'Romania and other Arabic words in Italian', in: *Medieval Arab Cookery: Essays and Translations*, ed. by M. Rodinson, A.J. Arberry, and C. Perry (Blackawton 2001), 167–82.

RTT H. Rabin, 'Toledot Targum Sefer ha-Qanun le- 'Ivrit', *Melilah* 3–4 (1950): 132–47.

SCP F. Steingass, *A Comprehensive Persian-English Dictionary* (Repr., London 1984).

SDA M. Sokoloff, *A Dictionary of Jewish Babylonian Aramaic of the Talmudic and Geonic Periods* (Ramat Gan 2002).

SHS 1 Shem Tov Ben Isaac, *Medical Synonym Lists from Medieval Provence: Shem Tov Ben Isaac of Tortosa, Sefer ha-Shimmush, Book* 29, pt. 1: *Edition and Commentary of List 1* (*Hebrew—Arabic—Romance/Latin*), ed. by G. Bos, M. Hussein, G. Mensching and F. Savelsberg (Leiden 2011).

SLN I. Stirling, *Lexicon Nominum Herbarum, Arborum Fructicumque Linguae Latinae*, 4 vols. (Budapest 1995–8).

SN D. Sontheimer, 'Nachricht von einer arabisch-medicinischen Handschrift, vermutlich des Ibn-Dschezla,' *Janus* 2 (1847): 246–72, repr. in: idem, *Beiträge zur Geschichte der arabisch—Islamischen Medizin. Aufsätze I* (*1819–1869*), ed. by F. Sezgin, in collab. with M. Amawi, D. Bischoff, E. Neubauer (Frankfurt 1987), 92–128.

SRP C. Singer and C. Rabin, *A Prelude to Modern Science being a Discussion of the History, Sources and Circumstances of the "Tabulae Anatomicae Sex" of Vesalius* (Cambridge 1946).

UW M. Ullmann, *Wörterbuch zu den griechisch-arabischen Übersetzungen des neunten Jahrhunderts* (Wiesbaden 2002).

UWS 1 M. Ullmann, *Wörterbuch zu den griechisch-arabischen Übersetzungen des neunten Jahrhunderts*, Suppl. 1: A–O (Wiesbaden 2006).

UWS 2 M. Ullmann, *Wörterbuch zu den griechisch-arabischen Übersetzungen des neunten Jahrhunderts*, Suppl. 2: Π-Ω (Wiesbaden 2007).

VL I. A. Vullers, *Lexicon Persico-Latinum Etymologicum*, 2 vols. (Repr., Graz 1962).

WA E. Wiedemann, *Gesammelte Schriften zur arabisch-islamischen Wissenschaftsgeschichte*, 3 vols. = Veröffentlichungen des Institutes für Geschichte der Arabisch-Islamischen Wissenschaften, Reihe B: Nachdrucke, ed. by D. Girke and D. Bischoff (Frankfurt 1984).

WI D. Waines, *In a Caliph's Kitchen* (London 1989).

WKAS *Wörterbuch der klassischen arabischen Sprache*, ed. by Deutsche Morgenländische Gesellschaft, in Verbindung mit A. Spitaler, ed. by J. Krämer, H. Gätje and M. Ullmann (Wiesbaden 1957–).

Introduction

The current volume[1] is part of a wider project aiming at mapping the novel[2] Hebrew[3] technical medical terminology as it features in medieval Hebrew medical works translated both from the Arabic and Latin.[4] In this way I hope to facilitate the consultation of these and other medical works and the identification of anonymous medical material. The terminology discussed below has been derived from three primary sources and seven secondary ones. The primary sources are:

1. *Sefer Ṣedat ha-Derakhim*; i.e., Moses Ben Samuel Ben Judah Ibn Tibbon's translation of Ibn al-Jazzār's *Zād al-musāfir wa-qūt al-ḥādir* (*Provisions for the Traveller and the Nourishment for the Sedentary*), bks. 1–2.[5] The basic Hebrew manuscript consulted is Ms London, British Library Ar. Or. 26 (cat. Margoliouth 1024[6]), which consists of 168 leaves and was copied in a Sephardic script in the fifteenth century. This manuscript generally has good, reliable readings. For the sections missing and for significant variant readings I consulted Ms Oxford, Bodleian, Poc. 353, Uri Heb. 314 (cat. Neubauer[7] 2111), which was copied in a Sephardic script in the

1 I thank Felix Hedderich and Jessica Kley for proofreading the manuscript.

2 With 'novel', I mean those terms that do not feature in the current dictionaries of the Hebrew language at all, or that feature in these dictionaries but without proper explanation or in a later period. Occasionally I include terms that have already been mentioned in the first three volumes dealing with novel Hebrew medical terminology in order to show the wider distribution of a certain term.

3 In addition to the Hebrew terms, the volume also includes Aramaic ones. I also added some Hebrew-Romance words and loan words from Romance and Arabic, especially concerning dishes and drinks that were common throughout medieval medical, culinary literature. Some loan words from the Arabic derived from the field of anatomy feature in the list as well.

4 Earlier volumes published are: NM 1–3; cf. also BMZ 7–8.

5 Moses Ibn Tibbon's translation probably dates from the year 1259. On Moses Ibn Tibbon, a member of the famous dynasty of translator(s) known as the 'Tibbonides', who was active as a physician, merchant and translator in Lunel, see NM 1:47–51, and the bibliography listed there. For the Arabic compendium consisting of seven books, see IJZ 1–6.

6 Cf. G. Margoliouth, *Catalogue of the Hebrew and Samaritan Manuscripts in the British Museum*, vols. 1–3 (London 1899–1915); and *Catalogue of the Hebrew and Samaritan Manuscripts in the British Museum*, vol. 4: *Indexes, Brief Descriptions of Accessions and Addenda and Corrigenda*, with an Introduction by J. Leveen (London 1935), 3:353–4. For the data concerning all Hebrew Mss mentioned in this study, I consulted also the Online Catalogue of Microfilmed Hebrew Mss at the National Library.

7 Cf. A. Neubauer, *Catalogue of the Hebrew Manuscripts in the Bodleian Library* (Oxford 1886, repr. 1994), and *Supplement of Addenda and Corrigenda*, comp. under the direction of M. Beit-Arié and ed. by R. A. May (Oxford 1994).

© KONINKLIJKE BRILL NV, LEIDEN, 2019 | DOI:10.1163/9789004382626_002

mid-fifteenth century, and Ms London, British Library Add. 27542,[8] which was copied in a Sephardic script in the fourteenth century.[9] The Arabic terms are derived from Ms Izmir, Millī 50/470 (26636).[10] The text is partly vocalised and was copied by Zayn al-ʿābidīn on Tuesday, 4. Shawwāl 972 H (1564).[11] In a few cases I will also mention Latin parallels for which I consulted the forthcoming critical edition by Long-McVaugh.

2. *Sefer ha-Shimmush*; i.e., Shem Tov Ben Isaac's Hebrew translation of the *Kitāb al-taṣrīf li-manʿağiza ʿan at-taʾlīf* (*The Arrangement of Medical Knowledge for One Who is Not Able to Compile a Book for Himself*), composed in the tenth century by the Andalusian physician al-Zahrāwī.[12] The discussion of the novel terminology is derived from bk. 27, *On the Powers of Foods and the Properties of Remedies*.[13] The basic Hebrew Manuscript consulted for the analysis is Ms Paris, BN 1163, which was copied in the

8 Cf. Margoliouth, *Catalogue of the Hebrew and Samaritan Manuscripts*, 4:152–3.

9 One entry, i.e., כתר מלכות, hails from Ms Munich, Bayerische Staatsbibliothek 19.

10 For the manuscript, cf. A. Dietrich, *Medicinalia Arabica: Studien über arabische medizinische Handschriften in türkischen und syrischen Bibliotheken*, = Abhandlungen der Akademie der Wissenschaften in Göttingen, Philologisch-Historische Klasse, vol. 3.66 (Göttingen 1966), 63; the manuscript was published in a facsimile edition by F. Sezgin, *Provisions for the Traveller and Sustenance for the Resident: Zād al-musāfir wa-qūt al-ḥāḍir by Ibn al-Jazzār, Abū Jaʿfar Aḥmad ibn Ibrāhīm ibn Abī Khālid (d. 979 AD)*, 2 vols., repr. from the Izmir manuscript, in collab. with M. Amawi and E. Neubauer, = Publications of the Institute for the History of Arabic-Islamic Science, Series C: Facsimile Editions, vols. 59.1–2 (Frankfurt 1996).

11 A critical edition of the first two books of the Arabic text of the *Zād al-musāfir*, Ibn Tibbon's Hebrew translation Constantine the African's Latin translation, and a Greek translation is currently being prepared by a team consisting of G. Bos, F. Käs, B. Long, M. McVaugh and P. Bouras-Vallianatos, with financial support of the Deutsche Forschungsgemeinschaft (DFG).

12 Shem Tov started his translation in 1254 and completed the work at an unknown date. On Shem Tov, see G. Bos, 'The Creation and Innovation of Medieval Hebrew Medical Terminology: Shem Tov Ben Isaac, Sefer ha-Shimmush', in *Islamic Thought in the Middle Ages: Studies in Text, Transmission and Translation, in Honour of Hans Daiber*, ed. by A. Akasoy and W. Raven (Leiden 2008): 197–202. This introduction is an adaptation of that which features in SHS 1:10–1. On an earlier occasion, I analyzed the novel terminology featuring in Shem Tov's adaptation of bk. 29 of al-Zahrāwī's *Kitāb al-taṣrīf* in the form of two lists of medical synonyms, in NM 1:73–120.

13 Cf. Arabic: المقالة السابعة والعشرون في معرفة قوى الأغذية وخواصّ الأدوية. The Hebrew translation has a more extensive version: מאמר שבעה ועשרים העתקת שם טוב בר יצחק זלה״ה בכחות המזונות והסמים ותקונם מה שצריך אליהם במלאכת הרפואה (Chapter twenty-seven translated by Shem Tov Ben Isaac, of blessed memory, on the powers of foods and remedies, and their correction, as far as needed for the art of medicine).

fourteenth century in a Sephardic script (= א);[14] and in the case of mistakes and/or significant variant readings: Ms Oxford, Bodleian Hunt. Donat 2, which was copied in a Sephardic script in 1369 (= ב).[15] For the Arabic terminology I used Ms Istanbul, Süleymaniye Library, Beşirağa 502, which was copied in 1497.[16] In the case of corruptions, I consulted Ms Istanbul, Süleymaniye Library, Beşirağa 503.

3. *Sefer ha-Qanun*[17] (Nathan); i.e., Nathan ha-Me'ati's Hebrew translation of the first book of Ibn Sīnā's *K. al-Qānūn*,[18] the section dealing with anatomy.[19] The Ms I consulted is Ms Oxford, Bodleian Library Can. Or. 43 (= cat. Neubauer 2098), which was copied in a Sephardic semi-cursive script by Joseph Ben Hayyim.[20] Some of the terms also feature in the glossary which Nathan compiled as a supplement to his translation (cf. NM 2:95–164). In addition to the terms hailing from Nathan's translation I mention the parallel terms featuring in the revisions of this translation

14 For an extensive description of the manuscript, see SHS 1:52–5.

15 For an extensive description of the manuscript, see ibid. 1:58–60.

16 Facs. ed. by F. Sezgin, *A Presentation to Would-Be-Authors On Medicine: Al Taṣrīf li-man ʿajiza ʿan al-Taʾlīf by Abūʾl-Qāsim al-Zahrāwī, Khalaf ibn ʿAbbās* (*d. ca. 1010* AD), 2 vols. (Frankfurt 1986).

17 *Sefer ha-Qanun*: The title I adopted for the Hebrew translation is part of the title mentioned by M. Steinschneider, *Die hebräischen Übersetzungen des Mittelalters und die Juden als Dolmetscher* (Berlin 1893, repr. 1956), 680: *Sefer ha-Qanun Be'uro Sefer ha-Kolel*. Ms Oxford, Bodleian Can. Or. 43 only has a title that was added by a later hand: *Sefer Refu'ah le-Ibn Sina*. On Nathan ha-Me'ati, who was active as a translator in Rome in the second half of the thirteenth century and completed the *Sefer ha-Qanun* in the year 1279, cf. NM 2:95–9.

18 For the *K. al-Qānūn* I consulted the edition Bulaq 1877, repr. in 5 vols., Beirut n.d.

19 As for secondary literature regarding the medieval Hebrew terminology of the section on anatomy in Ibn Sīnā's *K. al-Qānūn*, SRP has been consulted throughout.

20 For Nathan's translation of the *K. al-Qānūn*, see NM 2:95–9, and for an edition of his glossary to its translation, see NM 2:99–164. A small part of Nathan translation (bk. 1, ch. 2: *On the Anatomy of the Skull*) has been edited in RTT 139–45, with references to the translations by Zeraḥyah Ḥen and Joseph Lorki and a discussion of some anatomical terms.

by Zeraḥyah Ḥen[21] and by Joseph Ben Joshua Lorki,[22] (ca. 1400).[23] For Zeraḥyah Ḥen I consulted Ms Cesena, Biblioteca Malatestiana, Pluteo Sinistro XXVIII,1, which was copied in a Sephardic script in the fourteenth century and only covers bk. 1.[24] For Joseph Lorki I used Ms Paris, BN 1136, which was copied in Villalón de Campos in a Sephardic script in the year 1487 by the copyist Abraham Ibn Qarsaf.[25]

The secondary sources used for the composition of this study are:

1. *Sefer Issur ha-Qevurah le-Galienus* (ספר אסור הקבורה לגאליינוס קצור יושע האשורי טרם שבעים ושתים שעות) (Yoshaʿ the Syrian's Summary of Galen's *On the Prohibition to Bury [Someone] within Seventy-two Hours*), by Judah Ben Solomon al-Ḥarizi (around 1200).[26] The Hebrew title reflects the Arabic كتاب تحريم الدفن لجالينوس تفسير الشيخ أبي سعيد عبيد الله بن جبريل بن عبيد الله بن بختيشوع (The book *Prohibition of Burial* by Galen [in a] Commentary by the master Abū Saʿīd ʿUbaidallāh ibn Ǧibrīl ibn ʿUbaidallāh ibn Buḫtīšūʿ),[27]

---

21 On Zeraḥyah Ḥen, active as a translator in Rome at the same time as Nathan ha-Me'ati, see NM 1:122–7. As to the supposition that Zeraḥyah's translation is a revision of that by Nathan, see RTT 134; G. Freudenthal and M. Zonta, 'Avicenna among Medieval Jews: The Reception of Avicenna's Philosophical, Scientific and Medical Writings in Jewish Cultures, East and West,' in *Arabic Sciences and Philosophy* 22 (2012): 271; and G. Tamani, *Il Canon medicinae di Avicenna nella tradizione ebraica. Le miniature del manoscritto 2197 della Biblioteca Universitaria di Bologna* (Padova 1988), 61. The terms hailing from Zeraḥyah's translation are introduced by *Sefer ha-Qanun* (Zeraḥyah) and will only be discussed when they differ from those featuring in Nathan's translation.

22 On Joseph Ben Joshua Lorki's translation, see Steinschneider, *Hebräische Übersetzungen des Mittelalters*, 680–1; RTT 134; L. Ferre, 'Avicena Hebraico: La Traducción del *Canon* de Medicina', in *MEAH* 52 (2003): 175; and Freudenthal/Zonta, 'Avicenna among Medieval Jews', 271. As to the theory that Lorki's translation is a revision of that by Nathan, see Steinschneider, *Hebräische Übersetzungen des Mittelalters*, 681–2; A. Neubauer and E. Renan, *Les Écrivains Français du XIVe Siècle* (Paris 1893, repr. 1969), 770–1; RTT 134–5; B. Richler, 'Manuscripts of Avicenna's *Kanon* in Hebrew Translation: A Revised and Up-to-date List,' *Korot* 8.1–2 (1981): 147; Tamani, *Canon medicinae di Avicenna*, 61; and Freudenthal/Zonta, 'Avicenna among Medieval Jews', 271. The terms hailing from Joseph Lorki's translation are introduced by *Sefer ha-Qanun* (Joseph Lorki) and will only be mentioned in case they differ from those by Nathan ha-Me'ati.

23 These parallel terms will only be mentioned in case they differ from those by Nathan ha-Me'ati.

24 In my survey this translation is referred to as: *Sefer ha-Qanun* (Zeraḥyah).

25 Cf. H. Zotenberg, *Catalogues des Manuscrits hébreux et samaritains de la Bibliothèque Impériale* (Paris 1866), 211; Richler, 'Manuscripts of Avicenna's *Kanon*', 162, no. 71; and Ferre, 'Avicena Hebraico', 170, n. 14.

26 On Judah al-Ḥarizi (1165–1225), see EJ^{2} 1:655–7.

27 For this pseudo-Galenic treatise, see the forthcoming edition of the Arabic text and English translation by O. Kahl.

as it appears at the beginning of the treatise; however, whether original or added by a later hand, the Hebrew designation is likely to be corrupt, as it pretends to be a translation of the commentary by ʿUbaidallāh while in fact it only covers the pseudo-Galenic treatise itself. In the preface Judah al-Ḥarizi apologizes for the poor translation of the treatise due to a very corrupt Arabic Vorlage making the translation almost useless, and remarks that he only did so because of the insistence of the prominent physician Maistre Bonfos.[28]

2. *Hanhagat ha-Beri'ut le-Abu ʿAli Ben Zuhr*; i.e., Jacob ben Machir Ibn Tibbon's Hebrew translation of a *Regimen of Health* by Abū 'l-Alā' Ibn Zuhr (forthcoming ed. by G. Bos, M. McVaugh and J. Shatzmiller).[29] The original Arabic text of this treatise is lost, however, in addition to the Hebrew translation it survives in a Latin translation, of which we have two recensions, an earlier and a later one. The Latin translation was prepared in the year 1299 in the university town of Montpellier by the combined effort of Jacob ben Machir and a Christian surgeon named Bernat Honofredi. Ben Machir could read Arabic, and translated what he saw, orally, into the Romance vernacular that both men shared; then Honofredi wrote down the Latin meaning of the words he had just heard from his partner.
3. *Shemot ha-Mashqim*; i.e., Estori ha-Parḥi's Hebrew translation of the *Tabula Antidotarii*, composed by Armengaud Blaise (d. 1311). Estori ha-Parḥi (1280–1355?)[30] completed his translation in Barcelona at some time before 1306, in which year Armengaud left Barcelona and moved to Avignon to become physician to Pope Clement V.[31]

---

28 My quotations are derived from my forthcoming edition that will be part of the edition of the Arabic text by O. Kahl. The basic Ms consulted for the edition is Vatican Urbinati ebr. 41, fols. 136a–139a, copied in a Sephardic semi-cursive script in the city of Bologna in the year 1422. Secondary Mss consulted are: Ms Berlin Fol. 1057, possibly copied from the Ms tradition represented by the Vatican copy, in the fifteenth century in a square Sephardic script, and Ms. Leeuwarden, Tresoar Fr. 23, copied in the fifteenth–sixteenth century in an Ashkenazic semi-cursive script.

29 The Hebrew translation is based on Ms Bologna 3574B, fols. 139a–147b, which was copied in the fourteenth century in a Sephardic script; a second Ms Jerusalem, National Library MS Heb. 8°85, fols. 133v–122r, has been used for variant readings.

30 On Estori ha-Parḥi, see EJ² 6:522.

31 I consulted the edition of the Latin text and Hebrew and English translations by M. McVaugh and L. Ferre, *The Tabula Antidotarii of Armengaud Blaise and its Hebrew Translation*, = Transactions of the American Philosophical Society, vol. 90.6 (Philadephia 2000).

4. *Pirqei Arnauṭ de Vilanova*; i.e., Arnau de Vilanova's *Medicationis Parabole*, translated into Hebrew (probably in 1388) by Abraham Avigdor of Arles.[32]
5. *Sefer Hanhagat ha-Beri'ut* (*On the Regimen of Health*), composed by Judah Ben Jacob at an unknown date.[33]
6. *Sammim Libbiyim*, i.e., Anonymous translation (from the Arabic) of Ibn Sīnā, *K. al-adwiya al-qalbiya* (*On Cardiacs*),[34] Ms Munich, Bayerische Staatsbibliothek, Cod. hebr. 280, fols. 109–36, copied in a Sephardic script in the fifteenth century.[35]
7. *Sefer ha-Refu'ot ha-Libbiyot*; i.e., Anonymous translation (from the Latin) of Ibn Sīnā, *K. al-adwiya al-qalbiya* (*On Cardiacs*); Ms Munich, Bayerische Staatsbibliothek, Cod. hebr. 373, fols. 236b–254 (incomplete), copied in a Sephardic script in the fifteenth century.[36] In the introduction to the list of simple remedies featuring on fols. 247a–251b, the anonymous translator remarks that since the order of the Latin alphabet is different from the Hebrew alphabet he has rearranged the Hebrew terms according to the order of the Hebrew alphabet, for the benefit of the reader.

In addition, the list contains a number of terms in the field of materia medica drawn from anonymous unpublished glossaries which mostly feature parallel names of remedies in Arabic, Hebrew and Romance. My colleague, Guido Mensching, a specialist in Romance languages, and I have been doing research

32 I consulted the edition of the Latin text and Hebrew translation by J. A. Paniagua, L. Ferre and E. Feliu, *Arnaldi de Villanova Opera Medica Omnia*, vol. 6.1 (Barcelona 1990). For Arnau de Villanova (c. 1240–1305), one of the most prominent physicians in his day because of his writings, his university instruction and his professional activity, see the wonderful website of the research project 'Arnau DB: Corpus Digital d'Arnau de Vilanova' (http://grupsderecerca.uab.cat/arnau/en). On Abraham Abigdor of Arles, see EJ² 2:731–2.

33 For the otherwise unknown author and this treatise that was possibly composed in the first half of the fourteenth century, see the edition by R. Allgaier-Honal (Hamburg 2013). All my quotations are from this edition.

34 On this text composed by Ibn Sīnā (880–937), cf. M. Ullmann, *Die Medizin im Islam* (Leiden 1970, 155–6. For the Arabic text I consulted Ms Paris BN Arabe 5966. An edition of the text in this Ms will be published as a supplement to the edition of Arnau de Villanova's Latin translation by M. McVaugh.

35 Cf. M. Steinschneider, *Die hebräischen Handschriften der K. Hof- und Staatsbibliothek in München*, 2nd rev. enl. ed. (Munich 1895). In addition to this Ms, I used Ms Munich, Cod. hebr. 87, fols. 121–7, and Ms Leiden, Or. 4719. fols. 163–7. For the Arabic text I consulted Ms Paris BN Arabe 5966.

36 Cf. Steinschneider, *Hebräische Handschriften der K. Hof- und Staatsbibliothek*. In addition to this Ms I consulted the incomplete Ms Vienna, Hebr. 59, cat. Schwarz 175, fols. 128–149, copied in a Sephardic script in the fifteenth century. For the Latin version I consulted the forthcoming critical edition by M. McVaugh.

in these glossaries for several years now and have published some of them. These unpublished lists include: (1) Ms Vatican 361, fols. 176–81; copied in mid-late fourteenth century in Sephardic cursive script. The names of the drugs are in Arabic; it includes a very brief description in Hebrew and sometimes translations into other languages;[37] (2) Ms Oxford, Bodleian, Mich. Add. 22 (cat. Neubauer 2129). The Ms was copied in a Sephardic-Provencal semi cursive script in the Provence, c. 1400. The list featuring on fols. (5v)–(16r), is a glossary of medical terms, mostly arranged alphabetically according to the Arabic. It gives parallel terms in Hebrew, Latin, and the vernacular, i.e., Occitan;[38] (3) Ms Leiden, Universiteitsbibliotheek, Cod. Or. 4732/1 (SCAL 15);[39] fols. 1a–17b; copied in the fifteenth–sixteenth century in an Ashkenazi script. It contains two lists of drug names, alphabetically arranged, the first running from fols. 1a–11b also gives the powers of the drugs.[40] Two pharmaceutical terms, i.e., קנה הטוב and עטרת המלך (see below) do not hail from an anonymous source. The former features in the *Hanhagat ha-Beri'ut le-Abu ʿAli Ben Zuhr*; the latter term in Zeraḥyah Ḥen's translation of Maimonides, *Medical Aphorisms* (forthcoming ed. by G. Bos).

1 General Note

My references to a term featuring in a translation of Hippocrates' *Aphorisms* by Moses ibn Tibbon, Zeraḥyah Ḥen, or an anonymous translator always refer to the term as it features in their translations of Maimonides' Arabic *Commentary on Hippocrates' Aphorisms*. In the case of Nathan ha-Me'ati, the term in question hails from his translation of the Arabic version of Galen's *Commentary*

37 Cf. B. Richler, *Hebrew Manuscripts in the Vatican Library: Catalogue*, comp. by the staff of the Institute of Microfilmed Hebrew Manuscripts, Jewish National and University Library, Jerusalem, Palaeographical and Codicological Descriptions by M. Beit-Arié, 304. For a study of the glossary featuring on fols. 131v–166v, see G. Bos and G. Mensching, 'Arabic-Romance Medico-Botanical Synonym Lists in Hebrew Manuscripts from the Iberian Peninsula and Italy (Vatican Library, Fourteenth–Fifteenth Century)', in *Aleph* 15.1 (2015): 34–42.

38 For a description of some entries, see G. Bos and G. Mensching, 'The Literature of Hebrew Medical Synonyms: Romance and Latin Terms and their Identification', in *Aleph* 5 (2005): 177–84.

39 Cf. M. Steinschneider, *Catalogus Codicum Hebraeorum Bibliothecae Academiae Lugduno-Batavae* (Leiden 1858), 372; and A. van der Heide, *Hebrew Manuscripts of Leiden University Library* (Leiden 1977), 64.

40 An edition of the two lists by G. Bos and K. Fischer is forthcoming.

on Hippocrates' Aphorisms. In the case of Hillel of Verona the terms hail from his translation of Hippocrates' *Aphorisms* (based on Constantine the African's Latin version) that was incorporated in the commentary on the *Aphorisms* by Moses Rieti. And finally when referring to Judah Shalom, the term hails from Judah's commentary on Hippocrates' *Aphorisms* that was based on an unknown Latin or Hebrew Vorlage. In all these cases the commentary includes an integral translation of the *Aphorisms* themselves.[41]

41 For a detailed account of these translations, see NM 3:3–13.

List of Terms

אבן (Anonymous glossary; Ms Vatican 361) = 'mineral'; cf. fol. 181b: תותיאה היא טוטיאה והיא אבן דומה למרתק אבל היא יותר אדומה (TWTY'H; i.e., ṬWṬY'H (tutty); it is a mineral similar to MRTQ (litharge), but it is more red). Hebrew אבן is not attested in the current dictionaries in the sense of a 'mineral'.

אבק (*Sefer Ṣedat ha-Derakhim*) = Arabic سفوف 'powder' (FAQ 262–3); Latin 'pulvis'; cf. bk. 1, ch. 23 (fol. 36a): תאר אבק חברו יצחק לפלג והרפיון וכאיבי הפרקים והרעש ומותר העב (Recipe for a powder that was composed by Isaac against hemiplegia, feebleness, arthritis, tremors, and thick residues). Hebrew אבק features in BM 35 in attestations from the *Sefer ha-Qanun*,[1] and from the *Sefer Livyat Ḥen*.[2]

אבק מקרר (*Sefer Ṣedat ha-Derakhim*) = Arabic برود 'cooling remedy' (cf. FAQ 180); cf. bk. 2, ch. 2 (Ms London, British Library, Add. 27542, fol. 24b): תאר אבק מקרר חברו בן מאסויה יסיר הלובן וירפאהו (Recipe of a cooling remedy composed by Ibn Māsawayh that removes and cures leucoma). Hebrew אבק מקרר does not feature in the current dictionaries. Conform to the Arabic the Hebrew term not only refers to cooling powders but to any cooling remedy.

אבר: האבר הישר, Plur. האברים הישרים (*Shemot ha-Mashqim*)[3] **I.** = Latin 'membra spiritualia' (the spiritual members (organs))[4]; cf. 2 (25): משקה אסיטוס מעט החמוץ ... משקיט הצמא מלחלח פותח מבשל[5] האברים הישרים כמו שהוא בשלישית מהנהגות החדות (Mild vinegar syrup ... It lessens thirst, moistens, opens and concocts[6] [in] the spiritual members, as [can be seen] from *Regimen acutorum* 3). Hebrew האבר הישר does not feature in the current dictionaries; **II.** = Latin 'membra nobilia' (The noble members (organs)); cf. 7 (35): משקה רושאד ורדים הפרח נודע קר בא' יבש בב' מטהר האדומה בהיות לחה. מטהר האדומה והדם מחזק הלב והאברים הישרים (Rose syrup, roses, a well-known flower, cold in the first [degree] and hot in the second, drawing out yellow bile when it is fresh. It draws out red bile and blood, strengthens the heart and the noble members (organs)).

---

1 I.e., the medieval Hebrew translations of Ibn Sīnā's *K. al-Qānūn* as discussed above.

2 Ben Yehuda's suggestion that the specific translation of Ibn Sīnā's *K. al-Qānūn* he consulted is that by Nathan ha-Me'ati (cf. BM 1:274), is not always correct, as we shall see in the case of עין הכתף (see below).

3 In addition to האברים הישרים, Estori ha-Parḥi translates Latin 'membra spiritualia' as האברים הנפשיים (see entry), האיברים הרוחיים (see entry), האברים הרוחניים (see entry), and איברי הרוח (see entry).

4 'the spiritual members (organs)': In his *Speculum medicine*, Arnau uses 'membra spiritualia' to refer to the bodily members (organs) involved in breathing (and so in taking in air and spirit), namely the lungs, the trachea, and the epiglottis. I thank my friend and colleague Michael McVaugh for this information.

5 dissolvit L :מבשל.

6 'concocts': 'dissolves' L.

© KONINKLIJKE BRILL NV, LEIDEN, 2019 | DOI:10.1163/9789004382626_003

האבר המגדל, Plur. האברים המגדלים (*Shemot ha-Mashqim*) = Latin 'membra nutritiva' (nutritive members (organs)); cf. 33 (87): גיראופילאטום ... מועיל לרוע העכול וחולשתו ולסתום האברים המגדלים והרוחניים (Gariofilatum ... It is good against a bad and weak digestion, and for obstructions in the nutritive and spiritual members (organs)). Hebrew האבר המגדל, Plur. האברים המגדלים, does not feature in the current dictionaries. The verb גידל features in the related sense of 'to cause to grow' (BDB 152); 'to raise, to rear, train' (JD 212); cf. BM 701.

האבר הנפשי, Plur. האברים הנפשיים (*Shemot ha-Mashqim*)[7] = Latin 'membra spiritualia' (the spiritual members (organs))[8]; cf. 62 (145): פאולינום: אם ינתן לעצור הגרת השעול אל האיברים הנפשיים יותכו ששה או ארבעה בבשול (זנב) סוס נקי ופפאברי לבן (Paulinum. If given to[9] quell a cough and a flow of humours to the spiritual members (organs), dissolve six or four in a decoction of pure licorice and white poppy ...). Hebrew האבר הנפשי, Plur. האברים הנפשיים, does not feature in the current dictionaries.

האבר הקטן (*Sefer Hanhagat ha-Beri'ut*) = 'penis' (lit., 'small member'); cf. 8.1 (145): והכליות מושכות המים הרעים אשר בדם ומתפרנסות ממעט האדמימות הנשאר בו ושולחות המותר אל כיס המים והוא מזומן לקבלו ולהוציאו לחוץ על פי האבר הקטן והוא השתן (The kidneys attract the bad watery part of the blood and feed themselves with the small amount of the remaining red part and send the residue to the bladder which is ready to receive it and to expel it through the penis (lit., 'small member'), and this (i.e., what is expelled) is the urine). Hebrew האבר הקטן features as a euphemism for the penis in Rabbinic literature (cf. LW 1:15); cf. tb*Sanhedrin* 107a: אבר קטן יש באדם משביעו רעב מרעיבו שבע (there is a small organ in man which satisfies him in his hunger but makes him hungry when satisfied) (trans. *The Soncino Talmud*).

האבר הרוחי, Plur. האברים הרוחיים (*Shemot ha-Mashqim*)[10] = Latin 'membra spiritualia' (the spiritual members (organs))[11]; cf. 6 (33): משקה ויאולד ויאוליש: הפרח נודע קר בסוף הא' לח בראש הג' מלחלח [המעים] ומניע האדומה ישקיט ההתלהבות ובפרט מהכבד ואיברים הרוחיים (Violet syrup, violets: A familiar

---

7 In addition to האברים הנפשיים, Estori ha-Parḥi translates Latin 'membra spiritualia' as האברים הישרים (see entry), האיברים הרוחיים (see entry), האברים הרוחניים (see entry), and איברי הרוח (see entry).

8 'the spiritual members (organs)': See entry אבר: האבר הישר, Plur. האברים הישרים.

9 'to quell a cough and a flow of humours'; cf. Latin: 'ad conpescendum tussim et fluxum humorum' (144).

10 In addition to האברים הרוחיים, Estori ha-Parḥi translates Latin 'membra spiritualia' as האברים הישרים (see entry), האברים הנפשיים (see entry), האברים הרוחניים (see entry) and איברי הרוח (see entry).

11 'the spiritual members (organs)': See entry אבר: האבר הישר, Plur. האברים הישרים.

flower, cold at the end of the first [degree], wet at the beginning of the third, moistening the intestines and drawing out bile. It soothes inflammations, especially of the liver and the spiritual members …). Hebrew האבר הרוחי does not feature in the current dictionaries.

האבר הרוחני, Plur. **האברים הרוחניים** (*Shemot ha-Mashqim*)[12] = Latin 'membra spiritualia' (the spiritual members (organs))[13]; cf. 33 (87): … גיראופילאטום מועיל לרוע העכול וחולשתו ולסתום האברים המגדלים והרוחניים (Gariofilatum … It is good against a bad and weak digestion, and for obstructions in the nutritive and spiritual members). Hebrew האבר הרוחני does not feature in the current dictionaries.

איברי הרוח (*Shemot ha-Mashqim*)[14] = Latin 'membra spiritualia' (the spiritual members (organs))[15]; cf. 20 (61): דיאה פינידיאון פניד ברקות עשוי עם סוכר חם לח מועיל ליובש הריאה ולכל איברי הרוח (Dyapenidion, barley-sugar: A confection made from sugar, mildly[16] hot and wet. It is good for dryness of the lungs and all spiritual members …). Hebrew איברי הרוח does not feature in the current dictionaries.

אבש (*Sefer ha-Shimmush*) = Arabic برقوق 'apricot' (*Prunus armeniaca*); cf. fol. 138a, col. b: האבש יש ממנו פג בלתי מבושל כל צרכו ויש ממנו מבושל כל צרכו קוסס (Apricots: Some are green, not sufficiently ripe, and others are sufficiently ripe and [their taste is] sourish). Hebrew אבש is a Rabbinic term referring to 1) 'wild grapes', a species of grape of inferior quality (only featured in the plural ʾBŠYN = biblical Hebrew BʾWŠYM; cf. JD 21; BM 40; LF 1:78 and 2) 'quince', *Cydonia vulgaris* (ʾBŠ is ḤBWŠ); cf. FZ 118f.; LF 3:240; see also SHS 1:111–2 (Alef 25): אבש ב״ה משמש וב״ל אנפרישגש (BŠ, Arabic MŠMŠ, o.l. ʾNPRYŠGŠ).

(אדם) מאדם: See entry **סם**.

אֹדֶם: אודם (*Sefer Ṣedat ha-Derakhim*)[17] = Arabic طرفة 'blood-spot in the eye' (cf. MMT 252–3) (Greek ὑπόσφαγμα; cf. LSG 1897: 'a suffusion of blood in the eye'); cf. bk. 2, ch. 3 (fol. 43b): השער הג׳ באודם אשר באחת קצוות העין הנקרא בער׳ טרפא (Chapter three: On the blood-spot in one of the corners of the eyes called *al-ṭarfa* in Arabic). Hebrew אודם features in BM 65 in the sense

---

12 In addition to האברים הרוחניים, Estori ha-Parḥi translates Latin 'membra spiritualia' as האברים הישרים (see entry), האברים הנפשיים (see entry), האיברים הרוחיים (see entry) and איברי הרוח (see entry).

13 'the spiritual members (organs)': See entry אבר: האבר הישר, Plur. האברים הישרים.

14 In addition to איברי הרוח, Estori ha-Parḥi translates Latin 'membra spiritualia' as האברים הישרים (see entry), האברים הנפשיים (see entry), האיברים הרוחיים (see entry), and האברים הרוחניים (see entry).

15 'the spiritual members (organs)': See entry אבר: האבר הישר, Plur. האברים הישרים.

16 'mildly': Added according to the Latin 'temperata'.

17 In addition to אודם, Moses Ibn Tibbon uses the variant reading אדמימות (see entry).

of ‘redness in the eyes’, in an attestation from Moses Cordovero, *Elimah* [*Rabbati*].

אדמימות (*Sefer Ṣedat ha-Derakhim*)[18] = Arabic طرفة ‘blood-spot in the eye’ (Greek ὑπόσφαγμα; cf. LSG 1897: ‘a suffusion of blood in the eye’ (cf. MMT 252); cf. bk. 2, ch. 3 (fol. 44a): ואם לא יקבל תועלת ברפואות האלו יקח מרישארמה וישים אותה בקדרה וישפוך עליה מים וירתיחם ואחר כן יקח חתיכה מבגד פשתן ויטבול אותה במים ההם וישימה על העין כי זה יסיר האדמימות ההוא (If these remedies are not beneficial one should take hyssop, put it in a pot, pour water over it, boil it, then take a linen cloth, dip it in the water and put it on the eye for this will remove the blood-spot). Hebrew אדמימות features in BM 70 and is explained by Ben Yehuda as having the same meaning as אֹדֶם (see previous entry).

אוריטי (*Sefer ha-Qanun*, Nathan) = Arabic أوريطى ‘aorta’ (cf. DKT 606, 814; FAL 22, no. 385); cf. bk. 1 (fol. 61a): אמנם החלק העולה משני חלקי האוריטי הנה הוא מתחלק לשני חלקים (The ascending part of the two parts of the aorta divides into two parts). Hebrew אוריטי is a loan word from Arabic أوريطى, cf. SRP 14 (72).

אזן: אזנים: See entry **שרש**.

אָח (*Sefer ha-Shimmush*) = Arabic كانون ‘brazier’ (cf. RMA 62–3, n. 4: ‘Kohlenpfanne’)[19] (brazier); cf. fol. 125a, col. 1: הלחם האפוי באח[20] הטמון בדשן רע מפני שנוי חלקיו כי חצונו נשרף כמו אש ותוכו בלתי מצטמק[21] (Bread baked on a brazier and buried in ashes is bad because of the different [quality] of its parts. For the outside is burned [as if by fire] and the inside is not cooked[22]). Hebrew אח features in BM 137 in the sense of ‘Feuertopf, réchaud, brasier, stove’ in attestations from the Bible and medieval Hebrew poetry (Samuel ha-Nagid). Ben Yehuda (ibid., n. 1) mentions كانونة as its Arabic equivalent.

אטם: אוטם (*Sefer Ṣedat ha-Derakhim*) = Arabic انسداد ‘blockage, obstruction’; Latin ‘opilatio’; cf. bk. 1, ch. 23 (fol. 33b): יסור תנועת הלשון ויתבטל הדבור אם מנפילת הכח המניע אותה אשר יבא מן המח ואם מפני סבה מאוטם או מורסא יקרה בעצב אשר ילך בו מן המח אל הלשון כח התנועה (The movement of the tongue disappears and speaking is abolished either because of a collapse of the power that moves [the tongue and] that comes from the brain or because of the illness[23] of an obstruction or tumor occurring in the nerve through

18 In addition to אדמימות, Moses Ibn Tibbon uses the variant reading אודם (see entry).

19 Mielck refutes the opinion of Dozy (D 2:491) that it refers to an ‘oven’ (fourneau); cf. WKAS 1:11: ‘brazier, stove’; FL 4:61 ‘foculus’ (a little hearth, a fire-pan, chafing-dish, brazier); NA 684: ‘portable brazier used for heating purposes and cooking’.

20 באח: בכירה א[1]ב.

21 מצטמק: מבושל ב.

22 Translated after Ms ב; but cf. entry (צמק) הצטמק.

23 ‘illness’: Translated after the Arabic علة, which can mean both, ‘illness’ and ‘cause’.

which the moving power streams from the brain to the tongue). Hebrew אֹטֶם is attested for Rabbinical literature as אוטם בריאה in the sense of 'an obstruction in the lungs' (cf. JD 24; BM 168).

אילן השועל: אִילָן (*Sefer Ṣedat ha-Derakhim*) = Arabic عنب الثعلب 'black nightshade' (*Solanum nigrum* L.) (cf. DT 4:63); Latin 'solatrum'; cf. bk. 1, ch. 5 (fol. 11b): או יקח ממי אילן השועל הוא שולטרי שתים עשרה אוקיות ומירבולנש סיטרינש עשר אוקיות ויערבם עם מי אילן השועל (Or take twelve ounces of black nightshade, i.e., ŠWLṬRY juice and ten ounces of yellow myrobalan and mix these with the black nightshade juice). Hebrew אילן השועל does not feature in the current dictionaries and secondary literature. The standard Hebrew translation (calque) for the Arabic equivalent عنب الثعلب is ענב השועל (cf. BM 5574). The Romance equivalent ŠWLṬRY features as ענבי השועל הוא שולטרי in an additional entry in Ms Munich, Bayerische Staatsbliothek 302, containing Nathan ha-Me'ati's glossary to the *Sefer ha-Qanun* (cf. NM 2:118, n. 211).

אישרוב (*Sefer ha-Shimmush*) = Arabic شراب 'syrup' (cf. D 1:740–1); cf. fol. 142b, col. a: ויש שעושין מהם אישרוב להועיל מהשלשול (Some [doctors] make syrups from them (i.e., chestnuts) as a remedy for diarrhea). Hebrew אישרוב is a non-attested loan word from Romance (Occitan) 'exirop' (syrup).

אישרוב אסיטוש (*Sefer ha-Shimmush*) = Arabic سكنجبين 'oxymel'; cf. fol. 141a, col. b: והמתילדים בארצות חזקות הקרירות הם בהפך ממה שזכרתי שהם לא יוכלו להתבשל ותתגבר עליהם הקביצות ותקונם ודחיית נזקם לבעלי החמימות למהר תכף אכילתם למצוץ מן הרמונים הקוססים ולשתות מן האישרוב אסיטוש ([Dates] that grow in very cold countries [have opposite properties] to those that I mentioned (i.e., those which grow in very hot countries), for they cannot ripen and are dominated by astringency. To improve [their quality] and undo their harm people with a hot temperament should immediately after eating them suck [the juice] of sweet and sour pomegranates and drink oxymel …). Hebrew אישרוב אסיטוש is a loan word from Romance (Occitan) 'exirop acetos'.

אישרוב ג׳לאבי (*Sefer ha-Shimmush*) = Arabic جلّاب 'julep' (rose water syrup) (cf. FL 1:290; NA 597); cf. fol. 145a, col. b: ואם תתעורר אחריו חמימות וצמא חזק צריך לשתות עליו אישרוב ג׳לאבי או אישרוב אסיטוס במים קרים (And if [its consumption] (i.e., that of jerked[24] meat) causes heat and severe thirst, one should drink after it julep or oxymel with cold water …). Hebrew אישרוב ג׳לאבי is a non-attested loan word from Romance (Occitan) 'exirop' and Arabic *ǧullābī*.

אכול השנים: אִכּוּל (*Sefer Ṣedat ha-Derakhim*) = Arabic تأكّل الأسنان 'corrosion of the teeth (caries)'; cf. bk. 2, ch. 18 (fol. 59a): וכאשר יכאבו ויפסדו יחסר פעולתם ויראו בהם חליים מתחלפים ומהם חליים נראה אותם לעין כמו אכול השנים ונקובם

24 Cf. entry הבשר המליח המתובל.

ועפושם ותנועתם ולכלוכם אשר יהיה עליהם ומה שדומה לזה (When the teeth hurt and decay, they function less well and different illnesses become visible; some of them visible to the eye, such as caries, cavities, and decay, and when they move or become dirty, and the like). Hebrew אכול features in BM 205 in the sense of 'combustion, digestion, itching, and abscess'. See as well NM 1:77 for אכול in the sense of 'gangrene' (Shem Tov Ben Isaac), and ibid. 128 in the sense of 'corrosion' (Zeraḥyah Ḥen) (for the same meaning cf. NM 2:28–9).

אכחל: האכחל (*Sefer ha-Qanun*, Nathan) = Arabic الأكحل 'median vein' (cf. DKT 634–5, 814; FAL 6, no. 100); cf. bk. 1 (fol. 66a): והרביעי והוא הגדול שבהם והוא אותו אשר יראה ויעלה וישתלח ענף מאסף עמו שריג מן הקיפאל ויתהוה ממנו האכחל ושאריתו הוא הבאסליק (The fourth [branch of the axillary vein], the largest of all, is the one that goes up along the outer part and sends out branches that join a branch of the cephalic vein and from these branches the median vein is formed. The remaining part is the basilic vein). Hebrew האכחל is a non-attested loan word (with the Hebrew definite article) from Arabic الأكحل. Zeraḥyah Ḥen renders the Arabic الأكحل as גיד הראש הנקרא אכחל (see entry).

(אכל) נֶאֱכָל (*Sefer Ṣedat ha-Derakhim*) = Arabic متآكل 'being affected by caries'; cf. bk. 2, ch. 19 (fol. 61b): ואם היה האיכול בשרשי השנים נקח עפץ בלתי נקוב וישחוק אותו ויולש בליציאום או בטרבנטינה או בקטרן ואחר כן יחבש בה השן הנאכלת (If the caries affects the roots of the teeth we take unperforated gallnut, pound and knead it with buckthorn or mastic from the terebinth or tar and then apply this to the tooth affected by caries). Hebrew נאכל features in the Bible in the sense of 'to be consumed, to be wasted, to be destroyed' (of the body); cf. BDB 37; BM 213.

מְאַכֵּל: See entry **סם**.

מתאכל (*Pirqei Arnauṭ de Vilanova*) = Latin 'corrosivus' (corrosive); cf. 5.96 (110): הנגעים המתאכלים אשר יתרחבו ויתפשטו אל העומק מעצמם ראוי לרפאם עם דברים קובצים ומיבשים בלתי עוקצים ואם יהיו ארסיים כמו חולי הזאב יצטרך שיהיו בזהריים (Corrosive wounds that spontaneously spread and become deeper, should be treated with astringent, drying ingredients that do not bite. But if they (i.e., the wounds) are poisonous, as in the case of lupus,[25] [the ingredients] should have the property of the bezoar[26] (i.e., be antidotal)). Hebrew מתאכל features in Rabbinic literature in the sense of 'to be consumed, burnt up, digested' and 'to be worn off, spent' (cf. JD 63; BM 214).

---

25 Cf. entry זאב: חולי הזאב.

26 'have the property of the bezoar': Cf. entry בזהרי.

אלכסוני (*Sefer ha-Qanun*, Nathan) = Arabic مورّب 'oblique, diagonal'; cf. bk. 1 (fol. 46a): ואיזה שנים מצד אחד שיכווצו יטה הראש אליהם נטיה בלתי אלכסונית (When two [of the four muscles of the head] contract from one side, the head is inclined towards them with an inclination that is not oblique). Hebrew אלכסוני is attested as a modern term in EM 71.

אלכסוניות (*Sefer ha-Qanun*, Nathan) = Arabic توريب 'going in an oblique, diagonal line (obliqueness, diagonality)' (cf. D 1:16 (s.v. أرب)); cf. bk. 1 (fol. 46a): וסגולתו[27] שהוא מקיים נטיית הראש בעת התהפכו אל הענין הטבעי לאלכסוניותו (Because of its oblique (diagonal) position its specific function (i.e., of the third pair of the muscles of the head) is to return the head when it is bent to its natural position). Hebrew אלכסוניות is not attested in the current dictionaries. Zeraḥyah Ḥen translates the Arabic لتوريبه as באלכסוניו, and Joseph Lorki as אלכסון.

אלף עלים :אלף (Anonymous glossary; Ms Oxford, Bodleian, Mich. Add. 22, fol. 6v) = possibly 'yarrow' or 'milfoil' (*Achillea millefolium* L.) (Greek στρατιώτης ὁ χιλιόφυλλος) (cf. PDA 4:102, 293), or 'water milfoil' (*Myriophyllum spicatum* L.) (Greek μυριόφυλλον) (cf. PDA 4:114, 297). The Hebrew term is possibly a non-attested loan translation of the Arabic equivalent *ʾalf waraqa* (cf. DT 4:91 and 103[28]) or Latin 'millefolia' (cf. SLN 3:174).

אלפס: See entry **לחם**.

אַמָּה (*Sefer Issur ha-Qevurah le-Galienus*) = Arabic إحليل 'urethra' (Greek οὐρήθρα; cf. UW 483); cf. par. 31: והמקום השלישי העורק בין צדי האמה והאמה כשיהודקו הדוק חזק ירגיש האדם כמו התלהבות האש ואם תראה זה הנה הוא חי (Third, there is an artery between ureter and urethra which, when firmly palpated, feels to the (investigating) person as if a fire were burning [inside it]—if this is what you find, then (the patient) is alive). In the sense of 'urethra', Hebrew אַמָּה is a non-attested semantic borrowing from Arabic إحليل which can mean both 'penis' and 'urethra' (cf. UW 822). The same Hebrew term for Arabic إحليل already features in the Hebrew translation of Hippocrates' *Aphorisms* 4.82 by Moses Ibn Tibbon (cf. NM 3:25).

אמיצה (*Sefer ha-Qanun*, Nathan) = Arabic تقوية 'strengthening'; cf. bk. 1 (fol. 55b): ואותה שהיא במקרה הוא חוזק הבשר ואמיצת הגוף (The accidental [usefulness of the nerves] is that they strengthen the flesh and the body). Hebrew אמיצה features in BM 278 only in the sense of 'closing' (i.e., of the eyes). Zeraḥyah Ḥen and Joseph Lorki translate the Arabic تقوية as חיזוק.

---

27 a وخاصيته Ms וסכלה emend. ed. :וסגולתו.

28 The Hebrew term might also reflect Arabic *muryufullun* (= Greek μυριόφυλλον), the identity of which cannot be determined (cf. DT 4:103).

אמיצות המעים: אמיצות (*Sefer ha-Shimmush*) = Arabic حبس البطن 'constipation'; cf. fol. 124a, col. 1: ומי שנזרקו עליו מים מלוחים עד שתסור ממנו רוב לחותו הנותרת בו הבלתי מבושלת יהיה מזונו פחות ממזון המהובהב ויהיה דקותו יותר וימעטו רוחותיו ויסור ממנו העפוש ויתחזק על אמיצות המעים ועכולו יהיה קשה (And [the green toasted unripe wheat (KRML)] over which salt water has been sprinkled until most of the uncooked remaining moisture has gone provides less nutrition than the toasted [wheat]; it is finer, has less wind and no putrefaction, but it strengthens the constipation and is hard to digest). Hebrew אמיצות המעים does not feature in the current dictionaries. The verbal form אמץ את המעים is used in the sense of 'to cause constipation' by Shem Tov Ben Isaac in the *Sefer Almansur*; cf. NM 2:9.

אמצע החזה: אמצע I. (*Sefer ha-Qanun*, Nathan)[29] = Arabic قصّ 'sternum' (cf. FAL 123, no. 2697); cf. bk. 1 (fol. 36b): אמצע החזה מחובר מעצמות שבעה ולא נבראו עצם אחד כמו שנודע בשאר המקומות מן התועלת (The sternum is composed of seven bones. Because of its use it was not made from one bone as we know from other places). In the sense of 'sternum', Hebrew אמצע החזה features in MD 677 in addition to מפתח הלב and עצם החזה (cf. SRP 22 (121)). Zeraḥyah Ḥen renders the Arabic قصّ as עצם החזה (see entry); II. (*Sefer ha-Qanun*, Joseph Lorki) = Arabic لبّة[30] (emend. De Koning, cf. DKT 609, n. 1) (Greek σφαγή); cf. DKT 608–9, 826; WKAS 2.1: 84b: 'fossa iugularis, jugular fossa'; cf. bk. 1 (fol 18a): אמנם החלק העולה מחלקי אוריטי יחלק לשני חלקים היותר גדול שבהם אוחז למעלה כנגד אמצע החזה (The ascending part of the [two] parts of the aorta divides into two parts. The largest goes upwards towards the jugular fossa …). For the other translator(s), see entry העגול השחור שבבשר.

האסילם: אסילם (*Sefer ha-Qanun*, Nathan) = Arabic الأسيلم[31] (emend. De Koning, cf. DKT 637, n. 1) 'vena salvatella' (DKT 814; FAL 8, no. 135); cf. bk. 1 (fol. 66a): והולך ענף שני ממנו והוא האסילם ומתפרד במה שבין האמה והקמיצה (A second branch [of the median vein], the vena salvatella goes and spreads out between the middle finger and the ring finger). Hebrew האסילם is a non-attested loan word (with the Hebrew definite article) from Arabic الأسيلم.

אספידבאג׳ה (*Sefer ha-Shimmush*)[32] = Arabic إسفيدباجة cf. NA 608: 'white stew'. The name of the dish is an arabized form of Persian *ispīdbā* or *isfīdbā* (VL 1:92b, 99a), which is composed of the words *ispīd* 'white' (VL 1:92a) and *bāh*

29 Cf. entry צלעות אמצע החזה.

30 a لبّة: لثة.

31 a الأسيلم: الأسليم.

32 In addition to אספידבאג׳ה, Shem Tov has הבשר השלוק for Arabic إسفيدباجة (cf. entries אשכנז and הבשר השלוק).

'soup, broth, meat, victuals' (SCP 153, cf. 233 *pāh*)[33]; cf. fol. 148a, col. a: ותקונם לבשלם אספידבאג׳ה פשוטה וכל שכן השחורים מהם (To improve their quality (i.e., that of starlings) one should cook them as part of a simple white stew, especially in the case of black [starlings]). Hebrew אספידבאג׳ה is a non-attested loan word from Arabic إسفيدباجة, that occurs throughout bk. 27 of the *Sefer ha-Shimmush*.

אספלנית (*Sefer Ṣedat ha-Derakhim*) = Arabic مرهم 'salve; plaster' (cf. FAQ 240–1); cf. bk. 1 (fol. 10b) (Ms Oxford, Bodleian, Poc. 353, Uri Heb. 314): יתקן מהם אספלנית בדונג ויעשה בו (Prepare a salve of these [ingredients] with wax and apply it to the spot). Hebrew אספלנית (from Greek σπληνίον; Latin *splenium*; cf. HM 28) is attested for Rabbinic literature only, cf. JD 95–6; SDA 122 (Aram. אספלניתא). In his commentary to mShab 19.2 and mKel 28.3, Maimonides identifies אספלנית as Arabic مرهم (cf. SHS 1:125 (Alef 46)). Shem Tov Ben Isaac identifies it as Arabic لصوق 'sticking ... sticking plaster' (WKAS 2:664–5) and defines it as כל דבר מתדבק על האבר המושם (anything that adheres to the limb it is put onto) (cf. SHS 1:125 (Alef 46)).

אסתניסות (*Sefer ha-Shimmush*)[34] = Arabic غثيان 'sickness in the stomach, nausea'; cf. fol. 142a, col. b: ופעולתם על דרך הסם שהם מפסיקים האסתניסות והקיא ומו־ עילים אל המעי הצם ומוציאים התולעים הגדולים והקטנים מבטן המרבה באכילתם (As a drug they (i.e., chestnuts) are effective to stop nausea and vomiting; they are good for the jejunum and expel round worms and tapeworms from the stomach of someone who eats them frequently). Hebrew אסתניסות (noun formed from אסתנים, variant reading אסטנים (from Greek ἀσθενής 'weak'; cf. HM 44–5) features in BM 335 without further explanation in attestations from Judah Ibn Tibbon's Hebrew translation of Judah ha-Levi's *Kuzari* and from Meir Aldabi's *Shevilei Emunah*. Nathan ha-Me'ati renders Arabic غثيان as אסטנ(י)סות or חפץ (ה)קיא in his translation of Maimonides, *Medical Aphorisms* 9.55; 13.54; 23.86, 87 (forthcoming ed. by G. Bos); and Zeraḥyah Ḥen as קרבונקלי (cf. NM 2:30). A variant Hebrew reading אסטניסות (for Latin 'fastidium' (want of appetite)) features in Hillel[35] of Verona's translation of Hippocrates' *Aphorisms* 4.17 (cf. NM 3:26).

---

33 Cf. Maimonides, *On Asthma*, ed. and trans. by G. Bos (Provo, UT 2002), 1:19, 126, n. 2; idem, *On Hemorrhoids*, ed. and trans. by G. Bos (Provo, UT 2012), 12, 185–86, n. 90); MB 207–8; PI 263–6; MIG no. 100; and for some recipes, cf. ISW 159–60 (ch. 59) (Arabic); NA 282–4 (English); PD 340–2; AB 46; MWK 42–3.

34 In addition to אסתניסות for Arabic غثيان, Shem Tov renders the Arabic synonym تقلّب النفس as הפוך הנפש (see entry).

35 On Hillel of Verona (*c.* 1220–95), talmudic scholar, philosopher, physician and translator of medical works, see NM 1:9–15, 3:6–7, and the secondary literature there.

אֹפֶל (*Sefer Ṣedat ha-Derakhim*) = Arabic ظلمة 'dullness [of sight]' (amaurosis); cf. MMT, index 253; Greek ἀμαύρωσις; cf. LSG 78: 'complete hindrance to sight without any visible cause'; Latin 'continua tenebrositas oculorum'; cf. bk. 2, ch. 6 (fol. 45b): השער הו' באופל אשר יתחדש בעין. פעמים יחלש הראות מפני שנוי מזג העין או מפני עשן יעלה אליה מן האצטומכא (Chapter six: On the occurrence of dullness of sight. Sometimes vision weakens because of a change in the temperament of the eye or because of a vapour that arises to it from the stomach). Hebrew אֹפֶל features in the Bible in the sense of 'darkness' (cf. BDB 66 and BM 350); Masie (MD 26, s.v. 'amaurosis') has the following terms: עורון/כהיון/סנורים. The term סנורים features in this sense in the *Sefer Asaph ha-Rofe* (cf. MM 138).

אפרוחי הדבורים: אפרוח (*Sefer ha-Shimmush*) = Arabic فراخ النحل 'young bees'; cf. fol. 133a, col. a: והדבש החדש אשר יהיה מאפרוחי הדבורים הוא יותר רטוב וחומו יותר מועט (Fresh honey from young bees is moister and less hot). Hebrew אפרוח is only attested in the current dictionaries in the sense of 'the young of a bird'; cf. BDB 827; JD 108; BM 360.

אצבע (*Sefer ha-Qanun*, Nathan) = Arabic سبابة 'index finger'; cf. bk. 1 (fol. 50a): ואם יתנועע הראשון לבדו ירחיק בין הגודל והאצבע (When the first [muscle of the wrist] acts alone, it removes the thumb from the index finger). In the sense of 'index finger', Hebrew אצבע is attested for Rabbinic literature (cf. BM 365, LOW XXXVIII).

האצילי: אַצִּילִי (*Sefer ha-Qanun*, Nathan) = Arabic الإبطي 'the axillary vein' (cf. DKT 813; FAL 7, no. 1612); cf. bk. 1 (fols. 65b–66a): והשני פונה אל מקום כפיפת המרפק[36] בחיצוני הקנה ומתערב בעומק בשריג גם כן מן האצילי[37] (The second [branch of the branches of the cephalic vein] proceeds to the elbow pit (cubital fossa) at the outer part of the forearm and joins inside with a branch of the axillary vein). Hebrew האצילי features in BM 369 in an attestation form the *Sefer ha-Qanun*. Zeraḥyah Ḥen renders the Arabic الابطي as השחיי (see entry), and Joseph Lorki transcribes it as אבטי (cf. entry שטח המרפק).

ארון החזה: ארון (*Sefer ha-Shimmush*) = Arabic صندوق الصدر 'thorax' (cf. D 1:846); cf. fol. 145a, col. a: מקומות הבשר החשובים מגוף בעלי חיים: החשוב שבאיברי בעלי חיים הוא האבר שהוא תדיר התנועה כבשר הצואר והזרוע והכתף ודומיהם ומה שנמשך אל פני הבטן[38] ואל ארון החזה הוא יותר חשוב מן הנמשך בירך לקרבתו מן הלב (The best part of an animal for meat: The best part of an animal for meat is that which moves constanty, such as the neck, forelegs, shoulder and the

---

36 Ms המפרק emend. ed.: המרפק.

37 Ms האצלי emend. ed.: האצילי.

38 a البدن: הבטן.

like; and what lies close to the front part of the stomach[39] and chest is better than that which is near the haunch, because it (i.e., the former) is close to the heart). In the sense of 'thorax', Hebrew ארון החזה is a non-attested loan translation from Arabic صندوق الصدر.

ארכי: See entry **שלב**.

ארנבת (1) (*Sefer ha-Qanun*, Nathan) = Arabic أرنبة 'wing of the nostrils' (*ala nasi*) (cf. DKT 813; FAL 23, no. 415); cf. bk. 1 (fol. 43a): מה שידוע שעצלי הפנים הם כמספר האיברים המתנועעים בפנים והאיברים המתנועעים בפנים הם המצח ושתי[40] העפעפים התחתונים ושתי העפעפים העליונים והרקה[41] בשתוף עם השפתים <והשפתים> לבדם ושתי קצוות הארנבת והלחי התחתון (It is well-known that the muscles of the face correspond to the number of the parts of the face that can move. These are the forehead, lower[42] eyelids, upper eyelids, cheeks[43] in combination with lips, lips separately, ends of the wings of the nose, and lower jaw). Hebrew ארנבת features in BM 398 in an attestation from the *Sefer ha-Qanun* and is explained by Ben Yehuda as קצה האף (the tip of the nose); cf. Nathan's glossary to the *Sefer ha-Qanun*: ארנבת קצה החוטם נקרא כן (cf. NM 2:109 (Alef 20), 124). Zeraḥyah Ḥen translates the Arabic أرنبة as בתי השחי, and Joseph Lorki as ושתי קצוות הארנביות.

ארנבת (2): **הארנבת הימית** (*Sefer ha-Shimmush*) = Arabic الأرنب البحري (cf. D 1:19) (= Greek ὁ θαλάττιος λαγωός 'sea-hare' (shelled sea-slug; *Aplysia leporina*)), cf. LSG 1023); cf. fol. 146b, col. a: חלב הנשים יותר שוה מכל החלבים ... ולפיכך הוא מועיל מן העקיצה אשר תקרה באסטומ׳ ומשחין הריאה והמעים ומשתיית הארנבת הימית ומשתית הסם הנודע בהורג הזאב (Women's milk is the most balanced of all milks ... and for this reason it is good against a burning [sensation] in the stomach and against a tumor in the lung and intestines and against the comsumption of sea-hare and the poison known as aconite). Hebrew הארנבת הימית features in BM 398 without further explanation and in EM 119, s.v. ארנב ים, as a modern term in the sense of חלזון ים ערום (*Aplysia*).

אש: אש זרה (Anonymous glossary; Ms Leiden, Universiteitsbibliotheek, Cod. Or. 4732/1) = 'saltpeter'; cf. fol. 8a: שלניטרי הוא מלח אחר יתקנו ממנו אש זרה (ŠLNYṬRY (*sal nitri*); this is another [kind] of salt; 'artificial fire' (i.e., saltpeter) is made from it). In the sense of 'saltpeter', Hebrew אש זרה is not attested in the current dictionaries. The term features in the Bible in Num 3:4 in the

39 'stomach': 'body' a.
40 ושתי העפעפים התחתונים ושתי העפעפים העליונים: والمقلتان والجفنان العاليان a.
41 והרקה: والخدّ a.
42 'lower eyelids, upper eyelids': 'eye-balls, upper eyelids' a.
43 'cheeks': Translated acc. to Arabic خدّ; Hebrew רקה means 'temple'.

sense of 'illicit fire' (KB 1:92), and in modern Hebrew literature in the sense of 'evil inclination' (cf. EM 1:121).

האש הפרסי (*Pirqei Arnauṭ de Vilanova*) = Latin 'ignis sacer' (erysipelas)[44]; cf. 5.102: כמו שהקושי הנקרא אשקלירושיש כאשר יתישן שרשו יעתק אל החולי המכונה אירפיטים, כן בנגעים אשר יקרו באיברים החמים הבשר המת אם לא יעקר משרש, יוליד שם האש הפרסי בפתע (When the hardening that is called 'sclerosis' becomes chronic its root turns into the disease called 'herpes', in the same way, when the dead flesh of ulcers of hot organs is not removed in a radical way, it quickly causes erysipelas). Hebrew האש הפרסי is attested in BM 406 and defined by Ben Yehuda as 'a kind of ulcer' (אחד ממיני המורסות). The Hebrew term is possibly a loan translation of Arabic النار الفارسي, which can refer to both, 'erysipelas' and 'furoncle, carbuncle' (also called جمرة; Hebrew גחלת); cf. UW 112, s.v. ἄνθραξ; D 2:735. For this identification as both 'erysipelas' and 'carbuncle', cf. Ibn Sīnā, *K. al-Qānūn* 3 (118): 'Chapter on جمرة and النار الفارسية and other [afflictions]: These two names are sometimes applied to every corrosive, burning hot, blistering pustule that makes eschars, just like fire and cautering, and sometimes the term النار الفارسية is applied to a pustule that is of the kind of the corrosive, burning, blistering shingles …'.

אשך (*Sefer ha-Qanun*, Nathan) = Arabic خصية 'ovary' (cf. DKT 564, 817; FAL 81, no. 1784); cf. bk. 1 (fol. 52b): ואמנם הנשים יספיק להם אחד לכל אשך נפרד (In the case of women only one [pair of muscles] for each ovary is sufficient). Hebrew אשך only features in the current dictionaries in the sense of 'testicle'; cf. BM 416. Zeraḥyah Ḥen translates the Arabic خصية as ביצה (cf. entry); the same term is used by Joseph Lorki.

אשכי השועל (Anonymous glossary; Ms Oxford, Bodleian, Mich. Add. 22) = 'salep'[45]; cf. fol. 5b: אשכי השועל שטריאון ([Hebrew] ʾŠKY HŠWʿL; [Romance] ŠṬRYʾWN). Hebrew אשכי השועל is not attested in the current dictionaries. It is possibly a calque of the Arabic خصى الثعلب (lit., 'testicles of the fox'), which means 'salep'.[46] The Hebrew term also features in Judah ben Solomon (fourteenth century), *Kelal Qaṣar min ha-Sammim ha-nifradim*, i.e., his translation of Abū Ṣalt, *K. al-adwiya al-mufrada* (JNK 47, no. 105).

---

44 'ignis sacer' (erysipelas): Cf. D. Béguin, 'Un exemple d'exploitation de la base Esculape: Une liste des noms des maladies', in: *Nommer la maladie: Recherches sur le lexique gréco-latin de la pathologie*, ed. by A. Debru and G. Sabbah (Saint-Étienne 1998): 183.

45 A drug obtained from various species of orchids, esp. *Orchis morio* L. (= *Anacamptis morio*, green-winged orchid), *Orchis mascula* L. (early purple orchid), and *Orchis militaris* L. (military orchid).

46 Cf. DT 3:120 (480–1); MIG 1035. The Arabic translator of Diocurides, Iṣṭifān, applied the term خصى الثعلب to the species of orchid called in Greek σατύριον (Dioscurides, *Materia medica* 3.128, ed. by C. E. Dubler (Tetuan/Barcelona 1952–7), 2:296, 4).

אשכנז (*Sefer ha-Shimmush*), = Arabic الصقالبة 'the Slavs, the Skyths'; cf. fol. 145b, col. a: הבשר השלוק וקוראים אותו אנשי המזרח אספגדבאג'ה ואנחנו קוראים אותו גם כן שלוק האשכנז והוא חם בשוי ונאות ברוב העתים והענינים לכל בני אדם לבד מי שיגבר על מזגו החמימות ([The[47] dish with] boiled meat which is called by the people of the East ʾSPGDBʾĞH and which we also call the boiled [meat dish] from Ashkenaz; it is moderately hot and is at most times and in most cases good for all people, except for those whose temperament is dominated by heat). Hebrew אשכנז was used in medieval times first to designate the Kuzaris, then the Slavs and later the Jews of central Europe.[48] The equation of אשכנז with الصقالبة features explicitly in the travel account by Ibrahim Ibn Yaqub (tenth century).[49]

אתמולי (*Sefer Hanhagat ha-Beriʾut*) = 'pertaining to (from) yesterday'; cf. 6 (139): ומן הראוי לבלתי התעצל מהתיגע ומהתנועע יום יום קודם האכילה ואחר תום טחינת המאכל האתמולי באחת ממיני התנועות הראויות לו (One should not hesitate (be too lazy) to exert oneself and to move with an appropriate movement (to make appropriate exercises) every day before one eats and after yesterday's food has been digested). Hebrew אתמולי is a non-attested adjective coined from אתמול.

מביא דם (בא): See entry **סם**.

באסאליק: See entry **באסליק**.

הבאסליק: באסליק (*Sefer ha-Qanun*, Nathan) = Arabic الباسليق 'basilic vein' (cf. DKT 634–5, 814; FAL 31, no. 600, s.v. الباسليك); cf. bk. 1 (fol. 66a): והרביעי והוא הגדול שבהם והוא אותו אשר יראה ויעלה וישתלח ענף מאסף עמו שריג מן הקיפאל ויתהוה ממנו האכחל ושאריתו הוא הבאסליק (The fourth [branch of the axillary vein], the largest of all, is the one that goes up along the outer part and sends out branches that join a branch of the cephalic vein and from these branches the median vein is formed. The remaining part is the basilic vein). Hebrew הבאסליק is a non-attested loan word (with the Hebrew definite article) from Arabic الباسليق. Zeraḥyah Ḥen transcribes the Arabic الباسليق as הבאסאליק, and Joseph Lorki as בסליק.

---

47 '[The dish with] boiled meat which is called by the people of the East ʾSPGDBʾĞH': Cf. entry הבשר השלוק.

48 Cf. S. Krauss, 'Ha-shemot ʾashkenaz u-sefarad', in *Tarbiz* 3 (1931–2): 423–35; esp. 434.

49 Cf. F. Westberg (trans.), 'Ibrâhîm's-ibn-Jaʿḳûb's Reiseberight [für Reisebericht] über die Slawenlande aus dem Jahre 965', in: *Mémoires de l'Académie Impériale des Sciences de St.-Pétersbourg*, ser. 8, *Classe historico-philologique*, vol. 3.4 (St. Petersburg 1898), repr. in: *Studies on Ibrāhīm ibn Yaʿqūb (2nd Half 10th Century) and on His Account of Eastern Europe*, ed. by F. Sezgin et al., = PIHAIS: Islamic Geography, vol. 159 (Frankfurt 1994), 131–7, esp. 136. I thank Andreas Kaplony for this reference.

בגד (*Sefer Ṣedat ha-Derakhim*) = Arabic قرطاس 'papyrus'; Latin 'carta'; cf. bk. 1, ch. 7 (fol. 12a): או יקח בגד שרופה וישחקהו בחומץ חזק ויטוח אותו על הנגעים (Or take burned papyrus, pound it with strong vinegar and plaster it on the tumors). Hebrew בגד features in the current dictionaries in the sense of 'garment, clothing, raiment' (BDB 93–4); 'web, garment' (JD 137); 'web' (BM 458).

בדל: See entry **מבדיל**.

בדלי (*Sefer ha-Qanun*, Joseph Lorki) = Arabic غضروفي 'cartiliginous'; cf. bk. 1 (fol. 12a): העצה מחובר מחוליות ג׳ בדליים אין תוספת להם (The coccyx is composed of three cartiliginous vertebrae that do not have processes). Hebrew בדלי features in BM 467 with the same quotation[50]; however, instead of להם, Ben Yehuda has בהם. For the other translator(s), see entry שחוסי.

בהלה (*Sefer Ṣedat ha-Derakhim*) = Arabic غفلة 'unmindfulness, forgetfulness, neglectfulness, heedlessness, or inadvertence' (L 2276); cf. bk. 1, ch. 14 (fol. 21a): ונצוהו גם כן להתמיד לקיחת הרפואה הזאת כי כבר ניסינו אותה ושבחנוה והוא גרגרים חברם אצחק בן עמרם יועילו בע״ה מן הבהלה והשכחה וכאב הראש המתילד מן הליחה הלבנה (We also tell him (i.e., the patient suffering from forgetfulness) to frequently take the following medicine because we tried it and found it to be good; it is a pill that was composed by Isḥāq ibn ʿImrān and that is good, God willing, for unmindfulnes, forgetfulness, and headache caused by phlegm). Hebrew בהלה is attested for in the Bible and Rabbinic literature in the sense of 'terror' (BM 471); 'dismay, sudden terror or ruin' (BDB 96); 'suddenness, sudden calamity, shock' (JD 142); and 'a phenomenon, the characteristic of which is sudden death, a scare' (LOW XXXIX). The term also features in Ibn Tibbon's translation of Hippocrates' *Aphorisms* 7.5 for Arabic حيرة, 'confusion', and Zeraḥyah Ḥen uses it in his translation of Hippocrates' *Aphorisms* 7.14 for Arabic بهتة 'stupor' (cf. NM 3:30).

בֹּהַק: בהק שחור (*Sefer ha-Shimmush*) = Arabic بهق أسود 'black *bahaq*'; a kind of melanoderma[51]) cf. fol. 134b, col. b: והתמדת אכילתו גורמת השטות[52] והסרטן ומדוה השועל והדליות והטחורים והבהק השחור ודומיהם מן החליים השחוריים (Its frequent consumption (i.e., that of cabbage) causes melancholy, cancer, elephantiasis, varicose veins, hemorrhoids, black *bahaq* and similar black bile illnesses). Subsequent to Shem Tov Ben Isaac, Hebrew בהק שחור features in BM 475 in an attestation from the *Sefer ha-Qanun*; however, Ben Yehuda

50 In the survey of the sources he consulted for the compilation of his dictionary (cf. BM 1:274), Ben Yehuda is uncertain about the identity of the translation of Ibn Sīnā's *K. al-Qānūn* he was able to consult, and suggests that it is that by Nathan ha-Me'ati.

51 For an extensive discussion of this kind of *bahaq*, in addition to two others (white and dust-colored), see IJZ 108, esp. n. 196.

52 השטות: المالنخولية a.

does not define its meaning. The term בהק itself is defined by him as a 'dull white skin disease, vitiligo'. בהק already features in the Bible; cf. BDB 97: 'a harmless eruption on the skin'.

בורקי (*Pirqei Arnauṭ de Vilanova*)[53] = Latin 'nitrosus' (nitrous); cf. 4.13 (50): הדם הנוטה לצדדי העור בורקי או חלודי הנה יורק באופן נאות עם הנחת קרני המציצה וביחוד אם יהיה הדם עב או עמוק אמנם אם יהיה דק או שטחי הנה העלוקות יריקוהו (If the intercutaneous (lit., 'that tends to the sides of the skin') blood is nitrous or rust-like, it can be properly expelled by applying cupping glasses, especially when the blood is thick or deep. But when it is thin or superficial, it can be extracted by leeches). Hebrew בורקי is a non-attested loan word from Arabic بورقي 'alkaline' (cf. NM 2:30).

בזהרי (*Pirqei Arnauṭ de Vilanova*) = Latin 'theriacalis' (antidotal); cf. 5.96 (110): הנגעים המתאכלים אשר יתרחבו ויתפשטו אל העומק מעצמם ראוי לרפאם עם דברים קובצים ומיבשים בלתי עוקצים, ואם יהיו ארסיים כמו חולי הזאב יצטרך שיהיו בזהריים (Corrosive[54] wounds that spontaneously spread and become deeper, should be treated with astringent, drying ingredients that do not bite. But if they (i.e., the wounds) are poisonous, as in the case of lupus[55], [the ingredients] should have the property of the bezoar (be antidotal)). Hebrew בזהרי, lit., 'having the property of the bezoar (antidotal)', is a non-attested loan word from the Arabic بازهري.

בטול: ביטול הגוף (*Sefer Hanhagat ha-Beri'ut*) = 'paralysis'; cf. 8.5 (154): אז ינקה הגוף ממנה בסמים המנקים אותה נפרדים או מורכבים פן תוליד בו בטול כל הגוף או חציו ועקימת הפה (… then he should cleanse the body from it (i.e., the phlegm) with purgatives, simple or compound, so that they do not cause a total paralysis or a partial one (hemiplegia), and paralysis of the facial nerve). Hebrew בטול הגוף does not feature in the current dictionaries.

ביטול חצי הגוף (*Sefer Hanhagat ha-Beri'ut*) = 'hemiplegia'; cf. 8.5 (154): אז ינקה הגוף ממנה בסמים המנקים אותה נפרדים או מורכבים פן תוליד בו בטול כל הגוף או חציו ועקימת הפה. Hebrew ביטול חצי הגוף does not feature in the current dictionaries. An Aramaic synonym, פלג or פלגא (for Arabic فالج), features in the glossary to the *Sefer ha-Shimmush* composed by Shem Tov Ben Isaac; cf. SHS 1:409 (Pe 14).

בטנה: בטנים (*Sefer Ṣedat ha-Derakhim*) = Arabic صنوبر 'pine cone(s)'; bk. 2, ch. 8 (fol. 48b): או יקח סחיטת כרתי עם חלב אשה ויעורב עם שמן ורדים ויטיף ממנו באזן או יתיך מרישארמה הוא אישוף בשמן בטנים ויטיף ממנו בהם (Or take leek extract and women's milk, mix this with rose oil and drip it in the ear, or dissolve hyssop

53 Cf. entry מים: המים הגפריתיים והבורקיים.

54 'corrosive': See entry מתאכל (אכל).

55 'lupus': Cf. entry זאב: חולי הזאב.

in pine cone oil and drip it in it). Hebrew בטנה, Plur. בטנים features in the Bible and Rabbinic literature in the sense of 'pistachio' (*Pistacia vera*); according to some medieval authors, such as Sa'adya Gaon and Maimonides, it is the fruit of the terebinth tree; cf. SHS 1:130 (Bet 2). The first recorded identification of בטנים as a.o. 'pine cones' features in a list of plants by Kaleb Afendopolo (1464?–1525), according to whom בוטמים can be identified with בטנים and this term can also indicate 'pine cones' (*'ṣṭrobīlīn*), which are called *ṣanawbar* by the physicians (cf. LF 1:192; 4:225; SHS 1:113 (Alef 29), 130 (Bet 2).

ביצה (*Sefer ha-Qanun*, Zeraḥyah) = Arabic خصية 'testicle, ovary' (cf. DKT 564, 817; FAL 81, no. 1784); cf. bk. 1 (fol. 28a): אבל הנשים יספיק להן זוג לכל ביצה אחת (In the case of women only one pair [of muscles] for each ovary is sufficient). In the sense of 'testicle', or 'ovary', Hebrew ביצה is only attested for Rabbinic literature (cf. LOW XL). Ben Yehuda (BM 529) mentions it as synonymous with אשך (testicle), featuring in Rabbinic literature.

בית (*Sefer ha-Qanun*, Zeraḥyah) = Arabic بطن 'ventricle [of the brain]'; cf. bk. 1 (fol. 17b): ואמר גאלינוס ואי איפשר שיהיה לראש צורה רביעית בלתי טבעית עד שיהיה האורך יותר מחוסר מן הרוחב אלא אם יהיה חסור ממנו מבתי המוח או חלק אחד ממנו וזה הפך לכל חיי האדם נמנע מבריאות ההרכבה (Galen said that the head cannot possibly have a fourth unnatural shape whereby the length would be less than the breath, unless the ventricles of the brain or part of it would be reduced in size, and this is contrary to all human life [and] impossible with regard to a just composition [of the human body]). Hebrew בית does not feature in this sense in the current dictionaries. For the other trnaslator(s), see entry חדר.

בית הבליעה (*Sefer ha-Qanun*, Zeraḥyah) = Arabic حلق (cf. DKT 535–6, 816: 'gorge. 1. pharynx. 2. partie antérieure inférieure du cou'; FAL 68, no. 1505: 'Pharynx (+ Larynx)'; cf. bk. 1 (fol. 25a): האחד הוא הקלפיי אשר יבואנו החוש לפני בית הבליעה ותחת הזקן (The first (i.e., of the three cartilages of the throat) is the cartilage that can be seen at the anterior part of the throat beneath the chin). Hebrew בית הבליעה features in Rabbinic literature and is explained in the current dictionaries as 'esophagus' (JD 173, s.v. בליעה; BM 534; LOW XL) or 'pharynx' (LOW XL; MD 566). Nathan ha-Me'ati translates the Arabic حلق as גרון.

בית יד (*Sefer Issur ha-Qevurah le-Galienus*) = Arabic مقبض 'handle'; cf. par. 37: הרפואה הראשונה היא לזקנים ושוכני הארצות הקרות ומקבלי המקרה בסתיו. תרופתו שתצוה לקחת שתי לוחות ברזל כל לוח אר<ו>כה כמו אמה ויהיה לה בית יד וימשחנה בשמן אגוזים ותניחנה על האש ונפח במפוח (The first [kind of] treatment concerns the elderly and those who live in cold countries and those who suffer from the ailment [i.e., apoplexy] in winter. Its treatment is to take two slabs of steel, every slab a cubit by a cubit; they should have a handle that should be rubbed with walnut oil and put on a fire that should be fanned with bellows). In the sense of 'handle', Hebrew בית יד is attested in Rabbinic literature; cf. LW 1:226; EM 162; BM 535.

בליטה (*Sefer ha-Qanun*, Nathan) I. = Arabic نتوء 'prominence [of the head]'; cf. bk. 1, ch. 2 (fol. 29a): ואמנם תבניתי הראש הבלתי טבעיים הם ג׳ אחד מהם כשיחסר הבליטה הקודמת[56] (There are three non-natural shapes of the head, one [shape] is that where the frontal prominence is missing …). In the sense of 'prominence', Hebrew בליטה features in BM 549 in an attestation from Meir Aldabi, *Shevilei Emunah* only. The same Hebrew term is used by Shem Tov Ben Isaac for Arabic نتوء in the sense of 'protuberance [of flesh]' (cf. NM 2:80). Zeraḥyah Ḥen renders the Arabic نتوء as תוספת (see entry); II. = Arabic لقمة 'convex part of a vertebra, epiphysis' (cf. WKAS 2.2:1124b–1225a; DKT 488–9, 827; FAL 84, no. 1866); cf. bk. 1, ch. 13 (fol. 36a): ובהיות[57] שתי קצוות השדרה נוטים אל השכיבה[58] לא נוצר להם בליטות[59] אבל[60] נקרות (And since, [as[61] it were], the two ends of the spine incline to meet each other they were not provided with convex parts but with concave parts). Zeraḥyah Ḥen renders the Arabic لقمة as מקום רחב (see entry).

בליטת הרחם (*Sefer Ṣedat ha-Derakhim*) = Arabic نتوء الرحم 'prolapse of the uterus'[62]; cf. introduction (fol. 4a): השער הי״ד בבליטת הרחם (Chapter fourteen: On prolapse of the uterus). Hebrew בליטת הרחם does not feature in the current dictionaries. Masie (MD 601) mentions צניחת הרחם for 'prolapsus uteri'.

בליטת הרקה (*Sefer ha-Qanun*, Nathan) = Arabic وجنة (cf. DKT 830: 'upper part of the cheek, cheekbone'); cf. bk. 1 (fol. 44b): ואמנם יורדים מצד בליטת הרקה כי תנועתם אליהם (They (i.e., the muscles of the nose) come from [the region of] the cheekbones because their movement is directed towards these). Hebrew בליטת הרקה does not feature in the current dictionaries. Zeraḥyah Ḥen translates the Arabic وجنة as פנים, and Joseph Lorki as רקה.

בסליק: See entry **באסליק**.

---

56 Ms המאוחרת Ms[1] :הקודמת.

57 emend. De Koning (DKT 489, n. 4) وكأن a وكان :ובהיות.

58 a الالتقاء :השכיבה.

59 add. Ms ? בכובנא :בליטות.

60 Ms אצל emend. ed. :אבל.

61 '[as it were]': Trans. following emend. De Koning.

62 For Ibn al-Jazzār's discussion of this illness, cf. Ibn al-Jazzar, *On Sexual Diseases: A Critical Edition, English Translation and Introduction of Zad al-musafir wa-qut al-hadir (*Provisions for the Traveller and the Nourishment of the Settled*), bk. 6*, ed. and trans. by G. Bos (London 1997), 55–6; 177–80 (Arabic); 284–5 (English).

בקיעה (*Sefer Ṣedat ha-Derakhim*) = Arabic فتق 'hernia'[63]; cf. introduction (fol. 4a): השער הח׳ בבקיעה המתילד בביצים (Chapter eight: On scrotal hernia). Hebrew בקיעה features in the current dictionaries in Rabbinic literature in the sense of 'cleaving, cleft, that which is cloven' (JD 186; BM 594); in medieval literature as 'crossing' (of the Red Sea), and in modern literature as 'breaking' (of the egg by a bird) (EM 190–1). Masie (MD 351, s.v. hernia) mentions a variant reading: בקיע. Subsequent to Moses Ibn Tibbon, the term features in the same sense in the translations of Maimonides' *Medical Aphorisms* 9.123 by Nathan ha-Me'ati and Zeraḥyah Ḥen (cf. NM 1:131; 2:32). It also features in the same sense in the *Hanhagat ha-Beri'ut le-Abu 'Ali Ben Zuhr* (cf. Honofredi: 'ruptura'); cf. ch. 31: עוד השמר לבלתי תעלה עליך ותפחד בדפיקתה עליך מהמים שלה שזה יוליד הזק ולא תהיה יכול לדחות הזרע בכלל. וזה ממה שתפחד מזה הענין בקיעת הביצים (Take care [not to have coitus] while the woman is on top of you. If this happens and she presses on you you should fear for the harm caused by her moisture. Moreover, you will not at all be able to push your sperm inside her. And in this case you should [also] fear for a scrotal hernia).

בקיעת השפתים (*Sefer Ṣedat ha-Derakhim*) = Arabic تشقيق الشفتين 'lip fissures'; cf. introduction (fol. 2b): השער הי״ו בבקיעת השפתים (Chapter sixteen: On lip fissures). Hebrew בקיעת השפתים does not feature in the current dictionaries. For בקיעה, see previous entry.

הבריק (ברק) (*Sefer Issur ha-Qevurah le-Galienus*) = Arabic اصفرّ 'to turn yellow, to become pale'; cf. par. 142: ואות מי שיקרהו זה כי שיניו יהיו דופקות ועצביו יתקבצו וידיו ורגליו יזיעו ויבריק חוטמם (And the symptoms for those who are affected by this are: chattering teeth, contracting nerves, sweating hands and feet, and a nose turning yellow). Hebrew הבריק does not feature in this sense in the current dictionaries.

בְּשׂוּם (*Sefer ha-Shimmush*) = Arabic عطرية 'aroma'; cf. fol. 131a, col. b: ויש לו סגולה מופלאה איננה לשאר היינות כי כשישתה נודף ריחו ובשומו מבגדי שותהו (It (i.e., wine made from boiled honey) has a wonderful property which the other wines do not have, for if one drinks from it its fragrance and aroma spread from one's clothes). In the sense of 'aroma', Hebrew בְּשׂוּם features in EM 205 in an attestation from Naḥmanides' commentary on Ex 25:6.

מבשל (בשל): See entry **סם**.

בושמיות: בְּשָׂמִיּוּת (*Sammim Libbiyim*) = Arabic عطرية 'aroma'; cf. fol. 126a: ויש לו עם זה דקות והוא בסבת הבושמיות אשר בו נאות לעצם הרוח [ו]למה שיש בו מן הקביצות עם הדקות מקשר אותו מנקה לעצמיותו מפשיט אותו (… and it (i.e., the myrtle) has refining [power] and because of its aroma it is favorable to the substance of

63 For Ibn al-Jazzār's discussion, cf. ibid., 38, 118–25 (Arabic), 259–61 (English).

the pneuma. It strengthens, purefies and rarefies its substance (i.e., that of the pneuma) through its astringency and refining power). Hebrew בְּשָׂמִיּוּת features in EM 206 as a modern term, and in BM 643 as בְּשָׂמִיּוּת in an attestation from the *Sefer ha-Qanun*. The anonymous translator of *Sefer ha-Refu'ot ha-Libbiyot* renders Latin 'aromaticitas' as ריחניות (see entry).

בשר (*Sefer Ṣedat ha-Derakhim*) = Arabic شحم 'pulp (of fruit)'; cf. bk. 2, ch. 18 (fol. 60b): ואם היה כאב השנים מפני קור ... או יבשל בשר קולוקונטידא או עורקיו בחומץ ויגמא אותו (If the toothache is caused by cold ... or he (the patient) should boil pulp or roots of colocynth with vinegar and rinse [the mouth] with it). In the sense of 'pulp', Hebrew בשר features in BM 645, a.o. in an attestation from the *Sefer ha-Qanun*.[64]

הבשר המליח המתובל (*Sefer ha-Shimmush*) = Arabic اللحم المقدد; cf. L 2492, s.v. قديد: 'flesh-meat cut into strips, or oblong pieces, and spread in the sun, to dry'; NA 719: 'jerked meat made by slicing the meat into long and very thin strips and then marinating it in sour vinegar mixed with pure salt and spices such as black pepper, coriander, caraway, and *murrī* (liquid fermented sauce). It is left in this marinade for a day and then dried in the sun ...'; cf. fol 145a, col. a: הבשר המליח המתובל הנקרא בלשונם אלקדיד מיוחס אל הבשר החי אשר הומלח ממנו כי המלח יקנהו מותר יבשות וחמימות ואחור עכול (Jerked meat is a term used for fresh meat that is salted and spiced and that is called [in Arabic] *qadīd*, because the salt makes it extra dry and hot and slow to digest). Hebrew הבשר המליח המתובל (lit., 'salted, spiced meat') does not feature in the current dictionaries.

בשר נוסף (*Sefer Ṣedat ha-Derakhim*) = Arabic بواسير 'nasal polyps' (Greek πολύπους: cf. UWS 2:159); cf. bk. 2, ch. 13 (fol 53b): ואם יקרה בחוטם בשר נוסף (And if nasal polyps occur in the nose ...). Hebrew בשר נוסף does not feature in the current dictionaries. Shem Tov Ben Isaac renders Arabic بواسير in the sense of 'nasal polyps' as טחורים (cf. NM 2:12).

הבשר השלוק (*Sefer ha-Shimmush*) = Arabic اللحم المسلوق 'dish with boiled meat' (cf. D 1:676, s.v. مسلوق: 'du bouilli, chez Bc لحم مسلوق, portait en Espagne, entre autres noms, celui de مسلوق الصقالبة ...'; cf. fol. 145b, col. a: הבשר השלוק וקוראים אותו אנשי המזרח אספגדבאג׳ה ואנחנו קוראים אותו גם כן שלוק האשכנז והוא חם בשוי ונאות ברוב העתים והענינים לכל בני אדם לבד מי שיגבר על מזגו החמימות ובעתים החמים מאד ולמי שיש לו אסתניסות והפוך נפש ([The dish with] boiled meat which is called by the people of the East ʾSPGDBʾǦH and which we also call the boiled [meat dish] from Ashkenaz; it is moderately hot and is at most times and in most cases good for all people, except for

64 See also entry יבלת.

those whose temperament is dominated by heat or who suffer from sickness in the stomach or nausea and when the weather is very hot). Hebrew הבשר השלוק does not feature as the name for a dish in the current dictionaries.

בת: בת עין (*Sefer ha-Qanun*, Zeraḥyah)[65] = Arabic مقلة 'eyeball' (cf. DKT 518–9, 829; FAL 96, no. 2127); cf. bk. 1 (fol. 23b): הפרק הרביעי בנתוח המושקולו שלבת עין (Chapter four: The anatomy of the muscles of the eyeball). Hebrew בת עין features in biblical and modern literature in the sense of 'pupil of the eye' (cf. BDB 123; EM 208). For the other translator(s), see entry כלל העין.

גב: גב הערוה (*Sefer ha-Qanun*, Nathan) = Arabic عظم العانة '1. hip bone; 2. pubic bone' (cf. DKT 823; FAL 25, nos. 528–9); cf. bk. 1 (fol. 60a): ובעבור כי אין לעצלים הצומחים מצד עצבי גב הערוה דרך <אל> הרגלים מאחורי הגוף ומפנימי הפחדים לרוב מה שיש שם מן העצלים והעורקים (And because [the nerves for] the muscles that come from the region of the pubic bone cannot go to the legs through the posterior parts of the body, nor through the inner parts of the thighs, because of the large number of muscles and veins being there ...). Hebrew גב הערוה features in BM 668 in an attestation from the *Sefer ha-Qanun* (cf. NM 2:33). Zeraḥyah Ḥen renders the Arabic عظم العانة as עצם הערוה, and Joseph Lorki as עצם מקום שער הרגלים (see entry).

גבינה: הגבנה הטפלה בבצק (*Sefer ha-Shimmush*) = Arabic المجبّنة 'cheese pie, some are filled with cheese and fried and others baked in the oven' (cf. NA 570); see as well D 1:172: 'espèce de beignet fait avec de la farine et du fromage' (a pastry made from meal and cheese); cf. fol 147b, col. a: הגבנה הטפלה בבצק וקלויה[66] בשמן ראוי להיות בצקה שוה השאור (The dough of the cheese pie that is fried[67] in oil should be moderate in leaven). Hebrew הגבנה הטפלה בבצק does not feature in the current dictionaries.

גבנות (*Sefer Ṣedat ha-Derakhim*) = Arabic حدب 'hunchback'; Latin 'gibbositas'; cf. bk. 1, ch. 23 (fol. 35b): תאר גרגרי אבפורבי למה שתקנו יצחק מועיל מן הפלג שסבתו הקור והרעש ורוח הגבנות ולכל חולי יתילד בפרקים ממותר עב וניסיתיהו (Recipe of the euphorbium pill according to the improved version by Isaac and good for hemiplegia caused by cold, tremors, wind [causing?] hunchback, and every disease that arises in the joints and is caused by thick superfuities. I have tested it). Hebrew גבנות features as a modern term in EM 217. Subsequent to Ibn Tibbon, the term features in Zeraḥyah Ḥen's translation of Hippocrates' *Aphorisms* 6.46 (cf. NM 3:43). A variant derived from the

65 In addition to בת עין, Zeraḥyah translates Arabic مقلة as עין (see entry תחתית העין).

66 וקלויה: متّخذة a.

67 'fried': 'prepared' a.

same root, i.e. גבנינות, features in Nathan ha-Me'ati's translation of the same aphorism (cf. ibid.).

התגבר (גבר) (*Sefer Ṣedat ha-Derakhim*)[68] = Arabic فار 'to boil (over), to simmer, to bubble'; cf. bk. 1, ch. 18 (fol. 26a): ותתילד משתי סבות אחת מהן התלהבות מרה כרכומית והתלקח בחלקי המוח והאחרת מרתיחת דם הלב והתגברו כי דם הלב כשירתח ויתלהב בחום מרה אדומה יתגבר ויעלה חזקתו אל הראש (And it (i.e., phrenitis) is caused by one of two things: (1) the heat and burning of the yellow bile in the parts of the brain and (2) the boiling and bubbling of the blood of the heart; when the blood of the heart becomes boiling hot because of the heat of the yellow bile, it bubbles and its[69] burning heat arises to the brain). Hebrew התגבר does not feature in this sense in the current dictionaries.

הגיס (גוס) (*Sefer Ṣedat ha-Derakhim*) = Arabic ضرب 'to stir'; cf. bk. 2, ch. 13 (fol. 53a): ויגיס אותו עד שישוב אספלנית (And stir [these ingredients] until they turn into a salve). Hebrew הגיס does not feature in a medical context in the current dictionaries; cf. BM 724 with an attestation from Maimonides, *Mishneh Torah, Sefer Tohorah, Hilkhot Tum'at Okhalim.*

גיד: הגיד הדופק הורידי (*Sefer ha-Qanun*, Joseph Lorki) = Arabic الشريان الوريدي 'venous artery, pulmonary vein' (cf. DKT 604–5, 820; FAL 138, no. 2988); cf. bk. 1 (fol. 18a): ולכן נקרא הגיד הדופק הורידי (For this reason it is called 'venous artery' (pulmonary vein). Hebrew הגיד הדופק הורידי is not attested in the current dictionaries. For the other translator(s), see entry השריין הורידי.

הגיד הורידי (*Sefer ha-Qanun*, Zeraḥyah) = Arabic الشريان الوريدي 'venous artery, pulmonary vein' (cf. DKT 604–5, 820; FAL 138, no. 2988); cf. bk. 1 (fol. 32a): ועל כן נקרא הגיד הורידי. Hebrew הגיד הורידי is not attested in the current dictionaries. For the other translator(s), see entry השריין הורידי.

הגיד העליון (*Sefer Ṣedat ha-Derakhim*) = Arabic القيفال 'cephalic vein' (cf. DKT 825; FAL 123, no. 2710); cf. bk. 1, ch. 3 (fol. 8b): ויקיז הגיד העליון אם יעזור הזמן והשנים והמנהג והכח ויוציא מן הדם בשיעור כדי שיצא עמו מה שיהיה ממותר חד (He should bleed from the cephalic vein if the time [of the year], the age [of the patient], [his] habits and strength are conducive. He should extract a measure sufficient for the sharp residue to be removed together with [the blood]). Hebrew הגיד העליון does not feature in the current dictionaries. In addition to הגיד העליון, Ibn Tibbon has גיד הראש; see next entry. In his glossary to the *Sefer ha-Qanun*, Nathan ha-Me'ati uses the term הגיד העליון as an explanation for חבל הזרוע (cf. NM 2:113 (Ḥet 12) and 138 (Ḥet 12)).

גיד הראש (*Sefer Ṣedat ha-Derakhim*) = Arabic القيفال 'cephalic vein' (cf. DKT 825; FAL 123, no. 2710); cf. bk. 1, ch. 1 (fol. 5a): ואם היה מראה המקום אדום

---

68 See also entry התגברות.

69 'its burning heat': See entry חֲזָקָה.

נדע שהוא ממותר דם נפסד ואם עזר הזמן והשנים והמנהג והכח נקיז לו גיד הראש ונוציא מן הדם בשיעור הצורך והכח (If the colour of the [hairless] spot is red we know that it is caused by a residue of corrupt blood, and if the time [of the year], the age [of the patient], [his] habits and strength are conducive, we bleed from the cephalic vein and extract the necessary amount of blood). Hebrew גיד הראש does not feature in the current dictionaries. Masie (MD 763, s.v. 'vein, cephalic') has וריד הראש for 'cephalic vein'. In addition to גיד הראש, which also features in Shem Tov Ben Isaac's *Sefer ha-Shimmush* (cf. NM 1:82), Ibn Tibbon has הגיד העליון; see previous entry. Zeraḥyah Ḥen translates Arabic القيفال, featuring in Maimonides, *Medical Aphorisms* 12.23, as גיד הראש הנקרא קיפאל, and Nathan ha-Me'ati (ibid.) as הקיפאל הוא ספאליקא.

גיד הראש הנקרא אכחל (*Sefer ha-Qanun*, Zeraḥyah) = Arabic الأكحل 'median vein' (cf. DKT 634–5, 814; FAL 6, no. 100); cf. bk. 1 (fol. 34b): והרביעי הוא היותר גדול והוא אשר הוא נראה ויעלה וישתלח לשעיפים יתחבר שעיף מן הקיפל ויבא מהם גיד הראש הנקרא אכחל והנשאר הוא הנקר' באסאליק (The fourth [branch of the axillary vein], the largest of all, is the one that goes up along the outer part and sends out branches that join a branch of the cephalic vein and from these branches the median vein is formed. The remaining part is the basilic vein). Hebrew גיד הראש הנקרא אכחל does not feature in this sense in the current dictionaries. For the other translator(s), see entry אכחל.

הגידים הנחים (*Sefer Hanhagat ha-Beri'ut*) = 'veins'; cf. 2.1 (115): ועבדי הכבד הם הגידים הנחים היוצאים ממנו השולחים להם הדם הטהור והנקי להתפרנס בו (The veins are the servants of the liver. They issue from it and send it the pure, clean blood for nourishment). Hebrew גיד נח, Plur. גידים נחים, does not feature in the current dictionaries. The term also occurs in Shem Tov Ben Isaac's glossary to the *Sefer ha-Shimmush* for Arabic أوردة 'veins', cf. SHS 1:163 (Gimel 28).

גלגול (*Sefer Ṣedat ha-Derakhim*) = Arabic سدر 'dizziness'; Latin 'vertigo vel scotomia'; cf. bk. 1, ch. 13 (fol. 20a): הגלגול הוא שיתדמה לאדם שמה שיראה יתגלגל סביבו ויאבד הרגש הראות פתאום עד שיחשוב שכסה כל מה שהיה רואה חשך (Dizziness is [a condition] in which it seems to someone that what he sees is turning around him and in which his sense of vision is suddenly lost so that he thinks that all that he saw has been covered by darkness). Hebrew גלגול does not feature in this sense in the current dictionaries. Arabic دوار, a synonym of سدر, is translated by Ibn Tibbon as גלגול הראש (cf. entry below) and as סבוב (cf. NM 1:63). Subsequent to Ibn Tibbon, Zeraḥyah Ḥen translates Arabic سدر as גלגול as well (cf. NM 3:44–5).

גלגול הראש (*Sefer Ṣedat ha-Derakhim*) = Arabic دوار 'dizziness'; cf. bk. 1, ch. 23 (fol. 35b): תאר גירא בן מאסויה לניקוי הראש מליחה לבנה ומה שיתלד ממנה מן

השתוק והפלג ותרדמת האיברים וגלגול הראש (Recipe of a hiera[70] [composed by] Ibn[71] Māsawayh for cleansing the head from the phlegm and [the illnesses] caused by it, i.e., insensibility (apoplexy),[72] hemiplegia, numbness, and dizziness). Hebrew גלגול הראש does not feature in the current dictionaries. Subsequent to Ibn Tibbon, the term features in Zeraḥyah Ḥen's translation of Hippocrates' *Aphorisms* 2.37 (cf. NM 3:45).

גלגלת: See entry **מדוה**.

גמא (*Sefer Ṣedat ha-Derakhim*) = Arabic تمضمض (Greek διακλύζω) 'to rinse the mouth' (cf. UW 194–5); cf. bk. 2, ch. 18 (fol. 60b): ... ואם היה כאב השנים מפני קור או יבשל בשר קולוקונטידא או עורקיו בחומץ ויגמא אותו (If the toothache is caused by cold .... or he (the patient) should boil pulp or roots of colocynth with vinegar and rinse the mouth with it). Hebrew גמא only features in the current dictionaries in the sense of 'to take a draught, to quaff, to sip, to suck up' (JD 251; BM 793).

נגמר (גמר) (*Sefer Ṣedat ha-Derakhim*) = Arabic استحكم 'to become chronic (of an illness)' (cf. D 1:310); Latin 'morbi dominium'; cf. bk. 1, ch. 18 (fol. 27b): ונזכיר רפואת זה לפי דרך[73] הרפואה ונאמר כי ראוי שנקיז בעל מורסת הראש קודם שיגמר חליו ([Now] I will mention the treatment of this [illness] according to the medical rules and say that one should bleed a patient suffering from phrenitis before the illness becomes chronic). Hebrew נגמר does not feature in a medical sense in the current dictionaries.

גַּעַשׁ (*Sefer ha-Shimmush*) = Arabic جشاء 'belching, eructation'; cf. fol. 135a, col. b: וכבר נאמר שהוא מעפש המזון באסטו' והראיה על זה געשו (It has been said that it (i.e., radish) corrupts the food in the stomach and an indication for this is [that it produces] eructation). Hebrew געש is attested in medieval poetry in the sense of 'the activity of something that shakes' (פעולת דבר גועש), cf. BM 824, or of 'noise' (רעש) or 'gale, storm' (סער); cf. EM 260. Moses Ibn Tibbon translates the same Arabic term as קבסה in his translation of Hippocrates' *Aphorisms* 6.1 (cf. NM 3:198), Hillel of Verona and Nathan ha-Me'ati as פיהוק

70 'hiera' (from Greek ἱερά): Name used for a number of compound medicines; see Ullmann, *Medizin im Islam*, 296; the main ingredient of many of these was colocynth pulp (cf. O. Kahl, *Sābūr ibn Sahl's Dispensatory in the Recension of the 'Aḍudī Hospital* (Leiden 2009), 176–9).

71 'Ibn Māsawayh': I.e., Yaḥyā (Yūḥannā) ibn Māsawayh, the famous court physician and translator active in the ninth century, cf. Ullmann, *Medizin im Islam*, 112–5; and EI² 3:872–3.

72 'insensibility' (apoplexy): See entry שתוק below.

73 a דרך: القانون.

(cf. NM 3:187, 198), Zeraḥyah Ḥen as Romance רוטו (cf. NM 3:198), and Judah[74] Shalom as רוט (ibid.); see also SHS 1:151 (Gimel 8).

גפת (*Sefer ha-Shimmush*) = Arabic نوى 'kernels, stones'; cf. fol. 138b, col. a: וכשיבוקע יתפרד מן הגפת שלו (And if you cut them (i.e., peaches) open, they (i.e., their flesh) separate from their stones). Hebrew גפת features in Rabbinic literature in the sense of 'a pressed hard mass, peat, turf (of olive peels)' (JD 263; LW 1:353, 435–6 (Nachträge Fleischer)); cf. BM 828: 'husks of olives'. See also SHS 1:150 (Gimel 7).

גרגור: גירגורים (*Sefer Ṣedat ha-Derakhim*) = Arabic غراغر 'gargles'; cf. bk. 2, ch. 7 (fol. 48a): ויצוק המימות המבושל בהם הסמים החמים אשר יפתחו הסתומים ויעוטש בסמים הדקים המפתחים ויגרגר בגירא פיגרא עם דבש ובגירגורים אשר ימשכו הליחה וינקו הראש (He shall pour water [over his head] in which heating drugs have been cooked that open the obstructions and he shall let him sneeze with refining, opening drugs and gargle with hiera[75] picra with honey and with [other] gargles that draw the [obstructing] moisture and clean the head). In the sense of 'gargle', Hebrew גרגור features in EM 262 as a novel term; Ben Yehuda (BM 831) mentions it in the sense of 'gurgling' in an attestation from the *Sefer ha-Qanun*. According to Masie (MD 317), גרגור features in the sense of 'gargarism' in the *Sefer Asaph ha-Rofe*. The same Hebrew term is used by Moses Ibn Tibbon's contemporary Shem Tov Ben Isaac in the *Sefer ha-Shimmush* (cf NM 2:83–4).

גרגר: גרגרי הדלועים (*Sefer ha-Shimmush*)[76] = Arabic حبّ القرع 'tape-worms' (*Taeniidae*, esp. *Taenia solium* L. and *Taenia saginata* Goeze; cf. MIG 406); cf. fol. 141b, col. a: ורבוי אכילתם יוציא התולעים מהבטן הנקראים גרגרי הדלועים (Their frequent consumption (i.e., of walnuts) expels the worms called 'tape-worms' from the stomach). Hebrew גרגרי הדלועים features as גרגרי הדלעת in BM 832 in an attestation from Nathan ha-Me'ati's translation of Maimonides, *Medical Aphorisms* 7.31: התולעים הנקראים גרגרי הדלעת והם נקראים דלועיים אוכלים כל מה שיזון בו האדם לכן מרזים הגוף (cf. NM 2:91). In the glossary to the *Sefer ha-Qanun*, Nathan remarks: דלע: קראתי דלועים התולעים הדומים לגרגרי הדלעות (DLʿ. I called the worms that are similar to gourd seeds (i.e., tape worms) DLWʿYM) (cf. NM 2:112, 133 (Dalet 8)).

---

74 On Juda (Astruc) Ben Samuel Shalom, *c.* 1450, cf. NM 3:7–9.

75 'hiera picra': For the composition of this compound with aloe as main component, see 'Alī b. Rabban al-Ṭabarī, *Firdaws al-ḥikma*, ed. by M. Z. Siddiqi (Berlin 1928), 458; BAN 182–3. It is good, amongst others, for all dyscrasies of the head and for cold humours in eyes and ears.

76 In addition to גרגרי הדלועים, Shem Tov renders Arabic حبّ القرع as תולעים קטנים (see entry).

הגרגרים המוסרחים (*Sefer Ṣedat ha-Derakhim*) = Arabic حبّ المنتن 'malodorous pills'[77]; Latin 'fetidi pilluli'; cf. bk. 1, ch. 23: וזה[78] תאר הגרגרים המוסרחים לפי נסחת סאבור והוא מועיל בע"ה מן הפלג ועקום הפה וכאב הפרקים והנקרס והרוחות העבות והקולון והנאות וכאב העצבים והרפיון ויגיר הנדות והוא מנוסה עירובו יקח אלואי סיקוטרי ודיליום וקולוקונטידא וסרפי ואפופנק ואמוניאק וזרע סיקודא מ"א דרהם יקובצו אלה הסמים שחוקים ומנופים וישרה מהם מה שראוי לשרותו במי כרתי ויעשה ממנו גרגרים קטנים ויוצנעו והלקיחה מהם ב' דרהם וחצי במים חמים (This is the recipe of the 'malodorous pill' following Sābūr[79] [Ibn Sahl]; it is, God willing, good for hemiplegia, paralysis of the facial nerve, arthritis, podagra, thick winds, colic, crudeness [of the humours], neuralgia, feebleness; it makes the menstrual blood flow and has been tested: Its recipe is: Take one *dirham*[80] each of Socotrine aloe, bdellium, colocynth, sagapenum, opopanax, gum ammoniacum, and harmel seeds; pulverize and strain these ingredients together and steep an appropriate dosis in leek juice; prepare little pills from [this mixture] and store them, and [if needed] take two and a half *dirhams* with hot water). Hebrew הגרגרים המוסרחים does not feature in the current dictionaries. The anonymous *Sammim Libbiyim*, i.e., anonymous translation of Ibn Sīnā, *K. al-adwiya al-qalbiya* (*On Cardiacs*) renders the Arabic as גרגרי הסרוחים.

גרה (*Sefer Ṣedat ha-Derakhim*) = Arabic حبّة 'the weight of one barley corn', i.e., 0.05 grams[81]; cf. bk. 2, ch. 10 (fol. 50a): אם יגר מן האזן מוגלא והיה עם זה כאב חזק הנה ראוי שנתחיל במה שישקיט הכאב כמו שיקח משקל קיראט אופי ומשקל שתי גרות שעוה ויתיכהו במעט שמן ורדים ויטוח ממנו בפתילה וישים אותה באזן (If pus streams from the ear and it comes with a severe pain we should begin to [treat the patient with a remedy] that relieves the pain, [its composition is]: Take one

77 'malodorous pills' (pilulae foetidae): A compound remedy; for their composition see also Ibn Sīnā, *K. al-Qānūn fī l-ṭibb*, 5 bks. in 3 vols. (repr. Beirut n.d.), 3:390–1 (English translation: *The Canon of Medicine (al-Qānūn fī 'l-ṭibb): The Law of Natural Healing*, vol. 5: *Pharmacopeia*, comp. by L. Bakhtiar (Chicago 2014), 237–8).

78 וזה תאר הגרגרים המוסרחים לפי נסחת סאבור והוא מועיל בע"ה מן הפלג ועקום הפה וכאב: This passage is missing in the London Ms and has been copied after Ms Oxford, Bodleian, Poc. 353.

79 Cf. Sābūr Ibn Sahl, *Dispensatorium parvum* (*al-Aqrābādhīn al-ṣaghīr*), ed. by O. Kahl (Leiden 1994), 99 (Arabic text); and idem, *The Small Dispensatory: Translated from the Arabic together with a Study and Glossary*, trans. by O. Kahl (Leiden 2003), 84 (English translation).

80 The standard dirham is 3.125 grams; see W. Hinz, *Islamische Maße und Gewichte: Umgerechnet ins metrische System*, = Handbuch der Orientalistik, vol. 1, suppl. 1.1 (Leiden 1970), 3.

81 Cf. Ibn Sahl, *Dispensatorium parvum* (ed. Kahl, 226); Hinz, *Islamische Maße und Gewichte*, 12–3.

qīrāṭ[82] of opium and two barley corns (i.e., 0.1 grams) of wax, mix this with a small quantity of rose oil, put this on a tampon and insert it in the ear). As a medicinal weight, Hebrew גרה already features in the Bible as the smallest weight, being one twentieth of a *shekel* (cf. BDB 176). The term is defined by Ben Yehuda (BM 836) as the weight of one carob seed in an attestation from Solomon Ibn Gabirol, *Tikkun Middot ha-Nefesh*. According to Maimonides, *Mishneh Torah, Hilkhot Mishkalim*, ch. 1, *Halakhah* 3, the weight of a *gerah* is equal to that of a *maʿah*, namely, sixteen barley corns.[83]

גריסין: גריס (*Sefer ha-Shimmush*) = Arabic سويق **I.** 'the meal of the different kinds of grain, mostly barley, that was parched' (Greek ἄλφιτον 'meal, (barley) groats' (LSG 74)), or the dish prepared from this meal[84]; cf. fol. 124a, col. 2: גריסי החטה חמים במעלה הראשונה יבשים באמצעה זנין מעט מזער אלא שהם יותר זנין מגריסי השעורים (Meal from parched wheat is hot in the first degree and dry in the middle. They are only a little bit nutritious, but more than barley meal). Hebrew גריס is attested for Rabbinic literature in the sense of 'grits' (cf. DAS 3:251: 'Grütze') 1) esp. pounded beans, beans used for pounding; 2) a dish of pounded grains (cf. JD 268); Ben Yehuda (BM 841) states that its meaning is similar to גרש ('groats') (cf. BDB 176, s.v. גרש: 'groats; grits') or דבר גרוס (something that is crushed), and especially 'pounded beans'. Nathan ha-Me'ati translates Arabic سويق, featuring in his translation of Maimonides, *Medical Aphorisms* 5.16, 19 and of Hippocrates' *Aphorisms* 7.3 as גרש(י) כרמל (cf. NM 3:49, s.v. גֶּרֶשׂ: גרש כרמל); Zeraḥyah Ḥen renders the same term as גרישים in his translation of Maimonides, *Medical Aphorisms* 5.16, 19; **II.** 'the meal of parched or dried mealy fruits' (cf. L 1472, and 511, s.v. حتّى); cf. fol. 139a, col. a: וגריסי המנוגבים מהם עצירתם לבטן יותר חזקה (Their dried pulp (i.e., of the medlar) is stronger in binding the bowels).

גריש החטה: גריש (*Hanhagat ha-Beri'ut le-Abu ʿAli Ben Zuhr*) = 'pounded wheat; wheat groats'; cf. ch. 17: ועשית הקיא על המלוא מועיל מחולי המקוה מאד ואכילת המתיקה הידועה באכילתה והוא גריש החטה בלולה בחמאה טובה ולושה בדבש יש לה סגולה לחזק המקוה (Vomiting on a full stomach is very good for an illness of the bladder. The consumption of a well-known sweet dish, namely pounded wheat mixed with good butter and kneaded with honey is especially good for the bladder). Hebrew גריש is a variant reading of גריס; cf. previous entry.

גרם (*Sefer ha-Shimmush*) = Arabic جسم 'flesh, pulp' (cf. UW 266, s.v. σάρξ: 'Fruchtfleisch'); cf. fol. 137a, col. a: וגרם הצמוקים על הכלל חם ולח וחרצניהם קרים

82 One *qīrāṭ* is 0.2232 grams; cf. Hinz, *Islamische Maße und Gewichte*, 27.

83 Cf. J. G. Weiss, *Middot u-Mishkalot shel Torah* (Jerusalem 1985), 3.

84 Namely a thick kind of gruel, or ptisan, moistened with water, or butter, or fat of a sheep's tail etc.'; cf. L 1472; MMT 217, no. 284; IBF 2:308–9, no. 1255.

ויבשים (The flesh of raisins is generally hot and moist and their seeds are cold and dry). In the sense of 'flesh, pulp', Hebrew גרם is a non-attested semantic borrowing from Arabic جسم.

גת (*Sefer ha-Qanun*, Nathan) = Arabic معصرة 'confluence of sinuses, torcular Herophili, torcula' (cf. DKT 632–3, 828; FAL 89, no. 1961), cf. bk. 1 (fol. 65b): ואחר מתפרד ממנו במה שבין שתי המחיצות ונקרא מעצרה כלומר גת (Then it (i.e., blood from the branches of the jugular vein) spreads into the space between the two segments which is called [in Arabic] *maʿṣarah*; i.e., torcula). As an anatomical term, Hebrew גת features in BM 859 in an attestation derived from Joseph Lorki's version of this quotation. Referring to Masie (cf. MD 656), Ben Yehuda translates the term as 'sinus'.

(דבק) מדביק: See entry **סם**.

דבש: דבש רושד (*Sefer ha-Shimmush*)[85] = Arabic جلنجبين 'roses confected with honey' (M 85; FAQ 201–2); cf. fol. 132a, col. b: ואחר להרגיל אחד מן העסיסים החמוצים אם הוא בעל מזג חם ומן הדבש רושד אם הוא בעל מזג קר (Then he should take (as part of the treatment of inebriety) one of the sour robs if he has a hot temperament and roses confected with honey if he has a cold temperament). דבש רושד is an unattested term combined of Hebrew דבש (honey) and Old Occitan 'rosat'; cf. SHS 1:273–4 (Kaf 17): כבוש ורדים העשוי בדבש ב"ה ג'לנגג'בין וב"ל מאל רושד (rose conserve made with honey; Arabic ǦLNǦBYN; other language (Romance) M'L RWŠD).

דבשי: הדבשי (*Sefer ha-Shimmush*) = Arabic معسّل 'honey-dish'; cf. fol. 145b, col. a: הדבשי הנקרא בלשונם מעשל הוא תבשיל עשוי בדבש ובשר ותבלין ושקדים והוא חם וטוב לבעלי הקרירות ובזמן הקר (The honey-dish called in their language (i.e., Arabic) *muʿassal* is a dish made with honey, meat, spices, and almonds; it is hot and good for people with [a] cold [temperament] and in the cold season). Hebrew דבשי features in BM 884 only in the sense of 'of the nature of honey' (מטבע הדבש) in an attestation from the *Sefer ha-Qanun* and from Simeon Ben Zemah Duran, *Magen Avot*.

(דות) מדיית (*Sefer ha-Qanun*, Nathan) = Arabic مرشّح '1. transuding, sweating; 2. destined' (cf. L 1086); cf. bk. 1 (fol. 61a): אמנם נברא המדיית לירידה נוסף בשעורו על האחר כי הוא מנהיג אברים הם רבים יותר במספר והם יותר גדולים בשעורים והם האברים המונחים למטה מן הלב (The branch (i.e., of the two branches of the aorta) that is destined to descend has been made larger than the other [branch] because it leads to organs that are more numerous and larger,

---

85 The same Hebrew term is used by Shem Tov Ben Isaac for the synonymous ورد المربّى العسلي (cf. fol. 150, col. b).

namely those that are near the heart). In the sense of 'destined', מדיית (Part. Nitpa'el) is a non-attested semantic borrowing from Arabic مرشح. For מדיית in the sense of 'sweating, exuding', cf. NM 2:111, 132 (Dalet 2). Ben Yehuda discusses the term in this sense in the entry דיית (BM 933); for the root דות, cf. JD 299; SDA 323. Zeraḥyah Ḥen translates the Arabic مرشح as משולח. Joseph Lorki translates the Arabic وإنّما خلق المرشح للانحدار as נבראת להטפת המורד.

דיסא (Aramaic) (*Sefer ha-Shimmush*) = Arabic هريسة (*harīsa*)[86]; cf. fol. 124b, cols. 1–2: הדיסא היא גם כן מזה המין והיא בטבעה עבה וחלוקה ומתאחרת להתעכל ומולידה סתומים כהולדת הגריסין אלא שהיא כשתתעכל בגופי הבריאים תוליד דם יש בו לחות וחלוקה ותזון מזון רב (DYS' belongs also to this sort [of food]; it is by nature thick, viscous, and slow to digest. It produces obstructions, just like GRYSYN (grits, groats). However, when it is digested in the bodies of healthy people it produces moist, viscous blood and is very nutritious). Aramaic דיסא is attested for Rabbinic literature in the sense of 'coarsely pounded wheat or barley eaten alone or mixed with honey' (cf. SDA 329, s.v. דְּיְיסָא); cf. BM 930, s.v. דיס/דיסה 'barley or wheat that is pounded to remove the husks and then cooked'.

דליות: דלית (*Sefer ha-Shimmush*)[87] = Arabic دوالٍ 'varicose veins'; cf. fol. 134b, col. b: והתמדת אכילתו גורמת השטות[88] והסרטן ומדוה השועל והדליות והטחורים והבהק השחור ודומיהם מן החליים השחוריים (Its frequent consumption (i.e., of cabbage) causes melancholy, cancer, elephantiasis, varicose veins, hemorrhoids, black[89] BHQ and similar black bile illnesses). Hebrew דלית, Plur. דליות, features in Nathan ha-Me'ati's glossary to the *Sefer ha-Qanun*, where it is defined by him as: הוא חולי שהעורקים מן השוק ינפחו ויתראו ויתפשטו כדליות (An illness in which the veins of the leg become swollen and visible, and spread like vines (i.e., varicose veins)); cf. NM 2:112, 133 (Dalet 11). Ben Yehuda (BM 944) considers the plural דליות, as it features in the *Sefer ha-Qanun*, as a singular noun דָּלִיּוּת. In addition to דליות for Arabic دوالٍ, Shem Tov Ben Isaac

---

86 On *harīsa*, cf. FL 4:384: 'Spissi pulmenti species, quod ex cocto tritico, coctosque carnibus, simul contusis multum, conficitur' (A kind of thick dish, prepared from cooked wheat and cooked meats that are thoroughly pounded together); NA 606–7: 'smooth porridge cooked with meat and grains such as rice or wheat'. See also Maimonides, *On Coitus* 6 (forthcoming ed. and trans. by G. Bos): 'It is prepared from sheep's meat or cock's testicles, and spiced with the spices which we have mentioned; one may [also] strew cinnamon over it'; for a variety of recipes cf. ISW 128–40 (ch. 50) (Arabic); NA 256–8 (English).

87 Cf. entry דליות in NM 1:85.

88 השטות: المالنخولية a.

89 Possibly referring to a sort of melanoderma; see entry הבהק השחור.

uses the term זמורות (see entry). In his translation of Maimonides, *Medical Aphorisms* 23.47, Zeraḥyah Ḥen renders Arabic دوالٍ as חולי הנקרא גפנים.

דֶּמַע (*Sefer Ṣedat ha-Derakhim*) = Arabic دمعة 'persistent flow of tears (epiphora)' (cf. Greek ἐπιφορά (LSG 671); cf. bk. 2, ch. 4 (fol. 45a): כשיקרה לו הדמע ולא יהיה לו סבה מחוץ ידענו כי הגרת הלחות ההוא אל העינים מן הראש והגרתו תהיה אם בעורקים אשר למעלה מגולגולת הראש ואם בעורקים אשר תחת הגלגולת (If someone suffers from epiphora without any external cause we know that the flow of moisture to the eyes comes from the head, and that the flow happens either through the vessels that are on the skull or through the vessels that are below the skull). Hebrew דמע only features in the current dictionaries in the sense of 'tear' (cf. BM 965), not as a disease. For variant readings, cf. MD 263, s.v. 'epiphora': דמעת/דמוע/דמיעה. Shem Tov Ben Isaac translates Arabic دمعة as דמעה (cf. NM 2:11).

דפיקה (*Sefer Ṣedat ha-Derakhim*) = Arabic ضربان 'throbbing pain' (MMT 250–1); cf. bk. 2, ch. 1 (fol. 42b): ומזה תואר עגולים לבנים כוללים מועילים בע״ה לקצידה החמה והדפיקה (Recipe of white eye-salves (collyria) that are generally, God willing, good for hot ophthalmia[90] and throbbing pain). Hebrew דפיקה does not feature in this sense in the current dictionaries; cf. BM 977; EM 321; for דפיקה in the sense of 'pulse beat', featuring in Nathan ha-Me'ati's glossary to the *Sefer ha-Qanun*, see NM 2:112, 133 (Dalet 12).

דפיקת לב (*Sefer Ṣedat ha-Derakhim*) = Arabic خفقان 'cardialgia'[91]; cf. bk. 1; ch. 18 (fol. 26a): ויקרה לחולה עם עלות החולי וקרוב חזקתו מקרים מפחידים כמו צמא חזק ונגוב פה ושעירות לשון ושחרותה וסער ודפיקת לב (And when the illness becomes severe and burning hot, the patient suffers from frightening afflictions such as severe thirst, dryness of the mouth, roughness and blackness of the tongue, distress and cardialgia). Hebrew דפיקת הלב features, without further explanation, in BM 977 in an attestation from the *Sefer ha-Qanun*. The same Hebrew term is used by the anonymous translator of Hippocrates' *Aphorisms* 4.65 for Arabic خفقان في الفؤاد (cf. NM 3:53).

דק: See entry **סם**.

דקדק (*Sefer ha-Qanun*, Nathan) = Arabic تلطّف 'to act with grace, kindness'; cf. bk. 1 (fol. 42b): ודקדק הבורא והצמיח מן העצמות דבר דומה בעצבים נקרא עקבים[92]

---

90 'ophthalmia' (קצידה): See NM 3:206; and G. Bos, 'Two Notes on A Complete Dictionary of Ancient and Modern Hebrew', in *Ha-Lashon* (forthcoming).

91 'cardialgia' (Greek καρδιωγμός): I.e., palpitation of the heart or heartburn; Galen, *In Hippocratis Aphorismos commentarius* 4.65 (ed. Kühn, 17b:745–6) remarks that according to the ancients the term καρδία can mean both the heart and the cardia of the stomach, and that the term καρδιωγμός is explained by some in the sense of heartburn and by others in the sense of palpitation of the heart; cf. NM 3:27, n. 106.

92 corr. Ms בעקבים Ms בנקבים emend. ed. :עקבים.

וקשורים להתחברם עם העצבים ומסתבכים בו כדבר אחד (In his kindness the Creator made something grow on the bones resembling nerves, called [in Arabic] *aqabim*[93] and ligaments. He has attached them to the nerves and interlaced them with the nerves as if it is one thing). In the sense of 'to act with kindness', Hebrew דקדק is a non-attested semantic borrowing from the Arabic تلطّف. Joseph Lorki renders Arabic تلطّف as חשב.

מדקדק: See entry **סם**.

דרדני (*Sefer ha-Shimmush*) = Arabic لثة 'gums'; cf. fol. 141a, col. a: ומזיקים אל הדרדני ומחדדים שחין דק בפה ומולידים האפר בעינים (... and they (i.e., dates) are harmful for the gums and cause aphthae in the mouth and ophthalmia). Hebrew דרדני could not be identified, it is possibly a corruption of דרדר (Arabic دردر) 'the part of the jaws where the teeth of small children grow' (cf. FL 1:22a), or related to Persian *dandān* meaning 'teeth, mouth' (VL 1:844). See also SHS 1:175 (Dalet 11): דרדני ב"ה לתאת וב"ל ג'ינג'יבש and NM 1:85–6.

ההאצלות הנפשיות: האצלה (*Sefer Issur ha-Qevurah le-Galienus*) = Arabic القوة النفسانية 'the psychical faculties'; cf. par. 15: ויקרה מזה לאדם עד ו' או ז' שעות[94] שלא ישכיל ולא יאכל ולא ישתה אכן עורקיו דופקים ונשומו מתנועע וזה הסוג מן השעמום יסתום מעברי ההאצלות הנפשיות אשר לחושים (Then a person is without understanding, without eating and drinking for six or seven days,[95] whilst his blood vessels pulsate and his breathing is agitated—this kind of coma obstructs the passageways of the psychical faculty which is [responsible] for the senses). Hebrew ההאצלות הנפשיות features in BM 1023 without any further explanation or reference since, as Ben Yehuda remarks: נשמט מהפתקה המראה מקום.[96]

הברה (*Sefer ha-Shimmush*) = Arabic قراقر '[intestinal] rumblings' (borborygmus; Greek διαβορυγμός; cf. LSG 493); cf. fol. 124a, col. 1: החטה השלוקה כבדה מאד רבת הנפח וההברה ומתעכבת לרדת מן האצטומכא ומולידה חלט עב בתכלית העובי והחלוקה וכל שכן אם תהיה מן החטה הכבדה האדומה (Cooked wheat is very heavy and very flatulent and causes many [intestinal] rumblings; it is slow to descend from the stomach and produces a very thick and viscous humour, especially when it is made from the heavy red wheat). Hebrew הברה features in Rabbinic literature in the sense of 1) 'confused sound, noise', and 2) 'report, rumor' (JD 330) and in medieval linguistic literature in the sense of 'pronunciation' or 'syllable' (cf. BM 1029–30); see also NM 1:86.

---

93 'aqabim': Cf. entry עקב 'fibrous tissue, ligament'.

94 שעות: أيام a.

95 'days': Translated after the Arabic. The Hebrew text has 'hours'.

96 Cf. Bos, 'Two Notes', forthcoming.

הגרת הזרע מבלי רצון: הגרה (*Sefer Ṣedat ha-Derakhim*) = Arabic سيلان المني من غير إرادة 'an involuntary flow of sperm (spermatorrhea)'[97]; cf. introduction (fol. 4a): השער הג׳ בהגרת הזרע מבלי רצון (Chapter three: On an involuntary flow of sperm). Hebrew הגרת הזרע מבלי רצון does not feature in the current dictionaries.

הִדּוּק (*Sefer ha-Qanun*, Nathan) = Arabic وثاقة 'solidity, strength'; cf. bk. 1 (fol. 39a): וכן לא נבראו מפחות משלשה כמו שאם היה נברא משתי עצמות היה ההדוק נוסף והתנועות כחסרות מן המספיק (Neither have they (i.e., the fingers) been created from less than three [bones], for if they would have been formed from two bones they would have been more solid but their movements would not have been sufficient enough). Hebrew הִדּוּק is attested in Rabbinic literature in the sense of 'that which is squeezed in to fill a gap' (cf. JD 451, s.v. חידוק). Zeraḥyah Ḥen renders the Arabic وثاقة as חוזק, and Joseph Lorki as חזוק.

הִדֵּק (הדק) (*Sefer Issur ha-Qevurah le-Galienus*) = Arabic غمز 'to palpate'; cf. par. 31: והמקום השלישי העורק בין צדי האמה והאמה כשיהודקו הדוק חזק ירגיש האדם כמו התלהבות האש ואם תראה זה הנה הוא חי (Third, there is an artery between ureter and urethra which, when firmly palpated, feels to the (investigating) person as if a fire were burning inside it—if this is what you find, then [the patient] is alive). Hebrew הִדֵּק does not feature in this sense in the current dictionaries. Arabic غمز is rendered as כבש ביד by Nathan ha-Me'ati in his translation of Maimonides, *Medical Aphorisms* 4.36, and as כבש ועיסה in 6.66. Zeraḥyah Ḥen renders غمز as דחק in both 4.36 and 6.66.

פת הדראה: הדראה (*Sefer ha-Shimmush*) = Arabic خبز الخشكار 'whole wheat bread'[98]; cf. fol. 123a, col. b: המאמר בלחם. הלחם העשוי מן החטה הוא בטבעו על הכלל חם ויבש במעלה השניה לקנותו זה מן האש. והקמח הנלקח מן החטה לעשות ממנו הלחם שלשה מינים. הסלת והקמח הדק הנבדל מן הסלת הנקרא בלשונם דרמך ובל״ל פלור והקמח האדום אשר יעשה ממנו פת הדראה (On bread: Bread made from wheat is by its nature generally hot and dry in the second degree which it acquires from the fire. Flour derived from wheat which is used for bread consists of three [different] kinds: finest wheat flour (Arabic *samīdh*) and the fine [wheat] flour that is different (not as fine?) and that is called *darmak*[99] in Arabic and in Romance PLWR and the red flour from which whole wheat

---

97 This illness is called 'gonorrhea' in ancient literature (cf. Galen, *De locis affectis* 6.6 (ed. Kühn, 8:439–41)). For Ibn al-Jazzār's discussion of this illness, cf. Ibn al-Jazzar, *On Sexual Diseases* (ed. and trans. Bos, 33–4, 99–103 (Arabic), 25–2 (English)).

98 Cf. NA 565: 'Whole-wheat bread made with daqīq ḥinṭī 'whole wheat flour' from which nothing is removed (al-Isrā'īlī 2:20–1). It is said to go through the digestive system fast due to its high bran content.'

99 According to Mielck (RMA 38) and Nasrallah (NA 559), *darmak* is the equivalent to *samīdh* (Hebrew *solet*) in terms of the finest variety of fine wheat flour.

bread is made). Hebrew פת הדראה features in BM 5294 without any further explanation, and in JD 335 in the sense of 'bread made of seconds' (opp. פת נקיה); Löw (LF 1:717–8) explains the term, which is also attested as הרדאה (cf. KA 3:240, 9:156 (Krauss, *Addimenta*)), as 'Kleienbrot' (whole wheat bread) and relates it to Aramaic ח(י)זרא 'bran' (cf. SDA 448)[100]. פת הדראה also features in Moses Ibn Tibbon's translation of Maimonides, *Regimen of Health* 1:13 (forthcoming ed. and trans. by G. Bos) as a translation of خبز الحوّارى (bread made with fine bran-free flour, described as nourishing bread but slow to digest because it has no bran in it).[101]

הדרקון (*Sefer ha-Shimmush*) = Arabic قولنج 'colic'; cf. fol. 129b, col. b: המים ההולכים על מחצבי העופרת מולידים ההדרקון (Water that streams over lead ore causes colic). Hebrew הדרקון actually does not mean 'colic', but 'dropsy' (cf. SHS 1:187 (He 10), and NM 2:11). For some unknown reason, Shem Tov Ben Isaac translates Arabic قولنج as הדרקון or הדרוקן, while the Arabic term for 'dropsy', i.e., استسقاء, is translated by him as שקוי.

הווה: הוה (*Sefer ha-Shimmush*) = Arabic آفة 'affliction, disaster, harm'; cf. fol. 137a, col. a: אמנם מי שיקרה לו מאכילתו נפח ומשיכה בבטן או שיש בו הווה מההדרקון מתילד מן הרוח ראוי להזהר מאכילתו בזגו וחרצנו או עם לחם או לשתות עליו מים קרים (But if someone suffers as a result of their consumption (i.e., of grapes) from flatulence and stomach cramps or if he is afflicted by a flatulent colic he should be careful not to eat them with their skins and seeds, and not with bread, and not with a drink of cold water). Hebrew הוה features in the Bible as הַוָּה or הֹוָה in the sense of 'ruin, destruction, disaster' (cf. BDB 217; BM 1054); for הַוָּה in Rabbinic literature, see also JD 337: 'misfortune'. For medieval literature, cf. BM ibid., for an attestation from Solomon Ibn Gabirol (*Al Mot R. Yequtiel*). In his translation of Maimonides, *Medical Aphorisms* 3.22, 70; 9.15; 18.3; 21.6, 51; 23.21; 24.34, Nathan ha-Me'ati translates Arabic آفة as פגע, and Zeraḥyah Ḥen as חלי or מחלה.

הוראה (*Hanhagat ha-Beri'ut le-Abu 'Ali Ben Zuhr*) = 'indication, symptom' (cf. Honofredi: 'significo'); cf. ch. 28: וכאשר יהיה האדם רואה כאלו זבובים יפרחו נגד עיניו או שערות או יראה סביבו ענן או עשן פעמים יהיה הוראה לירידת המים בעין וישתדל ברפואתו (If someone sees as if flies or hairs are flying before his eyes or if he sees a cloud or smoke around him, it may be an indication for a cataract. One should try to treat it). Hebrew הוראה does not feature as a medical term in the current dictionaries; cf. BM 1060–1.

---

100 Saul Lieberman, *Tosefta kifshutah*, vol. 3: *Sefer Mo'ed* (New York 1992), 211, agrees to the opinion of Löw.

101 Cf. NA 565.

הורג הזאב: הורג (*Sefer ha-Shimmush*) = Arabic قاتل الذئب 'aconite' (*Aconitum napellus*) (cf. DT 4:68 (581–3)); cf. fol. 146b, col. a: חלב הנשים יותר שוה מכל החלבים ... ולפיכך הוא מועיל מן העקיצה אשר תקרה באסטומ׳ ומשחין הריאה והמעים ומשתיית הארנבת הימית ומשתית הסם הנודע בהורג הזאב ומשתית המאירות ועוד יועיל מאדמימות זנב[102] העין (Women's milk is the most balanced of all milks ... and for this reason it is good for a burning [sensation] in the stomach, for a tumor in the lung and intestines, for the consumption of sea-hare, for the poison known as aconite, and for the consumption of cantharides (Spanish flies); it is also useful for pterygium in the[103] canthi of the eyes). Hebrew הורג הזאב is a non-attested calque from Arabic قاتل الذئب. Subsequent to Shem Tov Ben Isaac, the Hebrew term also features in Nathan ha-Me'ati's translation of Maimonides, *Medical Aphorisms* 23.102 (cf. NM 2:39).

הזדככות (*Hanhagat ha-Beri'ut le-Abu 'Ali Ben Zuhr*) = 'cleansing; purification'; cf. ch. 2: ואמר אחד מן החכמים: התמדת הטיולים וההזדככות עבדי השכל (One of the sages has said that frequent walking and cleansing [the body] are the servants of the mind). Hebrew הזדככות does not feature in a medical context in the current dictionaries; cf. BM 1063 for attestations, a.o., from Judah ha-Levi, *Sefer Kuzari*; and Elazar Azikri, *Sefer Haredim* (= KTP 1:165 and EM 356).

הזמנה (*Sefer ha-Qanun*, Joseph Lorki) = Arabic استعداد 'disposition'; cf. bk. 1 (fol. 12b): והעמוד העליון מעוקל כאלו לוקח מן הצד הפנימי ונוטה מעט אל החיצוני בעקום וקפול[104] והתועלת בזה טוב[105] ההזמנה לתנועת הקפול (The radius is curved as if it comes from the inner side and turns somewhat to the outside; this is useful because in this way it is well-disposed for the movement of pronation). Hebrew הזמנה does not feature in this sense in the current dictionaries. Ben Yehuda (BM 1065) mentions it in the sense of 'being ready to' (מוכן ומזומן) in an attestation from David Kimḥi's commentary on Amos. For the other translator(s), see entry התעתדות.

הטחה (*Sefer ha-Shimmush*)[106] = Arabic تلطيخ 'dirtying, soiling, befouling' (cf. WKAS 2.2:692b); cf. fol. 144a, col. b: והמוח הצלוי מתעכב לרדת מן האסטומכא יותר מן המבושל אלא שהטחתו אל האסטומ׳ יותר מעוטה (Roasted brain is slower to pass through the stomach than boiled [brain], but its befouling effect on the stomach is less). Hebrew הטחה, coined from הטיח 'to plaster, to polish, to daub', is not attested in the current dictionaries.

---

102 זנב העין: العين a.
103 'the canthi of the eyes': 'the eyes' a.
104 Ms וכפול emend. ed.: וקפול.
105 Ms בהשר emend. ed.: טוב.
106 See also entry הטיח (טוח).

הטפה: הטפת השתן (*Sefer ha-Shimmush*) = Arabic تقطير البول 'strangury'; cf. fol. 141b, col. a: האגוזים ההודיים ... קשי להתעכל ומקלקלין האסטו' אלא שהם מועילים מהטפת השתן ומכאב הגב הישן (Coconuts ... are hard to digest and corrupt the stomach, but they are good against strangury and chronic back pain). Hebrew הטפת השתן does not feature in the current dictionaries. The same term features in *Sefer*[107] *Agur* in the translation of Hippocrates' *Aphorisms* 5.58 (cf. NM 3:64); and in *Hanhagat ha-Beri'ut le-Abu 'Ali Ben Zuhr*, cf. 20 it seems to occur in the sense of 'incontinence': וההליכה בטיט והליכת יחף מן הדברים יותר מזיקים אל המוח הקר ואל העינים החלושים ומי שעלול מרבמס הקר מאד וכל שכן בזמן הסתו, ויזיק מאד להטפת השתן מחולשת הכח המחזיק במקוה בסבת הקור (Walking in mud and walking barefoot are amongst the most harmful things for a cold brain and weak eyes and for someone suffering from a very cold rheum, especially in winter. It is also very harmful [as it causes] incontinence because of the weakness of the retentive force in the bladder because of the cold).

הכאה (*Sefer Ṣedat ha-Derakhim*) = Arabic ضربان 'beat [of the pulse]'; Latin 'percussio'; cf. bk. 1, ch. 20 (fol. 30a): ויהיו עיני בעליו בעבור זה עמוקים ממהרי התנועה בעבור סער הנפש במחשבה ותשוקתה להשיג מי שישתוקק אליו ויהיו עפעפיו כבדות ומראהו כרכומי לתנועת המרה האדומה בנדוד השינה ויהיה דפק עורקיו חזק ולא ימצא בו התפשטות הדפק הטבעי ולא ישפל[108] הכאתו (For this reason, the eyes of the person [suffering from lovesickness] are hollow, and move quickly because of the soul's anxious thoughts and desire to find the object of his desire. His eyelids are heavy and his colour yellowish because of the motion of the yellow bile during his sleeplessness. His pulse is strong and does not dilate naturally, nor does it keep[109] its beat). Hebrew הכאה does not feature in this sense in the current dictionaries. The regular Hebrew term for 'beat [of the pulse]', i.e., דפיקה, can be found in, e.g., the translations of Maimonides, *Medical Aphorisms* 25.19 by both Nathan ha-Me'ati and Zeraḥyah Ḥen. The term הכאה is used by them to render Arabic ضربة in the sense of 'blow' (cf. Maimonides, *Medical Aphorisms* 3.77; 6.70; 24.35).

המרצה (*Sefer ha-Qanun*, Nathan) = Arabic إحكام 'perfection, accuracy, precision'; cf. bk. 1 (fol. 61a): ואמנם נסתפק בשנים שאין שם מן הצורך אל המרצת התבנית[110] מה שיש הנה (Two (i.e., membranes for the venous artery) are sufficient

---

107 I.e., the Hebrew translation of the Hippocratic *Aphorisms* by Do'eg ha-Edomi (trans. betw. 1197–9); cf. G. Freudenthal, 'The Father of the Latin-into-Hebrew Translations: "Doeg the Edomite", the Twelfth Century Repentant Convert', in *Latin-into-Hebrew: Texts and Studies*, ed. by R. Fontaine and G. Freudenthal, vol. 1 (Leiden 2013), 105–21.

108 ישפל (= يخفض): يحفظ a.

109 'keep its beat': Translated after the Arabic. Ibn Tibbon has: 'lower its beat'.

110 התבנית: السكن a السكر emend. De Koning (DKT 607, n. 2).

because there is no need for an exact closure[111] [of this artery]). Hebrew המרצה features in BM 1119 without further explanation in an attestation from Nathan's translation of Maimonides, *Medical Aphorisms* 8.8 (where it stands for Arabic سرعة 'rapidity'), and of the *Sefer ha-Qanun*. Zeraḥyah Ḥen translates the Arabic إحكام as לשפוט, and Joseph Lorki as לתקן.

המתחה (*Sefer ha-Refu'ot ha-Libbiyot*) = 'extensio' (extension); cf. fol. 243b: והדבק הוא אותו אשר יסבול ההמתחה מבלי שיחתך (A viscous [drug] is that with can be extended without breaking). Hebrew המתחה only features as a modern term in EM 380. The anonymous author of *Sammim Libbiyim* (fol. 120a) renders the Arabic parallel term امتداد as המתח.

הנהגה (*Sefer ha-Shimmush*) = Arabic تدبير 'preparation'; cf. fol. 140a, col. a: הזתים ישתנו פעולותיהם כפי השתנות מיניהם ושנוי הנהגתם (The properties of olives vary according to the variation and difference in their species and preparation). Hebrew הנהגה does not feature in this specific sense in the current dictionaries, cf. JD 357; BM 1130–1; KTP 1:181–2.

הסתבכות (*Sefer ha-Shimmush*) = Arabic تشبّك 'cramps, spasms' (cf. D 1:722); cf. fol. 127b, col. b: ומין אחר רע מזיק לעצבים נזק גדול ויגרום למי שיישן עליו או יפרשהו תחתיו הסתבכות בשוקים עד שלא יכול בעליו ללכת (Another variety [of beans[112]] is bad, very harmful for the nerves; if someone sleeps on them or spreads them beneath him it causes spasms in the legs so that he cannot walk). Hebrew הסתבכות does not feature in this sense in the current dictionaries.

העמדה (*Sefer ha-Qanun*, Nathan) = Arabic وقوف 'maturity'; cf. bk. 1 (fol. 31b): והקצויות יצמחו ברוב באמצע זמן הגדול והוא אחר ההמרצה אל ההעמדה וזה כי ההעמדה קרובה מל' שנה ולכן נקראים שני אלחלם כלומ' החלימה (In most cases wisdom teeth appear during the time of growth, namely after reaching maturity. For one reaches maturity at about thirty years and therefore these teeth are called *shnei al-ḥilm*, i.e., *ha-ḥalimah* (wisdom teeth))[113]. Hebrew העמדה does not feature in this sense in the current dictionaries. Zeraḥyah Ḥen renders the Arabic وقوف as עמידה (see entry).

הפוך הנפש: הפוך (*Sefer ha-Shimmush*) = Arabic تقلّب النفس (Greek ἀσώδης; cf. UW 187) 'sickness in stomach, nausea'; cf. fol. 145b, col. a: הבשר השלוק וקוראים

---

111 'closure': Translated after the Arabic *al-sikr* (emend. De Koning); cf. L 1391 'the stopping up, or damming'.

112 'beans' (שעועית): The Hebrew term can refer to different species of beans, perhaps *Vigna sinensis, Vigna nilotica, Lathyrus cicera* or *Phaseolus vulgaris*; the Arabic original term جلّبان means 'vetch', for the equation of both terms, see also SHS 1:236. In addition to Hebrew שעועית, Shem Tov has טופח (*Lathyrus Cicera* L. or *Lathyrus sativus* L., 'everlasting-pea') for Arabic جلّبان (cf. SHS 1:246–7).

113 '*shnei al-ḥilm*, i.e., *ha-ḥalimah* (wisdom teeth)': Cf. entry שני החלימה.

אותו אנשי המזרח אספגדבאג׳ה ואנחנו קוראים אותו גם כן שלוק האשכנז והוא חם בשוי ונאות ברוב העתים והענינים לכל בני אדם לבד מי שיגבר על מזגו החמימות ובעתים החמים מאד ולמי שיש לו אסתניסות[114] והפוך נפש ([The dish with] boiled meat which is called by the people of the East ʾSPGDBʾĞH and which we also call 'the boiled [meat dish] from Ashkenaz'; it is moderately hot and is at most times and in most cases good for all people, except for those whose temperament is dominated by heat or who suffer from sickness in stomach or nausea and when the weather is very hot). Hebrew הפוך הנפש (lit., 'upsetting the soul') does not feature in the current dictionaries. In addition to הפוך הנפש, Shem Tov Ben Isaac renders the Arabic synonyms for تقلّب النفس, namely غثى and غثيان, as אסתניסות (cf. entry). Yet another Arabic synonym, namely تهوّع, features, a.o., in Maimonides, *Medical Aphorisms* 23.82 (ed. and trans. Bos, 5:59): 'Just as emesis (*qayʾ*) is preceded by nausea (*tahawwuʿ*), so too coughing is preceded and induced by distress. And just as someone's soul is upset and he is nauseous but does not vomit, so too he feels distress which may prompt coughing but he does not cough because the cause is [too] mild. *De [morborum] causis et symptomatibus* 5 (cf. ed. Kühn, 7:173)'. Nathan ha-Me'ati renders the term as קיא and Zeraḥyah Ḥen as רצון קיא הנקרא תהוע.

הִפֵּךְ (הפך) (*Sefer ha-Qanun*, Nathan) = Arabic نكس 'to bend (the head)'; cf. bk. 1 (fol. 45b): ואמנם העצלים המהפכים הראש ביחוד והם שני עצלים יורדים משני צדדים (The muscles that are specifically meant for bending the head are two muscles that descend from both sides [of the neck]). In the sense of 'to bend', Hebrew הִפֵּךְ is a non-attested semantic borrowing from the Arabic نكس, which can mean both 'to turn around, turn over, turn upside down' and 'to bend, incline (the head)' (cf. L 2851).

הִפֵּךְ על פניו (*Sefer ha-Qanun*, Zeraḥyah) = Arabic بطح 'to supinate'; cf. bk. 1 (fol. 27a): ואמנם המהפכת על פניו לזרוע הוא זוג אחד ממנו מונח מבחוץ (The supinator [muscles] of the forearm are one pair. One of these lies on the outer side [of the forearm]). Hebrew הִפֵּךְ על פניו does not feature in the current dictionaries. For the other translator(s), see entry (שטח) השטיח על ערפו.

מתהפך (*Sefer Ṣedat ha-Derakhim*) = Arabic متضادّ 'opposite'; Latin 'oppositus'; cf. bk. 1, ch. 15 (fols. 22a–b): ולכן אמר גאלינוס כי הכונה ברפואת החולי הזה הנקרא המוקץ נקוי המוח משתי אלו הליחות המתהפכות בעצמיהם ר״ל ליחה לבנה ומרה אדומה (For this reason Galen said that to heal this illness called 'being awake' one should aim to cleanse the brain from these two humours that are opposite in their substance, i.e., phlegm and yellow bile). In the sense of 'opposite', Hebrew מתהפך is attested in philosophical literature in an attestation

---

114 a غثّى :אסתניסות.

from Maimonides, *Millot ha-Higgayon*: משפטים מתהפכים 'iudicia contraria' (KTP 2:313). The term also features in this sense in Ibn Tibbon's translation of Maimonides' introduction to his *Commentary on Hippocrates' Aphorisms* (cf. NM 3:66).

הפרש (*Sefer ha-Qanun*, Nathan) = Arabic مسافة 'distance'; cf. bk.1 (fol. 36a): ואינם מתחברות מקדם אבל בהדרגה מעט מעט ההפסק שיהיו העליונות בהם יותר קרובות ההפרש מה שבין שתי קצותיהן היוצאות (They (i.e., the ribs) do not unite at the front but progressively decrease [in size] so that the distance between the ends of the upper [ribs] is shorter). Hebrew הפרש features in BM 1162–3 in the sense of 'difference; incommensurability', and in KTP 1:200 in the additional sense of 'distance in time and space' in an attestation from Samuel Ibn Tibbon's Hebrew translation of Maimonides, *Guide of the Perplexed* (cf. EP 39 (3): 'empty space, space interval (Arabic خلل)'. Zeraḥyah Ḥen does not translate Arabic مسافة. Joseph Lorki translates the Arabic term as מהלך.

הצטערות (*Sefer Ṣedat ha-Derakhim*) = Arabic قلق (Greek ταραχή; cf. LSG 1758: 'physiological disturbance or upheaval') 'disturbance, agitation, unrest' (cf. D 2:398: 'l'espèce d'irritation nerveuse que cause l'impatience, et qui empêche de durer en place, de dormir, etc.'); cf. bk. 1, ch. 17 (fol. 24a): ואם היה עם היובש חום יקרה עם התעורה הצטערות וערבוב[115] שכל ומחשב (And if the dryness is accompanied by heat [the patient suffers] in addition to sleeplessness from disturbance (unrest), mental[116] confusion, and worry). Hebrew הצטערות is mentioned in EM 400 in the sense of 'the feeling of sadness' (הרגשת צער/העצבות). The same Hebrew term features in an anonymous translation of Hippocrates' *Aphorisms* 2.13 for the synonymous Arabic اضطراب 'disturbance' (cf. NM 3:68, 170). In his translation of the same text, Ibn Tibbon renders اضطراب as הסתערות, while in Hippocrates' *Aphorisms* 7.33, he translates it as צער (cf. NM 3:65–6, 196–7). Hebrew צער also features for Arabic قلق in Zeraḥyah Ḥen's translation of Maimonides, *Medical Aphorisms* 23.86, while Nathan ha-Me'ati has מצוק.

הקעת הפרקים: הקעה (*Sefer Ṣedat ha-Derakhim*) = Arabic زوال المفاصل 'dislocation'[117]; cf. introduction (fol. 4b): השער הכ"ה בשבר והקעת הפרקים (Chapter twenty-five: On fractures and dislocations). Hebrew הקעת הפרקים does not feature in the current dictionaries. Subsequent to Moses Ibn Tibbon, a shortened form of הקעת הפרקים, namely הקעה features in the *Sefer ha-Qanun* (cf. BM 1173).

---

115 וערבוב שכל: وطيش وهذيان a.

116 'mental confusion': 'agitation and raving' a.

117 For Ibn al-Jazzār's discussion cf. IJZ 62–4 (Arabic text), 12–7 (English trans.), 165–7 (Hebrew trans.).

הרג: See entry **הורג**.

הרגל (*Sefer ha-Shimmush*) = Arabic استعمال 'use, application'; cf. fol. 133b, col. a: וסדר ההרגל החשוב יותר לבעלי החמימות לבשלם בחבושים או לתקנם במי רמונים קוססים (The best way to apply them (i.e., gourds) for people with a hot temperament is to boil them with quinces and to improve [their quality] with sweet and sour pomegranate juice). Hebrew הרגל only features in the current dictionaries in the sense of 'habit'; cf. BM 1182–3. Cf. the verb הרגיל in the sense of 'to take' (for Arabic تناول) in Judah Shalom's translation of Hippocrates' *Aphorisms* 4.45 (NM 3:215).

השפעה (*Sefer ha-Shimmush*) = Arabic نزف 'flow of menstrual blood; menstrual bleeding'; cf. fol. 142a, col. b: והקלפות הדקות אשר על הפרי עצמו מבפנים הנקראות בלשון הגרי ג׳פת אל בלוט קביצותם יותר חזקה מן הבטנים ולכן הם מועילים מרקיקת הדם וההשפעה אשר תקרה לנשים (And the thin arils that are on the fruit [of the oak] itself inside [the shell] and that are called *ǧaft*[118] *al-ballūṭ* in Arabic are more astringent than the fruit; therefore they are good for bleeding from the nose and for menstrual bleeding occurring to women). Hebrew השפעה only features in the current dictionaries in the sense of 'emanation, influence' (cf. BM 1209–10; KTP 1:220; EM 416).

השתוממות (*Sammim Libbiyim*) = Arabic توحّش 'anxiety'; cf. fols. 123a–b: עוד תועלת השלשול בהשתוממות למה שיש בו מנקוי הרוח יותר מתועלתו בחולשת הלב (Because of its cleansing effect on the pneuma purging is more useful in the case of anxiety than in the case of weakness of the heart). Hebrew השתוממות features in BM 1212 in an attestation from Shem Tov Falaquera, *Zori ha-Yagon*. For the meaning of the term, Ben Yehuda refers to השתומם in the sense of 'to be astonished'. In EM 417 we find the same attestation, whereby the term השתוממות is explained as היות משמים (desolateness) and as העגמות (anguish). השתוממות also features in the anonymous translation of Maimonides, *Regimen of Health* 0, 3.10, 15 (forthcoming ed. and trans. Bos) for Arabic استيحاش in the sense of 'loneliness, fear'. The anonymous translator of *Sefer ha-Refu'ot ha-Libbiyot* (fol. 246a) renders the Latin *tristitia* as יגון (sorrow).

ההשתוממות השחורי (*Sammim Libbiyim*) = Arabic التوحّش السوداوي 'atrabiblious anxiety' (anxiety caused by black bile); cf. fol. 133b: הסכנגבין אשר חברתיו לבעלי ההשתוממות השחורי והכפייה ינקה העלה לעט[119] (The oxymel

118 *'ǧaft al-ballūṭ'*; cf. MIG 202: جفت البلّوط، قال جالينوس في الأدوية المفردة: إنّه الغشاء المستبطن لقشر ثمرة البلّوط الملفوف على نفس جرم البلّوط (*Ǧaft al-ballūṭ* (acorn aril). Galen said in his 'Simple drugs' (*al-Adwiya al-mufrada*): 'It is the membrane, which lies beneath the shell of the oak fruit, and which envelops the fruit pulp of the acorn').

119 לעט: بالرفق a.

[remedy] which I composed for those suffering from atrabiblious anxiety and epilepsy removes the illness easily). Hebrew ההשתוממות השחורי does not feature in the current dictionaries.

השתנת הדם: השתנה (*Sefer Ṣedat ha-Derakhim*) = Arabic بول الدم 'urinating blood (hematuria)': cf. introduction (fol. 3b): השער הט״ו בהשתנת הדם (Chapter fifteen: On urinating blood). Hebrew השתנת הדם does not feature in the current dictionaries.

התגברות (*Sefer Ṣedat ha-Derakhim*)[120] = Arabic فوران 'boiling, simmering, bubbling'; cf. bk. 1; ch. 18 (fol. 26a): ויקרה לחולה עם עלות החולי וקרוב חזקתו מקרים מפחידים כמו צמא חזק ונגוב פה ושעירות לשון ושחרותה וסער ודפיקת לב ושלא[121] יראה ועלוף ושינוי תמונת הפנים מן הענין הטבעי אל ענין יוצא מהטבע אם אל האדמימות אם היתה סבת החולי רתיחת דם הלב והתגברותו או אל הכרכומות אם היתה סבת החולי התלהבות מרה כרכומית בגבול[122] המוח (And when the illness becomes severe and burning hot, the patient suffers from frightening afflictions such as severe thirst, dryness of the mouth, roughness and blackness of the tongue, distress, cardialgia, fatigue,[123] fainting, change from a natural complexion into an unnatural complexion; into [a red complexion] if the illness is caused by the boiling and bubbling of the blood or into a [yellow complexion] if the illness is caused by burning hot yellow bile in the major[124] part the brain). Hebrew התגברות features in EM 424 in the sense of (1) 'strengthening, increase' (התחזקות/התרבות); (2) 'boldness, audacity' (התנשאות/תקיפות) (cf. EP 44 and KTP 1:227).

התמגלות (*Pirqei Arnauṭ de Vilanova*) = Latin 'saniatio' (purulence); cf. 5.89 (108): התמגלות הפצעים מצד היותו בסבת חולשת הכח המשנה אינו מן הראוי אל הרופא שישתדל בהגעתו (When wounds are purulent because of the weakness of the transforming faculty, the physician should not attempt to treat it). Hebrew התמגלות features in EM 432 in attestation from the *Sefer ha-Qanun*; cf. NM 2:116, 146 (Mem 11).

התנערות ללכת: התנערות (*Sefer ha-Qanun*, Nathan) = Arabic نهوض 'standing up'; cf. bk. 1 (fol. 41b): ושם ישיגה הכבדות בעת ההתנערות ללכת והכריעה על הברכים (And there (i.e., at the front) [the knee] is severely affected when one stands up or kneels down). Hebrew התנערות features in BM 1237 in the sense of פעולת תנועה לקום וכדומה in an attestation from the *Sefer ha-Qanun*. Zeraḥyah Ḥen renders Arabic نهوض as התעוררות, and Joseph Lorki as הלוך.

---

120 See also entry (גבר) התגבר.

121 a שלא יראה (وعمى): والإعياء.

122 a בגבול: في حومة.

123 'fatigue': Translated after the Arabic.

124 'major part': Translated after the Arabic.

התעתדות (*Sefer ha-Qanun*, Nathan) = Arabic استعداد 'disposition'; cf. bk. 1 (fol. 38a): וזנאד העליון מעוקם כאלו לוקח מן הצד הפנימי ונוטה מעט אל החיצוני בקפול והתועלת בזה טוב ההתעתדות לתנועת הקפול והעקום (The upper bone (radius)[125] is curved as if it comes from the inner side and turns somewhat to the outside; this is useful because in this way it is well-disposed for the movement of pronation). Hebrew התעתדות features in EM 438 in the sense of 'preparation for the future' (הכנת עצמו לעתיד). Zeraḥyah Ḥen renders Arabic استعداد as שיהיה, and Joseph Lorki as הזמנה (see entry).

התפשטות: התפשטות הדפק (*Sefer Ṣedat ha-Derakhim*) = Arabic انبساط النبض 'dilation of the pulse'; cf. bk. 1, ch. 20 (fol. 30a): ויהיו עיני בעליו בעבור זה עמוקים ממהרי התנועה בעבור סער הנפש במחשבה ותשוקתה להשיג מי שישתוקק אליו ויהיו עפעפיו כבדות ומראהו כרכומי לתנועת המרה האדומה בנדוד השינה ויהיה דפק עורקיו חזק לא ימצא בו התפשטות הדפק הטבעי ולא ישפל[126] הכאתו (For this reason, the eyes of the person [suffering from lovesickness] are hollow, and move quickly because of the soul's anxious thoughts and desire to find the object of his desire. His eyelids are heavy and his colour yellowish because of the motion of the yellow bile during his sleeplessness. His pulse is strong and does not dilate naturally, nor does it keep[127] its beat). Hebrew התפשטות הדפק features in BM 1245–6 in an attestation from the *Sefer ha-Qanun*. Nathan ha-Me'ati uses the same term to render Arabic انبساط 'expansion' in his translation of Maimonides, *Medical Aphorisms* 4.2, while Zeraḥyah Ḥen uses the term פישוט.

התקבצות (*Sefer ha-Qanun*, Nathan) I. = Arabic انقباض 'flexion'; cf. bk. 1 (fol. 51a): והנה הושם הבהן מסתפק בהתקבצות על עצל אחד (For flexion the thumb only needs one muscle). Hebrew התקבצות does not feature in this sense in the current dictionaries. Zeraḥyah Ḥen translates the Arabic انقباض as קבוץ (see entry), and Joseph Lorki as מתקבץ; II. = Arabic انقباض 'contraction'; cf. bk. 1 (fol. 52a): ומהם שישענו הטרפשות ועוזרים אצל הנפיחה לבעל ההתקבצות (Another [use of the muscles of the abdomen] is that they support and assist the diaphragm during exsufflation and contraction [of the thorax]). For התקבצות in the sense of 'contraction', cf. BM 1246. In his translation of Maimonides, *Medical Aphorisms*, Nathan ha-Me'ati uses the same Hebrew term for Arabic انقباض in the sense of 'contraction', and for Arabic اجتماع in the sense of 'accumulation, contraction'. Zeraḥyah Ḥen translates انقباض as קיבץ האויר, and Joseph Lorki as קבוץ.

---

125 'The upper bone (radius)': Cf. entry זנד.

126 a يحفظ :(= يخفض) ישפל.

127 'keep its beat': Translated after the Arabic. Ibn Tibbon has: 'lower its beat'.

התקשרות (*Sammim Libbiyim*)[128] I. = Arabic متانة 'compactness, firmness, solidity'; cf. fol. 123b: הסמים הקובצים והמטיחים יכנסו ברפואות הלב להקנות עצם הרוח התקשרות והתדבקות נאות (Astringent and smoothing (agglutinant) remedies are part of (pertain to) the cardiacs as they give the substance of the pneuma appropriate (sound) compactness and continuity). Hebrew התקשרות does not feature in this sense in the current dictionaries. Nathan ha-Me'ati uses the same term to render Arabic انعقاد 'coagulation' in his translation of Maimonides, *Medical Aphorisms* 8.62; cf. NM 2:43. The anonymous translator of *Sefer ha-Refu'ot ha-Libbiyot* renders the Latin 'soliditas' as קיום (see entry); II. = Arabic تمتين 'strengthening, consolidation'; cf. fols. 130–131a: סוסן אראה[129] אותו קרוב הטבע מן הזעפראן קרוב המשפט ממשפטיו <ו>אבל הוא יותר חסר החום והיובש וזה יותר נאות לחיזוק הלב וזה ג"כ להיותו שמח כי בסוסן מהתקשרות הרוח קרוב ממה שהוא בזעפראן ואין בו התפשטות חזק והנעה מופלגת לרוח אל חוץ כמו שהוא בזעפראן (Wild[130] white iris (*Dietes grandiflora*): It is close to saffron in nature and properties. However, it is less hot and dry and thus better suited for strengthening, i.e., exhilarating, the heart. For in strengthening the spirit the iris is close to saffron, but it is not as strong as saffron in dilating the pneuma and moving it outward). Hebrew התקשרות does not feature in this sense in the current dictionaries. The anonymous translator of *Sefer ha-Refu'ot ha-Libbiyot* (fol. 250a) renders the Latin 'potentia dilettandi' as כח להמתיח (see entry מתח: המתיח הרוח).

הודאג הנגלה: ודאג (*Sefer ha-Qanun*, Nathan) = Arabic الوداج الظاهر 'the external jugular vein' (cf. DKT 830); cf. bk. 1 (fol. 65a): ואמנם הודאג הנגלה אחר התערב נפרדיו הנה מתחלק לשניח ונכנס בפנים חלק ממנו (The external jugular vein, once its parts have united, divides into two parts and one part goes inside). Hebrew הודאג הנגלה is a combined term, the first part ודאג is a non-attested loan word from Arabic وداج. Zeraḥyah Ḥen renders the Arabic الوداج الظاهر as העורקים הנראים הנקראים ודאג, and Joseph Lorki as הוריד הנראה.

הורד הסוכרי: ורד (*Hanhagat ha-Beri'ut le-Abu 'Ali Ben Zuhr*) = 'rose syrup' (cf. Honofredi: 'sirupum rosatum'); cf. ch. 10: ומשקה הורד הסוכרי ומשקה לינגא אלו־ בין ההנדי מועילים ושומרים הבריאות (A drink of rose syrup and Indian aloeswood are beneficial and preserve one's health). Hebrew הורד הסוכרי does not feature in the current dictionaries.

---

128 In addition to התקשרות, the anonymous author of *Sammim Libbiyim* renders Arabic متانة as עובי (see entry).

129 a אראה אותו: أزاد.

130 'Wild white iris (*Dietes grandiflora*)': Translated after the Arabic سوسن أزاد.

הוריד אשר על פי הטבעת :וריד (*Sefer ha-Qanun*, Joseph Lorki) = Arabic الوريد العجزي 'sacral vein'; cf. bk. 1 (fol. 19a): וכת יורד תחת העצל הישר ומתפזרים בו שריגים וסופם דבק בחלקים העולים מן הוריד אשר על פי הטבעת אשר נזכר אותו (One group [of branches of the vena cava] descends beneath the flat muscles and some of them spread and their ends join [the branches] that go upwards from the sacral vein that we shall mention later). Hebrew הוריד אשר על פי הטבעת is not attested in the current dictionaries. For the other translator(s), see entry הוריד העגזי.

הוריד הדופק (*Sefer ha-Qanun*, Zeraḥyah) = Arabic الوريد الشرياني 'arterial vein (pulmonary artery)' (cf. DKT 604–5, 830); cf. bk. 1 (fol. 32a): ואמנם הוריד הדופק אשר אנו זוכרים[131] אותו ואע״פ שהוא שכן לריאה אבל יעבור ממנו מאחורו מקום שהוא סמוך לגב (Although the arterial vein which I will mention [later on] is close to the lung, it passes at the back side [of this organ] near the spine). Hebrew הוריד הדופק is not attested in the current dictionaries. For the other translator(s), see entry הוריד השרייני.

הוריד הזקני (*Sefer ha-Qanun*, Zeraḥyah) = Arabic الوريد العجزي 'sacral vein'; cf. bk. 1 (fol 34a): וכת יורד תחת המושקולו הישר ויתחלק מהם שעיף וסופם מתדבק בחלקים העולים מן הוריד הזקני אשר אנו עתידים לזכרו (One group [of branches of the vena cava] descends beneath the flat muscles and some of them spread and their ends join [the branches] that go upwards from the sacral vein that I will mention later). Zeraḥyah's translation, resulting from reading Arabic عجزي as عجوزي (cf. entry עגז), is discussed in SRP 42 (326). For the other translator(s), see entry הוריד העגזי.

הוריד החלול (*Sefer ha-Qanun*, Zeraḥyah)[132] = Arabic الوريد الأجوف 'vena cava' (cf. DKT 604–5, 830); cf. bk. 1 (fol. 32a): ועל כן נקרא הגיד הורידי. אמנם נברא מקרום אחד למען היותו יותר[133] לח ויותר משועבד לפשיטות ולקביצות ולמען היות משועבד להזיע מה שיזיע ממנו אל הריאה מן הדם הדק העשני הניאות בעצם הריאה הקרוב לבשול השלם בלב ואינו צריך למותר בשול כצורך הדם ההולך בוריד החלול (For this reason it is called 'venous artery (pulmonary vein)'. It is made from one coat so that it would be more[134] soft and flexible, so that its dilation and contraction would be easier, and so that the transudation of thin, vaporous blood to the substance of the lung would be easier as well. [This blood] fits the substance of the lung because it has almost completely been concocted in the heart and does not need any more concoction, contrary to the blood

---

131 Ms דופקים emend. ed. :זוכרים .

132 In addition to הוריד החלול, Zeraḥyah has החלול (cf. entry) to refer to the 'vena cava', conform to Arabic الأجوف.

133 a ألين وأسلس :יותר לח.

134 'more soft and flexible': Translated according to ألين وأسلس a.

that flows through the vena cava). For Hebrew הוריד החלול as featuring in the *Sefer ha-Qanun*, cf. SRP 6 (37). For the other translator(s), see entry הוריד הנבוב.

הוריד הנבוב (*Sefer ha-Qanun*, Nathan)[135] = Arabic الوريد الأجوف 'vena cava' (cf. DKT 604–5, 830); cf. bk. 1 (fol. 60b): ולכן נקרא השריין הורידי. אמנם נברא מעור אחד שיהיה יותר רך ורפה ויותר נשמע להתפשטות והתקבצות ויותר נשמע להתדיית מה שיתדיית ממנו אל הריאה מן הדם הדק האדיי הנאות לעצם הריאה אשר כבר קדם לשלמות הבשול בלב ולא יצטרך ליתרון בשול כצורך הדם העובר בוריד הנבוב. Hebrew הוריד הנבוב features as הוריד הנבוב העליון (superior vena cava) and הוריד הנבוב התחתון (inferior vena cava) in MD 765; see also SRP 6 (37). Zeraḥyah Ḥen translates the Arabic الوريد الأجوف as הוריד החלול (see entry), and Joseph Lorki as הוריד הפנימי (see entry).

הוריד העגזי (*Sefer ha-Qanun*, Nathan) = Arabic الوريد العجزي 'sacral vein'; cf. bk. 1 (fol. 64b): וכת יורד תחת העצלים הישרים ומתפרד מהם שריגים ואחריתם[136] מתחברים בחלקים העולים מן הוריד העגזי[137] אשר נזכירהו (One group [of branches of the vena cava] descends beneath the flat muscles and some of them spread and their ends join [the branches] that go upwards from the sacral vein that I will mention later). Zeraḥyah Ḥen renders the Arabic الوريد العجزي as הוריד הזקני (see entry), and Joseph Lorki as הוריד אשר על פי הטבעת (see entry).

הוריד הפנימי (*Sefer ha-Qanun*, Joseph Lorki)[138] = Arabic الوريد الأجوف 'vena cava' (cf. DKT 604–5, 830); cf. bk. 1 (fol. 18a): ועל כן נקרא הגיד הדופק בהיותו יותר לח ויותר רך ויותר נקל אל הפשיטה והקבוץ ולהיותו[139] יותר נקל להטיב מה שנוסף ממנו אל הריאה מהדם הדקיק הקטורי הנאות לעצם הריאה אשר קרב בהשלמת הבשול בלב ואינו צריך ליתרון בשול כמו צורך הדם בוריד הפנימי (For this reason it is called 've nous artery (pulmonary vein)'. [It is made from one coat] so that it would be more soft and flexible, so that its dilation and contraction would be easier, and[140] so that the transudation of thin, vaporous blood to the substance of the lung would be easier as well. [This blood] fits the substance of the lung because it has almost completely been concocted in the heart and does

135 In addition to הוריד הנבוב, Nathan uses the adjective הנבוב (see entry) to indicate the 'vena cava', conform to Arabic الأجوف.

136 a Ms وأواخرها ואחרית הם emend. ed.: ואחריתם.

137 Ms העגזים emend. ed.: העגזי.

138 In addition to הוריד הפמימי, Joseph Lorki uses the adjective הפנימי (see entry) to indicate the 'vena cava', conform to Arabic الأجوف.

139 a وليكون أطوع لترشّح ما يترشّح: ולהיותו יותר נקל להטיב מה שנוסף.

140 'and so that the transudation of thin, vaporous blood to the substance of the lung would be easier as well': Translated after a.

not need any more concoction, contrary to the blood that flows through the vena cava). Hebrew הוריד הפנימי is not attested in the current dictionaries. For the other translator(s), see entry הוריד הנבוב.

הוריד הפנימי היורד (*Sefer ha-Qanun*, Joseph Lorki) = Arabic الأجوف النازل 'the inferior vena cava'; cf. bk. 1 (fol. 19b): פרק ה׳ בנתוח הוריד הפנימי היורד כבר השלמנו מאמרינו בחלק העולה הפנימי והוא היותר קטן שבחלקיו (Chapter five: On the anatomy of the inferior vena cava. We have finished the discussion of the ascending vena cava which is the smaller of the two). Hebrew הוריד הפנימי היורד is not attested in the current dictionaries. For the other translator(s), see entry הנבוב היורד.

הוריד השרייני (*Sefer ha-Qanun*, Nathan) = Arabic الوريد الشرياني 'arterial vein (pulmonary artery)' (cf. DKT 604–5, 830); cf. bk. 1 (fol. 60b): ואמנם הוריד השרייני אשר נזכירהו אע״פ שהוא שכן לריאה אמנם הוא עובר ממנו מאחורו במה שנלוה לשדרה (Although the arterial vein which I will mention later on is close to the lung, goes at the back side [of this organ] near the spine). Hebrew הוריד השרייני is not attested in the current dictionaries. Zeraḥyah Ḥen translates the Arabic الوريد الشراني as הוריד הדופק (see entry), and Joseph Lorki as הוריד הדופק הנקרא שריני.

ורידי: See entries **גיד** and **שריין**.

ושט (*Sefer ha-Qanun*, Zeraḥyah) = Arabic حلقوم 'throat' (cf. DKT 538–9, 816: 'gorge. 1. partie antérieure inférieure du cou. 2. larynx. trachée artère'; FAL 70, no. 1566: '1. larynx + trachea; 2. pharynx; 3. anterior and lower part of the neck); cf. bk. 1 (fol. 25b): המושקלו של הושט. אמנם הושט כולו יש לו שתי זוגות ימשכוהו למטה (The muscles of the throat. The throat as a whole has two pairs [of muscles] which pull it downward). Hebrew ושט features in the current dictionaries and secondary literature in the sense of 'gullet, esophagus' (JD 1:376; BM 1272; MD 269; LOW XLVII). Nathan ha-Me'ati translates the Arabic حلقوم as גרון, and Joseph Lorki as קנה (cf. NM 2:82–3; 3:203–4).

ותיקה (*Sefer ha-Shimmush*) = Arabic عصيدة 'pulmentum spissius' (anything dense eaten with bread) (FL 3:166); 'pultes' (a thick pap or pottage) (D 2:133);[141] cf. fol. 124b, col. 1: הותיקה העשויה מן הגריסין היא קרובה להוליד החלט העב והס־ תומים והרטט (WTYQH prepared from GRYSYN (coarse meal) can produce a thick humour, obstructions and arthritis). The term ותיקה is only attested in Rabbinic literature as Aramaic ותיקא; cf. JD 376: 'name of a certain pastry, tart; SDA 396: 'dish made with flour, olive oil and salt'; cf. KA 3:259–60.

---

141 See also L 2060: 'a sort of thick gruel, consisting of wheat-flour moistened and stirred about with clarified butter, and cooked'; DAS 3:282: 'Mehlbrei'; NA 604: 'a kind of soup *ḥasā*', rather dense in consistency. The main ingredients are flour, fat and water … However it may be a kind of dessert when made with mashed dates and clarified butter …'.

Maimonides, *On Asthma* 3.1 (ed. and trans. Bos, 1:12) states that it is something prepared from cooked flour. In *On Hemorrhoids* 6.3 (ed. and trans. Bos, 23), Maimonides mentions a liniment against hemorrhoids consisting of ʿasida made from fine white flour with sesame oil or chicken fat. He adds that 'if one adds some saffron to it, it has an [even] stronger alleviating effect.'

זאב: חולי הזאב (*Pirqei Arnauṭ de Vilanova*) = Latin 'lupus'[142]; cf. 5.96 (110): הנגעים המתאכלים אשר יתרחבו ויתפשטו אל העומק מעצמם, ראוי לרפאם עם דברים קובצים ומיבשים בלתי עוקצים, ואם יהיו ארסיים כמו חולי הזאב יצטרך שיהיו בזהריים (Corrosive wounds that spontaneously spread and become deeper, should be treated with astringent, drying ingredients that do not bite. But if they (i.e., the wounds) are poisonous, as in the case of lupus, [the ingredients] should have the property of the bezoar (i.e., they be antidotal)). Hebrew חולי הזאב features in BM 1276 in an attestation from Judah al-Ḥarizi, *Maḥberot Itiʾel*. The term is identified by Ben Yehuda as Arabic דא אלד׳יב, מחלת הזאב, והוא חולי של רעב חזק (the wolf's disease, i.e., a severe hunger) (cf. L 949).

זבל: זבל שטן (Anonymous glossary; Ms Leiden, Universiteitsbibliotheek, Cod. Or. 4732/1) = 'asafoetida'; cf. fol. 7a: מילשא היא גומ׳ והוא זבל שטן (MYLŠʾ; i.e., gum, i.e., 'Teufelsdreck'). Hebrew זבל שטן is a non-attested calque of German 'Teufelsdreck', i.e., asafoetida, i.e., the dried latex (gum) exuded from the rhizome of several species of *Ferula*. The common Hebrew term is חלתית (cf. SHS 1:209–10 (Ḥet 2)).

זהב: זָהוּב I. (*Sefer ha-Refuʾot ha-Libbiyot*) = Latin 'aureus' (aureus) (Arabic مثقال; i.e., a pharmaceutical weight of 4.46 grams; cf. NM 2:63–4); cf. fol. 252a: והרופאים הסכלים עדיין חושבים שיש למטרודיטוס ולתריאק חום גובר ומפני זה בורחים לתת ממנה שיעור חצי זהוב (Ignorant physicians still believe that both the Mithridates[143] and theriac are exceedingly hot and therefore refrain from administering [even] half an aureus). Hebrew זהוב only features in the current dictionaries as a gold coin; cf. BM 1294–5. The anonymous author of *Sammim Libbiyim* (fol. 132b) renders Arabic مثقال as משקל (cf. NM 2:63–4); II. (*Sefer ha-Shimmush*) = Arabic مثقال (i.e., 4.46 grams); cf. fol. 136a, col. b: ואם יקרה

142 'lupus': In the twelfth—thirteenth centuries, lupus was identified as a type of cancer (that affected the lower body); or as herpes esthiomenus (a slowly advancing corrosion of the skin); cf. L. Demaitre, *Medieval Medicine. The Art of Healing from Head to Toe* (Santa Barbara; CA 2013), 91–5.

143 An antidote ascribed to Mithridates VI. Eupator, king of Pontus (reg. 120–63 BC); see Ullmann, *Medizin im Islam*, 321; for its composition, see Ǧābir ibn Ḥayyān, *Das Buch der Gifte des Ǧābir ibn Ḥayyān. Arabischer Text in Faksimile (HS. Taymūr, Ṭibb 393, Kairo)*, trans. by A. Siggel (Wiesbaden 1958), 217.

מאכילת המין הרע מהם קצת מה שזכרתי בפטריות מן החניקה והגנוח[144] ראוי לשתות אחריהם מיד מים שנתבשל בהם שבת עם חמאת בקר או שמן שומשמין או לקחת מצואת התרנוגלות משקל שני זהובים ולצרף אותה באישרוב אסיטוס ומים חמין ולשתותם (If the consumption of the bad kind [of truffles] causes some of [the symptoms] which I mentioned in the case of mushrooms, namely suffocation and asthma,[145] one should after [eating] them immediately drink water in which anet with cow's butter or sesame oil has been cooked. One can also take two *zehubim* of chicken poop, mix it with oxymel and hot water and drink this).

זוהמת הצמר: זֻהֲמָה (Anonymous glossary; Ms Vatican 361)[146] = 'wool grease'[147]; cf. fol. 177b: זופ<ט>א רטב הוא אישוף לח יקראו זוהמת הצמר ([Arabic] *zūfā raṭb* is moist hyssop, called ZHMT H-ṢMR [Hebrew]). Hebrew זוהמת הצמר does not feature in the current dictionaries. The same Hebrew term can be found in Nathan ha-Me'ati's translation of the Arabic synonym *wadaḫ al-ṣūf*, featuring in Maimonides, *Medical Aphorisms* 23.89, and in Ms Florence, Biblioteca Medicea Laurenziana, Or. 17, that was copied in Anagni in the year 1464, fol. 77r: זופא רטב הוא איספו לח ונקר׳ כן זוהמת הצמר ונלקח בארמניאה מצמר הצאן בעודם חיים וזה גילה לנצרים בן מסואי (ZWP' RṬB, that is moist 'YSPW, and it is also called ZWHMT HṢMR (filth/grease of wool), and it is taken in 'RMNY'H, from the wool of the cattle, while alive, and this was revealed to the Christians by Ibn Māsawayh). For a Hebrew synonym of זוהמת הצמר, namely דשן הצמר, cf. SHS 1:174–5 (Dalet 10).

זוג (*Sefer ha-Qanun*, Nathan) = Arabic زوج 'zygomatic arch' (cf. FAL 30, no. 566); cf. bk. 1 (fol. 30a): ובכל אחד משני צדי הצדעים שתי עצמות קשות מסתירות העצבים העוברים בצדעים והנחתם באורך הצדע באלכסון ונקראים הזוג (On each side of the temples are two hard bones that protect the nerves that pass through the temples. They are situated in the lengh of the temples obliquely and are called 'zygomatic arch'). For Hebrew זוג, as featuring in the Hebrew *Sefer ha-Qanun*, cf. SRP 31 (213). Zeraḥyah Ḥen does not translate Arabic زوج.

זורקי (*Sefer ha-Qanun*, Nathan) = Arabic زورقي 'navicular or scaphoid [bone]'; cf. DKT 512–3, 818; FAL 173, no. 3701); cf. bk. 1 (fol. 41b): עצמות כף הרגל ששה[148]...

144 add. a והגנוח: والذبحة.

145 'asthma': 'and angina' add. a.

146 Cf. Ms Oxford, Bodleian, Mich. Add. 22, fol. 9a: זופא לח זוהמת הצמר.

147 Dioscurides described the substance in his entries ἔρια οἰσυπηρά (*Materia medica* 2.73) and οἴσυπος (2.74). Arabic *zūfā raṭb* literally means 'moist hyssop.' The term οἴσυπος was obviously confounded with ὕσσωπος the Greek name of hyssop. Cf. DT 2:60 (235–6); M 136; MIG 315.

148 a ששה: ستّة وعشرون.

וזורקי שבו יהיה החלל (The foot has six[149] bones … the navicular (scaphoid) bone through which the hollow [of the foot] is formed). For the term זורקי, a loan word from Arabic زورق, featuring in the *Sefer ha-Qanun*, cf. SRP lxxxi. Joseph Lorki translates the Arabic as העצם השוה (see entry).

זירבאג׳ (*Sefer ha-Shimmush*) = Arabic زيرباج; cf. FL 2:270: 'species cibi iusculenti' (a kind of broth);[150] cf. NA 620, s.v. *zīrbāja*: 'Delicate bird stew … The dish is cooked in several ways. The most common variety is made light with birds, golden with saffron, seasoned and spiced with a light hand (sometimes with cumin), and lightly soured with vinegar, with some sugar added to balance the taste …'[151]; cf. fol. 148a, col. b: והרוצה להשוות המזג ולהשקיט חמימות האסטומ׳ ראוי לבשלם תבשיל זירבאג׳ (If someone wants to balance the temperament [of the body] and to allay the heat of the stomach he should cook them (i.e., chickens) as part of the dish [called] ZYRB'Ǧ). Hebrew זירבאג׳ is a non-attested loan word from the Arabic زيرباج, that was adopted into Shem Tov Ben Isaac's Hebrew culinary vocabulary as it features in bk. 27 of the *Sefer ha-Shimmush*. The term also features in the Hebrew translations of Maimonides, *On Asthma* 4.4, 9.13 (ed. Bos, 2:255, 331, 399; 275, 350, 419). Moses Ibn Tibbon renders the Arabic زيرباج as מרק (see entry below).

זלוף הדם מן החוטם :זלוף (*Sefer Hanhagat ha-Beri'ut*)[152] = 'nosebleed'; cf. 8.5 (153): וצריך להקיז מיד ויוציא מן הדם כפי השיעור הצריך שאם ימנע מהקיז תאחזהו הקדחת התמידית וחולי הצלעות וזלוף הדם מן החוטם והמות הפתאומית והרבה חליים מלבד אלה (He should be bled immediately; blood should be extracted as much as needed, for if one does not do so he will suffer from continuous fever, illness of the ribs, nosebleed, sudden death and many other illnesses). Hebrew זלוף

149 'six': The Arabic text has 'twenty-six'.

150 The Arabized term is derived from Persian *zīr-bā*, "broth or spoon-meat" (SCP 633), respectively from *zīrah-bā*, "a dish made of the flesh of birds, with cumin-seed and vinegar" (ibid. 634).

151 See also MB 207–8; WI 14, 21, 40–1, 58–9; IJZ 112, n. 215; and the definition of the term in Nathan ha-Me'ati's glossary to the *Sefer ha-Qanun*: זירבאג הוא מטעם כרכומי עשוי בשמן וסוכר וכמון כי זיר בלשון פרס כמון ובאג מטעם כלומר מטעם הכמון (ZRYB'G. I.e., a saffron dish, prepared with oil, sugar and cumin, for ZYR means 'cumin' in Persian and B'G means 'dish', that is to say, the 'cumin dish') (NM 2:113, 136 (Zayin 5)); and in Ibn Ǧanāḥ, *Kitāb al-Talḫīṣ* (MIG 338): زيرباج معناه لون أصفر عن أبي الحجّاج، وأخبرني أبو الفتوح أنّ معناه لون كمّون، قال: واسم الكمّون بالفارسية زيرة. (*Zīrabāǧ*—the meaning of this term is 'yellow soup' (*lawn aṣfar*), according to Abū l-Ḥaǧǧāǧ. Abū l-Futūḥ told me that its meaning is 'cumin soup' (*lawn kammūn*). He said: The Persian name of cumin (*kammūn*) is *zīra*). Different varieties of the dish feature in ISW 152–4 (ch. 57) (Arabic); NA 274–7 (English); MWK 14, 52, 63, 70, 75, 226.

152 Cf. entries עריפת דם החוטם and עריפת דם הנחירים.

הדם מן החוטם does not feature in the current dictionaries. Synonyms featuring in medieval Hebrew medical literature are/צאת דם הנחירים/זוב דם הנחירים הגרת דם מהנחירים/רעיפת דם מן הנחירים/רעיפת דם מן החוטם (cf. NM 3:75).

זמורות: זמורה (*Sefer ha-Shimmush*)[153] = Arabic دوالي 'varicose veins'; cf. fol. 127a, col. a: הלחם העשוי מן העדשים יתילד מן ההתמדה עליו חליים שחורים כגון השטות והסרטנים והזמורות והטחורים והבהק השחור והספחת והדומה להם מן החליים (A frequent consumption of bread made from lentils causes melancholic diseases, such as melancholy,[154] [different] cancers, varicose veins, hemorrhoids, black[155] *bahaq*, eczema, and similar diseases). Hebrew זמורה, Plur. זמורות, does not feature in this sense in the current dictionaries. In addition to זמו־רות, Shem Tov Ben Isaac uses דליות (see entry).

הזנאד העליון: זנאד (*Sefer ha-Qanun*, Nathan)[156] = Arabic الزند الأعلى 'radius' (cf. FAL 172, no. 3683); cf. bk. 1 (fol. 38a): אמנם פרק המרפק[157] הנה הוא מחובר מן פרק הזנאד העליון ופרק הזנאד התחתון עם הזרוע (The elbow is formed by the articulation of the radius, ulna and humerus). For Hebrew זנאד עליון, featuring in the *Sefer ha-Qanun*, cf. SRP 24–5 (135, 143) and MD 618 (variant reading זנד עליון), s.v. 'radius'. Zeraḥyah Ḥen renders the Arabic الزند الأعلى as הזינד העליון, Joseph Lorki as העמוד העליון (see entry).

הזנאד התחתון (*Sefer ha-Qanun*, Nathan)[158] = Arabic الزند الأسفل 'ulna' (cf. FAL 172, no. 3684); cf. bk. 1 (fol. 38a): אמנם פרק המרפק[159] הנה הוא מחובר מן פרק הזנאד העליון ופרק הזנאד התחתון עם הזרוע. For Hebrew הזנאד התחתון, featuring in the *Sefer ha-Qanun*, cf. SRP 25 (144, 147) and MD 747 (variant reading זנד התחתון), s.v. 'ulna'. Zeraḥyah Ḥen renders the Arabic الزند الأسفل as העצם השפל (see entry), and Joseph Lorki as העמוד התחתון (see entry).

זנבות: זנב (*Sefer ha-Shimmush*) = Arabic مآقان 'the canthi (inner and outer angles) of the eyes' (cf. DKT 827); cf. fol. 136b, cols. a–b: וסחיטתו כשיוכחל בו העינים תחזק בת העין ותפסיק הלחויות העבות אשר בעפעפים ותועיל מגסות העין ומן החכוך אשר בראשי העינים וזנבותיהם (If one uses its juice (i.e., of grapes) for an eyewash (collyrium), it strengthens the pupil and stops the thick fluids in the eyelids, and is good for thickness of the eyes, and for itch in the eyes themselves and in their inner and outer canthi (i.e., corners, angles)). In the sense of 'canthus' (angle of the eye), Hebrew זנב is not attested in the current dictionaries. In the glossary to the *Sefer ha-Shimmush*, Shem Tov Ben

153 Cf. NM 1:89–90.
154 'melancholy': Cf. NM 1:117.
155 'black bahaq': 'a kind of melanoderma'; cf. entry בֹּהַק: בהק שחור.
156 Cf. entry זנד.
157 Ms המפרק emend. ed.: המרפק.
158 Cf. entry זנד.
159 Ms המפרק emend. ed.: המרפק.

Isaac uses זנב העין as a loan word from the Arabic parallel ذنب العين (SHS 1:201–2 (Zayin 8)). See as well NM 1:90.

שני הזנדים: זנד (*Sefer ha-Qanun*, Nathan)[160] = Arabic الزندان 'the two bones of the forearm (radius and ulna)' (cf. DKT 497, n. 6; SRP 24 (142); FAL 172, no. 3682)[161]; cf. bk. 1 (fol. 38a): הקנה מחוברת משני עצמים מדובקים באורך ונקרא שני הזנדים[162] (The forearm is composed of two bones that are attached to each other lengthwise and that are called the two *zand*). Hebrew זנד, a loan word from the Arabic, features in BM 1367 in attestations from the *Sefer ha-Qanun* and is explained by Ben Yehuda as עצם קצה הזרוע (a bone of the forearm); see also SRP 24–5 (143–4, 147); in his glossary to the *Sefer ha-Qanun*, Nathan defines the term זנד as אחד העצמות אשר בקצה הזרוע ושניהם נקראים זנדים (This is one of the [two bones] (i.e., radius and ulna) in the forearm; the two bones are called ZNDYM) (cf. NM 2:113, 135 (Zayin 2)). Zeraḥyah Ḥen renders the Arabic الزندان as זינדן, and Joseph Lorki as שני עמודים (see entry).

זָקָן (*Sefer ha-Qanun*, Nathan) = Arabic ذقن 'chin'; cf. bk. 1 (fol. 31a): ואמנם הלחי התחתון הנה צורת עצמיו ותועלתו ידוע כי הוא משתי עצמות יחבר ביניהם תחת הזקן פרק מהודק (The shape and usefulness of the bones of the lower jaw are well-known. [The chin] consists of two bones which are connected beneath the chin by means of a strong joint). In the sense of 'chin', Hebrew זקן features in the current dictionaries in attestations from the Bible only (cf. BDB 278; BM 1382).

זָקֵן (*Sefer ha-Qanun*, Zeraḥyah) = Arabic عجز 'sacrum' (cf. DKT 486–7, 821; FAL 6, no. 99); cf. bk. 1 (fol. 20a): הפרק האחד עשר בנתוח העצם הנקרא הזקן (Chapter eleven: On the anatomy of the sacrum). Zeraḥyah's translation results from reading Arabic عجز (sacrum) as عجوز (old man, woman). For the other translator(s), see entry עגז.

זרוע (*Sefer ha-Qanun*, Nathan) = Arabic عضد 'humerus; upper arm' (cf. DKT 823; FAL 5, no. 85); cf. bk. 1 (fol. 37a): ונוטה אל הצד החיצוני ומחוברת בראש הכתף ונקשרת בה הכתף ובהם יחדו נקשר הזרוע (Then it (i.e., clavicle) goes to the outside and articulates with the acromion process so that the scapula is joined to it, and the humerus to both of them). In the sense of 'humerus', Hebrew זרוע is a semantic borrowing from Arabic عضد. The Hebrew term features in the current dictionaries in the sense of 'arm' (BDB 283–4; JD 412; BM 1397–8); 'upper arm' (LOW XLIX). According to Singer-Rabin (SRP 24 (131)), the term זרוע is mostly applied to the forearm (cf. קנה הזרוע used by Nathan and

160 The term זנד also features as זנאד (cf. entries התעתדות, זנאד תחתון, זנאד עליון, and השטיח על ערפו).

161 Arabic *zand* originally means 'one of a pair of sticks used for producing fire' (cf. L 1257).

162 Ms הזכרים emend. ed.: הזנדים.

featuring in the glossary to the *Sefer ha-Qanun* (NM 2:119, 156 (Qof 3)); see also entry קנה).

זריקה: זריקות (*Sammim Libbiyim*) = Arabic زراقة, Plur. زراقات 'syringe, Plur. syringes'; cf. fol. 122a: ויספיק בזה המשך המימות המתאחרות בעת הזלת הקודמות וכן הרוחות וכן העורות בכוסות המציצה והמימות בזריקות (It is sufficient in this matter [to refer to the example of] flowing water which draws the water behind it, similar is the case of winds, and of skins during cupping and water through syringes). Hebrew זריקה, Plur. זריקות, features in Rabbinic literature in the sense of 'sprinkling the blood on the altar; thrusting' (JD 414).

זרע: זרעים קרים (*Sefer Ṣedat ha-Derakhim*) = Arabic مزوّرات lit., 'simulated dishes' or 'counterfeit dishes' (cf. NA 613: 'They are meatless dishes meant to give the semblance of the original version, commonly prepared with meat ... Cooks also make them for the sick since they are light and nourishing. Doctors prescribe them because they are easier to digest'[163]; cf. D 1:612, s.v. مزوّر: 'plat maigre, aux légumes, sans viande'); cf. bk. 2, ch. 1 (fol. 41a): ויהיה מאכלו זרעים קרים ויהיה משתהו מים ערבים צלולים (He should eat a vegetarian dish and drink sweet clear water). Hebrew זרע קר, Plur. זרעים קרים (lit., 'cold seeds'), does not feature in the current dictionaries.

חֶבֶל: חבל הזרוע (*Sefer ha-Qanun*, Nathan) = Arabic حبل الذراع (lit. 'cord of the fore-arm'), i.e., 'funis brachii, the median cephalic vein of the arm' (cf. DKT 634–5, 816; FAL 67, no. 1488); cf. bk. 1 (fol. 65b): ואחר בקרוב מפרק[164] המרפק מתחלק לשלשה חלקים אחד מהם חבל הזרוע (Then, near the elbow joint, it (i.e., the cephalic vein) divides into three branches. The first branch is the median cephalic vein). Hebrew חבל הזרוע features in MD 311. s.v. 'funis brachii'.

חֶבֶל: חבלים: See entry **ציר**.

חִבּוּשׁ (*Sefer ha-Shimmush*) = Arabic جَبْر 'setting (of bones)'; cf. fol. 143b, col. b: הראש הוא בכלל עב מחמם רב המזון ... ועוזר על חבוש שבירת העצמות ([The meat of] the head [of animals] is generally thick, heating and very nutritious ... and useful for setting broken bones). Hebrew חִבּוּשׁ features as a modern term in EM 495 in the sense of קשירה/אריזה (binding, packing) and כריכה בתחבושת (bandage, dress). Nathan ha-Me'ati translates Arabic جَبْر as חבישה or לחבוש, and Zeraḥyah Ḥen as דבקות or לדבק in their translations of Maimonides, *Medical Aphorisms* 15.46, 63, 64. Moses Ibn Tibbon, a contemporary of Shem Tov Ben Isaac, uses the term חִבּוּשׁ as a translation of Arabic تكميد 'vapour bath; fomentation'; cf. NM 3:78.

163 For some recipes, cf. ISW 46 (119–24) and 105 (281–4); NA 232–9, 433–7.
164 a من مفصل المرفق Ms מתפרק המפרק emend. ed.: מפרק המרפק.

חבש (*Sefer Ṣedat ha-Derakhim*) = Arabic كمّد 'to foment, to apply a fomentation; to make a warm poultice, to apply a warm pack' (D 1:488; WKAS 1:452; FL 4:58); cf. bk. 2, ch. 1 (Ms Oxford, Bodleian, Poc. 353, Uri Heb. 314, fol. 11b): ואם היה הכאב חזק ראוי שיחבוש העין במי בשול קורונא ריאל ופנגריג (If the pain is severe he should foment the eye with a decoction of melilot and fenugreek). In a medical context, Hebrew חבש only features in the current dictionaries in the sense of 'to bind, to bind up [a wound]'; cf. BDB 289–90; BM 1438–9; EM 500.

חיבש (*Sefer ha-Refu'ot ha-Libbiyot*) = Latin 'consolido' (to make firm, to strengthen) (= Arabic متّن); cf. fol. 247b: ולו עפיצות מעט ומפני זה מחבש[165] עצם רוח הלב (It (i.e., French lavender, *Lavandula stoechas* L.) has a little astringency, and therefore strengthens the substance of the pneuma of the heart). Hebrew חיבש does not feature in this sense in the current dictionaries. The anonymous author of *Sammim Libbiyim* renders Arabic متّن as קישר (see entry).

חדוש (*Sefer ha-Shimmush*)[166] = Arabic طراوة 'freshness' (cf. D 2:43); cf. fol. 144b, col. b: ולפעמים ישתנה החלב בפעולתו וכחו כפי מזג הבעל חיים אשר הוא ממנו ושניו ומדת זמן החלב מישנותו וחדושו (And sometimes the strength of the effect [of the consumption of] fat differs according to the temperament of the animal from which it hails, or its age or that of the fat, whether it is old or fresh). Hebrew חדוש does not feature in this sense in the current dictionaries.

חדר (*Sefer ha-Qanun*, Nathan) = Arabic بطن 'ventricle' (of the brain, heart); cf. bk. 1 (fol. 56a): הנה יצמח מן המוח מן העצביים <שבעה> זוגות הזוג הראשון התחלתו מעומק שני החדרים המוקדמים מן המוח אצל שכונת שתי התוספות הדומות לשתי פטומות (Seven pairs of cranial nerves originate from the brain. The first pair originates deep in the frontal ventricles, near the nipple-like (mastoid) processes). In the sense of 'ventricle' (of the brain), Hebrew חדר features in MD 769, s.v. 'ventricle'. Ben Yehuda (BM 1454) only refers to it in the sense of 'ventricle' (of the heart); cf. NM 3:80. Zeraḥyah Ḥen translates the Arabic بطن as בית (see entry).

חדש (*Sefer ha-Shimmush*)[167] = Arabic أخضر 'green, fresh' (cf. L 756); cf. fol. 126a, col. a: הפול: יש ממנו חדש אשר לא נגמר בשולו ויש ממנו יבש והחדש הלח קר באמצע המעלה הראשונה לח בסופה (Broad beans (*Vicia faba* L.): There are fresh broad beans that are not completely ripe and there are those that are dry. The fresh [and] moist ones are cold in the middle of the first degree and moist at the end of it). In the sense of 'fresh', Hebrew חדש features in JD 427 as 'new,

165 Ms Munich 373, fol. 247b יערב Ms Vienna 59, fol. 144a :מחבש.
166 See also entry חדש.
167 See also entry חדוש.

fresh, additional' and in BM 1455 as 'fresh' (טרי) in an attestation from Jacob Zahalon (second half of the seventeenth century), *Ozar ha-Hayyim*.

חוג (*Sefer ha-Shimmush*) = Arabic دوار 'dizziness'; cf. fol. 132a, col. b: והחוג והרעישה וכבדות כל הגוף וצרות הנשימה הממית בעליו באורך הזמן (... and dizziness, trembling, heaviness of the whole body, and orthopnea which will be fatal when it lasts for a long time). Hebrew חוג only features in the current dictionaries in the sense of 'circle' (cf. BM 1459–60). The term features in the combination גרם חוג for Arabic أسدر (to cause dizziness) in Shem Tov Ben Isaac's *Sefer Almansur* (cf. NM 1:12).

חוט (*Sefer Ṣedat ha-Derakhim*) = Arabic خطّ (lit., 'line, streak, stripe'); h.l., 'cerebral (longitudinal) fissure'; Latin 'linea'; cf. bk.1, ch. 11 (fol. 18b): המוח יחלק תחלה[168] באורך לשני חלקים: ימין ושמאל וביניהם חוט נמשך באמצע המוח מבדיל בין מדוריו (The brain is first[169] of all divided lengthwise in two halves: right and left, and between these [halves] is a fissure that divides between its ventricles (h.l., hemispheres?)). Hebrew חוט does not feature in this sense in the current dictionaries.

חוט השדרה (*Sefer Ṣedat ha-Derakhim*) = Arabic نخاع الفقار 'spinal chord'; cf. bk. 1, ch. 23 (fol. 33b): ואם יהיה הסתום באחד מפלחי חוט השדרה ימין ושמאל יהיה הפלג במה שלמטה מן הצואר מן הפלח ההוא האטום (If the obstruction is in one side of the spinal cord, right or left, the hemiplegia will be in that obstructed side below the neck). In the sense of 'spinal cord', Hebrew חוט השדרה is attested for Rabbinic literature in JD 431 and EM 510 (cf. LOW XLIX). Ben Yehuda mentions the term under the entry שדרה (BM 6919–20) without a clear definition.

חוטי הבצים (*Sefer Hanhagat ha-Beri'ut*) = 'spermatic cords'; cf. 10.2 (167): צריך אדם להזהר אם רצה לחיות בטובה שלא יבעול אלא כשימצא גופו בריא וחזק והוא מתקשה מאליו שלא מדעתו וימצא כובד ממתניו ולמטה כאילו חוטי הבצים נמשכים למטה (When a man wants to live well he has to be careful only to have sexual intercourse when his body is healthy and strong and he has a spontaneous unintentional erection and he feels a heaviness from his hips downwards as if the spermatic cords are drawn downwards). Hebrew חוטי הבצים features in Rabbinic literature and is mentioned in LOW XLIX: 'cordae spermaticae'. In medieval literature it features, e.g., in Maimonides, *Mishneh Torah, Sefer Qedushah, Hilkhot Issurei Bi'ah*, ch. 16, and is defined by Maimonides as השבילין שבהן תתבשל שכבת זרע (the channels in which the sperm is ripened).

חולב: החולבים (*Sefer ha-Qanun*, Nathan) = Arabic الطالعان (read: الحالبان, emend. De Koning, DKT 638–9) 'the [two] renal veins'; cf. bk. 1 (fol. 66b): ואחר יתענף

168 om. a :תחלה.

169 'first of all': om. a.

מהם שני עורקים גדולים נקראים החולבים פונים אל הכליות לזכך מימיות הדם (Then two large veins detach from [the inferior vena cava] called 'the [two] renal veins' which go into the kidneys to purify the watery part of the blood). Hebrew החולב, Plur. החולבים, is not attested in the current dictionaries. The term features in the sense of 'groins' (for Arabic الحالبان)[170] in Nathan's translation of Maimonides, *Medical Aphorisms*. Zeraḥyah transcribes the Arabic حالبان, Genitive حالبين, as האליבין, and Joseph Lorki as חלבון (read: חלבין).

חוליא: החוליא ההולכת באורך (*Sefer ha-Qanun*, Zeraḥyah) = Arabic الدرز الطولي 'the longitudinal suture'; cf. bk. 1 (fol. 17a): ותהיה החוליא ההולכת ברוחב באמצע הרחב מן האוזן אל האוזן כמו שהחוליא ההולכת באורך הוא באמצע האורך (The transverse suture is in the middle of the width, from ear to ear, just as the longitudinal suture is in the middle of the length). The term החוליא ההולכת באורך does not feature in the current dictionaries. For the other translator(s), see entry השלב הארוכיי.

החוליא ההולכת ברוחב (*Sefer ha-Qanun*, Zeraḥyah) = Arabic. الدرز العردي 'the transverse suture'; cf. bk. 1 (fol. 17a): ותהיה החוליא ההולכת ברוחב באמצע הרחב מן האוזן אל האוזן כמו שהחוליא ההולכת באורך הוא באמצע האורך. Hebrew החוליא ההולכת ברוחב is not attested in the current dictionaries. For the other translator(s), see entry השלב הארוכיי.

חוליה: חליה, Plur. חליות (*Sefer ha-Qanun*, Zeraḥyah) = Arabic شأن, Plur. شؤون 'cranial sutures' (cf. DKT 456–7; FAL 137, no. 2968); cf. bk. 1 (fol. 17a): ולכמו זאת הצורה שלשה חליות אמתיות ושני חליות כזביות (A skull with such a shape has three 'true' sutures and two 'false' sutures). As a medical term, Hebrew חוליה features in the current dictionaries in the sense of 'vertebra' (cf. JD 434; BM 1465–6); see also LOW L. The term features in SRP 38 with a reference to its occurrence in the *Sefer ha-Qanun*. Nathan ha-Me'ati renders the Arabic term as שלב, Plur. שלבים (see entry).

חולית הארכובה (*Sefer ha-Qanun*, Joseph Lorki) = Arabic رضفة 'patella' (cf. DKT 570–5, 818; FAL 126, no. 2777); cf. bk. 1 (fol. 16a): ולו שתי ראשים האחד מהם בשרי וידבק בחולית[171] הארכובה קודם שישוב יתר והאחר קרומי דבק בקצה השמאלי מקצוי הירך ([This muscle] (i.e., of the kneejoint) has two ends, one is fleshy and inserted on the patella before becoming a tendon, and the other which is membranous is inserted on the left end of the thigh bone). Hebrew חולית הארכובה is not attested in the current dictionaries. For the other translator(s), see entry עגול הארכובה.

---

170 Arabic حالبان represents the Greek βουβῶνες as it features in Galen, *De methodo medendi* (e.g., 11.4; ed. Kühn 10:744). Note that Fonahn (FAL 68, no. 1508 and 168, no. 3617) and Ullmann (UWS 1:815, s.v. οὐρητήρ) only mention this term in the sense of 'ureters'.

171 Ms בחוליות emend. ed.: בחולית.

החוליה הקלפית (*Sefer ha-Qanun*, Zeraḥyah) = Arabic الدرز القشري 'the squamosal suture'; cf. bk. 1 (fol. 17b): ושני השרשים[172] שהם ימין ושמאל הם שתי העצמות אשר בהם האזנים ונקראות שתי האבנים מפני קשים כאבן וגבול[173] כל אחד מהם מלמעלה לחוליה הקלפית (The walls[174] on the right and left side [of the skull] are the petroid bones which are called like that because they are hard as a stone. They are bounded above by the squamosal suture ...). Hebrew החוליה הקלפית does not feature in the current dictionaries. The term קלפי features in BM 5971 in an attestation from Simon Ben Zemah Duran, *Magen Avot*. For its occurrence in the *Sefer ha-Qanun*, see RTT 147. For the other translator(s), see entry השלב הקלפיי.

חוצץ (*Sefer ha-Qanun*, Nathan) = Arabic حاجز 'spine of the scapula' (cf. DKT 548–9, 816; FAL 67, no. 1500); cf. bk. 1 (fol. 49a): וחמשה עצלים צמיחתם מעצמות הכתף מהם עצל תולדתו מעצם הכתף ומתחבר[175] מה שבין החוצץ והצלע העליון לכתף (There are five [other] muscles [of the arm] which arise from the scapula. One of them arises from the scapula and occupies[176] the [space] between the spine of the scapula and its superior border). Hebrew חוצץ does not feature in this sense in the current dictionaries. Zeraḥyah Ḥen translates the Arabic حاجز as מבדיל (see entry); Joseph Lorki has מבדיל as well.

חזוק (*Sefer ha-Qanun*, Joseph Lorki) = Arabic عَقَب 'ligament, fibrous tissue' (cf. DKT 516–7; 823; FAL 22, no. 395; FL 3:190): 'nervi seu tendines, quibus chordae conficiuntur'; cf. bk. 1 (fol. 13b): ועל כן חשב[177] הבורא והצמיח מהעצמות דבר דומה בעצב נקרא חזוק וקשרים והוא נאסף מהעצב ונסתבך בו כדבר אחד (In[178] his kindness the Creator made something grow on the bones that resembles nerves—and is called 'fibrous tissue'—and ligaments. He has attached them to the nerves and interlaced them with the nerves). Hebrew חזוק does not feature in this sense in the current dictionaries. For the other translator(s), see entry עקב.

(חזק) מחזק: See entry **סם**.

חֲזָקָה (*Sefer Ṣedat ha-Derakhim*) = Arabic وهج 'burning heat'; Latin 'fumus'; cf. bk. 1, ch. 18 (fol. 26a): ותתילד משתי סבות אחת מהן התלהבות מרה כרכומית והתלקח בחלקי המוח והאחרת מרתיחת דם הלב והתגברו כי דם הלב כשירתח ויתלהב בחום מרה אדומה יתגבר ויעלה חזקתו אל הראש (And it (i.e., phrenitis) is caused by one of two things: (1) the heat and burning of the yellow bile in the parts of the

---

172 a الجداران Ms¹ השרשים: הגדרים.
173 Ms¹ וגבול: ונאחז.
174 'walls': Translated after Ms¹.
175 a ומתחבר: وتشغل.
176 'and occupies': Translates after Arabic وتشغل.
177 a וחשב: وتلطّف.
178 'In his kindness the Creator made': Translated after a; cf. entry דקדק.

brain, and (2) the boiling and bubbling of the blood of the heart; when the blood of the heart becomes boiling hot because of the heat of the yellow bile, it bubbles[179] and its burning heat arises to the brain). Hebrew חָזְקָה only features in the current dictionaries as a biblical and modern term (cf. BDB 306; BM 1493–4; EM 520) in the sense of 'strength, force, violence'.

הליחה המחטיאה: מחטיא (חטא) (*Pirqei Arnauṭ de Vilanova*) = Latin 'vitiosus humor' (peccant humour)[180]; cf. 4.1 (48): רוע מזג אם יקרה בלי ליחה הנה יתוקן ענינו עם הדברים המשנים המזג אך אם יהיה עם ליחה לא יתוקן ענינו אלא עם נקוי הליחה המחטיאה (If a bad temperament (dyscrasy) occurs without a [corrupt] humour, it should be cured with ingredients that change the temperament, but if it occurs with a [corrupt] humour, it can only be corrected by purging [the body] from the peccant humour). Hebrew הליחה המחטיאה does not feature in the current dictionaries.

חטים: חטה (*Sefer Ṣedat ha-Derakhim*) = Arabic لوزتان 'tonsils'; cf. introduction (fol. 3a): השער הג׳ בכאיבי האונקלי והשפוי כובע והחטים (Chapter three: On pains of the uvula, larynx, and tonsils). The unattested Hebrew חטים corresponds to Aramaic חיטי, Sing. חיטתא, the meaning of which is uncertain, but which is traditionally explained as 'a cartilage on the trachea'; cf. SDA 453. The term can also be found in Shem Tov Ben Isaac's *Sefer ha-Shimmush* as a translation of Arabic لوزتان (cf. NM 1:92), and in Nathan's translation of Arabic نغانغ (tonsils) in Maimonides, *Medical Aphorisms* 22.19. The term also features as חטי (מקדם המוח) in Ṭodros Ṭodrosi's Hebrew translation of Ibn Sīnā's *K. al-Najāt* (ed. by G. Elgrably-Berzin) for Arabic زائدتي (?), and is translated by the editor as 'the two protuberances [of the front part of the brain]'[181]. In his glossary to the *Sefer ha-Qanun*, Nathan ha-Me'ati remarks: שקד. קראתי שקדים החטים שבגרגרת כי קראום כן הערביים (ŠQD (almond). I called the tonsils (ḤṬYM) in the throat ŠQDYM, because this is the name that the Arabs have given to them) (cf. NM 2:120, 162 (Shin 5)).

מחכך (חכך): See entry **סם**.

---

179 'bubbles': See entry התגבר (גבר).

180 '(peccant humour)': Cf. F. Wallis, *Medieval Medicine. A Reader* (Toronto 2010), 548, s.v. 'peccant (humor)': 'a bodily humor that has become excessive or corrupt (e.g., by being adust (burnt or scorched)), and hence transformed into morbific matter, which leads to (literally, is 'guilty of') disease. The doctor aims to evacuate peccant humors.'

181 G. Elgrably-Berzin, *Avicenna in Medieval Hebrew Translation. Ṭodros Ṭodrosi's Translation of Ibn Sīnā's K. al-Najāt on Psychology and Metaphysics* (Leiden 2015), 30, 194. In her commentary on this term (117–8), Elgrably-Berzin relates the term to Hebrew *ḥute* (threads), *ḥate* (canine teeth, or Arabic خطي (two lines)). She does not relate it to Aramaic חיטי in the sense of tonsils, although such an identification seems logical since the Avicennian text compares these protuberances to the 'two nipples of the breast' (פטומתי השדים), whose shape is similar to that of tonsils.

חלאה (*Sefer ha-Shimmush*) = Arabic رغوة 'foam'; cf. fol. 127a, col. b: וכשיקרבו השעורים אל הבשול וישגו ויתפחו להסיר חלאתם ולרחצם במים חמין (When the barley is almost done and swells and becomes larger, remove the foam, and wash it in hot water). Hebrew חלאה features in BM 1552 in the sense of 'filth'. In the sense of 'waste matter' (פסולת של דבר), it features (ibid.) as חלאת הקצף (the waste of the foam) in an attestation from Rabbenu Gershom Me'or ha-Golah.

חָלָב: See entry **מִיץ**.

החלב החמוץ (*Sefer ha-Shimmush*) = Arabic الدوغ 'sour buttermilk' (cf. NA 585: 'thick sour *makhīḍ* (buttermilk)[182], made by draining it of its whey'); cf. fol. 147a, col. a: חחלב החמוץ הנקרא אלדוע'[183] קר יבש קשה להתעכל רחוק לרדת כבד על האצטומ' (The sour milk called *al-dūġ* is cold and dry, hard to digest, far from going down and heavy on the stomach ...). Hebrew החלב החמוץ features in BM 1552 in attestations subsequent to Shem Tov Ben Isaac, namely from the *Sefer ha-Qanun* and Me'ir Aldabi's *Shevilei Emunah*.

החלב הקרוש (*Sefer ha-Shimmush*) = Arabic للبن الرائب 'thick curdled milk' (cf. FL 2:205: 'crassum (lac) cuius cremor ablatus est ...')[184]; cf. fol. 147a, col. a: החלב הקרוש הנקרא אלראיב יותר קר מן החמוץ ויותר נאות אל האצטומ' החמה ולבעלי החמימות (Thick, curdled milk called *al-rā'ib* is colder than sour buttermilk and better for a hot stomach and for people with a hot temperament ...). Hebrew החלב הקרוש features in Rabbinic literature, a.o., *Tosefta* 11.8 (cf. BM 6223, s.v. קרש).

חֵלֶב: חלב החטה (*Sefer ha-Shimmush*) = Arabic نشاء الحنطة وهو النشاستج 'starch' (Greek ἄμυλον) cf. UW 102; NA 570; cf. fol. 124b, col. 1: חלב החטה קר ויבש והראיה על קרירותו החמיצות המועטת אשר בו והמזון המתילד ממנו יש בו חלוקה ולפי כך יועיל

182 Cf. Maimonides, *Medical Aphorisms* 23.107 (trans. Bos, 5:69): 'Among the names of [different] types of milk are the following: if milk is churned and its butter removed, the rest is called 'buttermilk' (*makhīḍ*). It is also called *dūgh*'; MIG 245: الدوغ هو مخيض البقر كان حامضًا أو غير حامضٍ عن مسيح، وهو عند الإسرائيلي الرائب، وقد أشار الرازي فيه إلى مثل هذا في المنصوري، وقال يحيى بن ماسويه: هو اللبن الحامض المنزوع الزبد المتّخذ من لبن الغنم (*Al-dūġ* is—according to Masīḥ—cow's buttermilk (*maḫīḍ*), be it sour or not. According to al-Isrā'īlī it is curdled milk (*rā'ib*). Al-Rāzī held a similar view about it in his *Manṣūrī*. Yaḥyā ibn Māsawayh: It is the sour milk from which the butter has been extracted. It is made from ewe's and goat's milk (*laban al-ġanam*)); see also entry מיץ החלב.

183 Mss אללדוע emend. ed. :אלדוע.

184 In the *Medical Aphorisms* 23.107 (trans Bos, 5:69), Maimonides states regarding the term 'rā'ib': 'If the milk congeals completely either by rennet or by leaving it [standing] for days until it becomes thick, it is called *rā'ib* (thick, coagulated)'; cf. n. 183 above.

מנחרת החזה והריאה ועיצום[185] המעים והפשטתם ומשחין כיס מקוה המים (Starch is cold and dry; an indication for its coldness is that it has only little acidity. The nutrition it provides is viscous and for this reason it is good for roughness of the chest and lungs, for abrasion of the intestines and for a tumor in the urinary bladder). Hebrew חלב החטה features in the Bible (e.g., Ps 81:17), and is translated as 'the best, choice part of the wheat' (KB 316; BDB 317). The term also features in Maimonides, *Mishneh Torah, Sefer Zemannim, Hilkhot Ḥameṣ u-Maṣah*; cf. BM 1553. In their translations of Maimonides, *Medical Aphorisms* 6.17 and 20.17 (forthcoming ed. Bos), Nathan ha-Me'ati renders Arabic نشاستج and its synonym نشاء as Latin אמידום, and Zeraḥyah Ḥen as אמידו.

חלודה (*Hanhagat ha-Beri'ut le-Abu 'Ali Ben Zuhr*) = 'filth' (cf. Honofredi: 'sordicies'); cf. ch. 20: ואמרו חכמי׳: כאשר ירחץ הבלן הגוף במרחץ בדבש יוציא מן הגשם מה שהוא דבק בין עור ובשר מן המותרות הלחות העשניות ויפתח הסתומים וימרק מה שעליו מן החלודה והדומה אליו (The learned doctors said: When the bath attendant washes one's body in the bathhouse with honey; it extracts the moist, smoky residues that are stuck between the skin and the flesh and opens the blocked pores and cleanses [the body] from filth and the like). Hebrew חלודה features in the current dictionaries in the sense of 'rust; mould' (BM 1559; JD 465) and in a medical context in Rabbinic literature as a skin affliction which looks like mould or rust (LOW LI; JD 465). Ben Yehuda (BM 1560), quoting Maimonides, *Medical Aphorisms* 24.10 (trans. Nathan ha-Me'ati), mentions חלודה in the sense of 'blood serum'. In his translation of Maimonides, *Medical Aphorisms* 15.54 (forthcoming ed. Bos), Nathan ha-Me'ati uses the same term to render Arabic صديد (fluid, watery moisture); cf. NM 2:46. Hillel of Verona has חלודה for Latin 'limositas', Plur. 'limositates' (viscous matters) (cf. NM 3:82).

חלוחלת I. (*Sefer Ṣedat ha-Derakhim*) = Arabic مقعدة 'buttocks'; cf. introduction (fol. 3b): השער הכ׳ ברפיון החלוחלת ויציאתה (Chapter twenty: On the weakness [of the muscles] of the buttocks and anus); II. (*Sefer ha-Qanun*, Nathan) = Arabic سرم 'rectum' (cf. DKT 819, FAL 145, no. 3132); cf. bk. 1 (fol. 40b): וגם הונחו על העצם הזה איברים נכבדים כמו המקוה והרחם וכלי הזרע מן הזכרים והשת והחלוחלת (Also placed on these bones (i.e., of the pelvis) are noble organs such as the bladder, the uterus, the spermatic cord in males, the anus and the rectum). Hebrew חלוחלת features as חלחולת in secondary literature in the sense of 'mesentery' or 'rectum' (JD 466; KA 3:390, 9:183; BM 1568; LOW LI). Hebrew חלוחלת also features in Shem Tov Ben Isaac's glossary to the

185 a עיצום המעים והפשטתם: سحوج المعاء.

Sefer ha-Shimmush as an equivalent to Arabic مبعر (rectum, intestine or gut); cf. SHS 1:229 (Ḥet 34). A translation of the Arabic term is missing in Zeraḥyah Ḥen.

חלול: החלול (*Sefer ha-Qanun*, Zeraḥyah)[186] = Arabic الأجوف 'vena cava' (cf. DKT 830, s.v. الوريد الأجوف); cf. bk. 1 (fol. 34b): הפרק החמישי בניתוח החלול היורד הנה חתמנו המאמר בחלק העולה מן החלול והוא היותר קטון שבחלקיו (Chapter five: On the anatomy of the inferior vena cava. We have finished the discussion of the ascending part of the vena cava which is the smaller of the two). For Hebrew החלול, featuring in the *Sefer ha-Qanun*, cf. SRP 6 (37). For the other translator(s), see entry הנבוב.

החלול היורד (*Sefer ha-Qanun*, Zeraḥyah) = Arabic الأجوف النازل 'the inferior vena cava'; cf. bk. 1 (fol. 34b): הפרק החמישי בניתוח החלול היורד הנה חתמנו המאמר בחלק העולה מן החלול והוא היותר קטון שבחלקיו. Hebrew החלול היורד is not attested in the current dictionaries. For the other translator(s), see entry נבוב: הנבוב היורד.

חלוק (*Sefer ha-Shimmush*) = Arabic لزج 'viscous'; cf. fol. 124b, col. 1: סובין של חטה חמים יבשים מעטי המזון מאד ומנגבים ולוטשים לטישה רבה יותר מלטישת קמח החטה[187] וכשיעשה מהם שרף ימהר לרדת מן האסטומ׳ ולוטש מה שיש בחזה והריאה מהלחויות החלוקות (Wheat bran is hot [and] dry, it provides very little nourishment, it is drying and has a stronger cleansing effect than wheat flour. A broth prepared from it quickly descends from the stomach and cleanses the chest and lungs from the viscous moistures). Hebrew חלוק does not feature in this sense in the current dictionaries. In the Bible we find the term in the sense of 'smooth' in חַלֻּקֵי אֲבָנִים 'smooth stones' (1 Sam 17:40; cf. BDB 325).

חלי: החולי הנופל (*Sefer Ṣedat ha-Derakhim*) = Arabic صرع 'epilepsy'; cf. introduction (Ms Oxford, Bodleian, Poc. 353, Uri Heb. 314, fol. 1b)[188]: השער הכ״ב בחולי הנופל (Chapter twenty-two: On epilepsy). Hebrew החולי הנופל does not feature in the current dictionaries.[189] The term features in the *Sefer Agur*; in Moses Ibn Tibbon's translation of Hippocrates' *Aphorisms* 2.45 we find חולי הנופל (cf. NM 3:85).

חלימה (*Sefer ha-Qanun*, Nathan) = Arabic حلم 'intelligence, understanding, wisdom'; cf. bk. 1 (fol. 31b): והקצויות יצמחו ברוב באמצע זמן הגדול והוא אחר ההמרצה

186 In addition to החלול, Zeraḥyah has הוריד החלול (see entry) to indicate the 'vena cava' conform to the Arabic الوريد الأجوف.

187 החטה: א¹.

188 Note that in the header to the text itself, the term does not feature as החולי הנופל but as חולי הכפיה.

189 MD 262 mentions—next to the standard term כפיה—the following synonyms: חלי נפל/נפילה/נופלים.

אל ההעמדה וזה כי ההעמדה קרובה מל׳ שנה ולכן נקראים שני אלחלם כלומ׳ החלימה
(In most cases wisdom teeth appear during the time of growth, namely
after reaching maturity. For one reaches maturity at about thirty years and
therefore these teeth are called 'wisdom teeth'). Hebrew חלימה features in
BM 1575 in a quotation of the same text. Ben Yehuda derives the term from
the root חלם in the sense of 'to be sane' (cf. BM 1584). Zeraḥyah Ḥen renders the Arabic حِلْم as חלומות, reading Arabic حِلْم as حُلْم (dream); cf. entry שן:
שני החלומות.

חלל (*Sefer ha-Shimmush*) = Arabic أَحْشَاء 'intestines'; cf. fol. 129a, col. a: ויזיקו למי
שיש בתוך חללו מורסא (It (i.e., water from snow) is harmful for those suffering
from intestinal ulcers). Hebrew חלל only features in the current dictionaries in the sense of 'cavity, empty space, hollow' (JD 470; BM 1580). Zeraḥyah
Ḥen uses the term חלל for Arabic مُقَعَّر (concave [part]) in his translation of
Maimonides, *Medical Aphorisms* 7.57 (cf. NM 1:148–9), and Nathan ha-Me'ati
for Arabic تَجْوِيف (ventricle) in his translation of Maimonides, *Medical
Aphorisms* 1.53 (cf. NM 2:48).

חללות (*Sammim Libbiyim*) = Arabic تَجْوِيف 'cavity'; cf. fol. 120b: והפותח הוא אשר
יניע החומר אשר נופל בחללות המעברים ויוציאהו לא בפיותיהם לבד (An opening
[drug] is one that moves and expels the matter that is not only in the openings but in the cavities of the passages as well). Hebrew חללות features in BM
1583 in an attestation from Ḥasdai Crescas, *Or Adonai*, in the sense of 'the
property of something that is hollow' (סגולת מה שהוא חלול) and is then taken
up by Klatzkin (KTP 1:305) and rendered as 'Volumen, Rauminhalt'. The
same Hebrew term features in Judah Shalom's translation of Hippocrates'
Aphorisms 7.51 (cf. NM 3:88). The anonymous translator of *Sefer ha-Refu'ot
ha-Libbiyot* (fol. 243a) renders Latin 'concavitates' as חלל (cf. NM 3:87–8).

חלץ :חלצים (*Sefer Ṣedat ha-Derakhim*) = Arabic شَرَاسِيف 'costal cartilages' (cf.
DKT 820; FL 2:411); cf. bk. 1, ch. 18 (fol. 26b): הדרך הראשון כשיהיה החולי משוקע
במוח עצמו והשני כשיהיה באסטו׳ ומה שקרוב ממנה כמו חולי החלצים הנפוחים אשר
צבותם מן המרה השחורה והשלישי כשיבא מן הידים והרגלים ([Phrenitis occurs in
three ways (manners)]: (a) when the illness is settled in the brain itself; (b)
when [the illness] is in the stomach and the adjacent parts, as the illness of
the costal cartilages that are swollen because of the black bile; (c) when [the
illness] comes from the hands and feet). Hebrew חלץ, Plur. חלצים, features
in the current dictionaries and secondary literature in the sense of 'flanks,
loins' (cf. JD 473; BM 1590; LOW LI).

החליץ (חלץ) (*Sefer Hanhagat ha-Beri'ut*) = 'to strengthen, to invigorate'; cf. 4.5
(134): ולפיכך ראוי לאדם שלא ישתה ממנו לתענוג ולשעשוע כדרך הסובאים אלא כדי
להבריא גופו ולהחליץ אבריו (Therefore one should not drink it (i.e., wine) for

pleasure and amusement as boozers do, but only to make the body healthy and strengthen its organs). In the sense of 'to strengthen', Hebrew החליץ features in the Bible in Is 58:11: עצמותיך יחליץ (he will brace up, invigorate, thy bones; trans. BDB 323). Ben Yehuda (BM 1592, esp. n. 3) renders the term החליץ את העצמות as 'to fatten the bones' (i.e., to increase their marrow) (עשה אותן דשנות) while referring to Ibn Janāḥ, *K. al-Uṣūl* (cf. IJ 230).

מחליק (חלק): See entry **סם**.

חֲלַקָּה: חלוקה (*Sefer ha-Shimmush*) = Arabic لزوجة 'viscosity'; cf. 124b, cols. 1–2: הדיסא היא גם כן מזה המין והיא בטבעה עבה וחלוקה ומתאחרת להתעכל ומולידה סתומים כהולדת הגריסין אלא שהיא כשתתעכל בגופי הבריאים תוליד דם יש בו לחות וחלוקה ותזון מזון רב (DYS' (coarsely pounded wheat or barley eaten alone or mixed with honey)[190] belongs also to this sort [of food]; it is by nature thick, viscous, and slow to digest. It produces obstructions, just like GRYSYN (grits, groats). However, when it is digested in the bodies of healthy people it produces moist, viscous blood and is very nutritious). In the sense of 'viscosity', Hebrew חלוקה is a non-attested verbal noun (derived from חלק in the sense of 'to be soft, smooth' (cf. BM 1600–1). It is thus a variant to חֶלְקָה, which features in the current dictionaries in the sense of 'smoothness' (ibid. 1601–2).

חלקות: חלקות המעים הוא זלק אל מעא (*Sefer Ṣedat ha-Derakhim*) = Arabic زلق الأمعاء 'lientery'; cf. introduction (fol. 3b): השער הי״ד בחלקות המעים הוא זלק אל מעא (Chapter fourteen: On lientery, i.e., [Arabic] *zilq al-miʿāʾ*). Hebrew חלקות המעים does not feature in the current dictionaries. The same term features as חליקות המעים in an anonymous translation of Hippocrates' *Aphorisms* 3.30 (cf. NM 3:87).

חם: החם הנכרי (*Sefer Hanhagat ha-Beriʾut*) = 'unnatural heat'; cf. 2.1 (116): ומן הראיות הגדולות על זה כי כשיצא החום הטבעי מן הקו האמצעי באיכותו או בכמותו ויתערב עמו חום נכרי תראה הרגשת הראות והרגשת השמע ושאר ההרגשות משובשות (Conclusive proof for this is that when the natural heat declines from a moderate measure in its quality or quantity and is mixed with unnatural heat the senses of sight, hearing, and the other senses become clearly defective). Hebrew חם נכרי features in BM 1607 in an attestation from Jacob Ben Machir Ibn Tibbon's *Kol Melekhet Higgayon*, i.e., his translation of Ibn Rushd's commentary on Aristotle's *Organon*. Ben Yehuda does not provide an explanation for the term. It also features in KTP 38 in a quotation from Meir Aldabi, *Shevilei Emunah*. The Arabic parallel term حرارة غريبة or حرارة خارجة عن الطبيعة features, e.g., in Maimonides, *Medical Aphorisms* 3.49 (ed.

190 Cf. entry דיסא.

and trans. Bos, 1:45), and is translated by Nathan ha-Me'ati as חום נכרי and חום יוצא חוץ מן הטבע.

חמאיי (*Sefer ha-Shimmush*) = Arabic سمني 'buttery'; cf. fol. 146b, col. a: חלב הבקר יותר עב מכל החלבים ויותר רחוק מן העכול והירידה ויותר כבד על האסטומ׳ ושלשולו הבטן יותר מועט אלא שהוא זן יותר מכל החלבים ועל כן חלבם מועיל מן השלשול המררי והעיצום הכרכומי (Cows' milk is thicker than all the other [kinds of] milk, but it is slower to digest and to go down and it is heavier on the stomach and is not so good for relieving the bowels, but it is more nutritious than all the other [kinds of] milk. For this reason [cow's] milk is good for bilious diarrhea and for tenesmus and [discharge of] yellow bile). Hebrew חמאיי only features as a modern term in EM 550.

חמוץ: See entry ירק.

חמיצות האתרוג :חמיצות (*Sefer Ṣedat ha-Derakhim*) = Arabic حماض الأترج 'citron pulp' (cf. NA 641); cf. bk. 1, ch. 19 (fol. 29b): ויהיה מזונו פיישאן הנקרא בערב׳ דראג׳ ותרנוגלים קטנים ומאכלים חמוצים עשויים בקני הלגלוגות ומי בוסר ומי חמיצות האתרוג (He should feed himself with francolin called in Arabic *durrāǧ*, young chickens, sour dishes prepared with purslane stems, sour grape juice and citron pulp juice). Hebrew חמיצות האתרוג does not feature in the current dictionaries.

חנגרי (*Sefer ha-Qanun*, Nathan)[191] = Arabic خنجري 'xiphoid [cartilage]' (cf. DKT 824; FAL 64, no. 1425); cf. bk. 1 (fol. 52b): וקצה שנים האחרים אצל החנגרי [192] (The ends of the other [muscles of the abdomen meet at] the xiphoid [cartilage]). For Hebrew חנגרי, a loan word from Arabic خنجري, featuring in the *Sefer ha-Qanun*, cf. SRP 23. Zeraḥyah Ḥen translates the Arabic خنجري as חלצים(?), Joseph Lorki as השנים הגרונים.

חפירה (*Hanhagat ha-Beri'ut le-Abu 'Ali Ben Zuhr*) = 'cavity'; cf. ch. 28: ואם תרצה שלא יהיה בשיניך חפירה ולא שנוי יהיה חכוכך בעץ האפרסק (If you want your teeth to be free of cavities and to [remain healthy], you should rub them with peach wood). Hebrew חפירה does not feature in this sense in the current dictionaries. The same term features in the sense of 'cavity' in Shem Tov Ben Isaac's *Sefer Almansur* (cf. BMZ 68 (Qof 1)): קיסום: קר יכנס בסמי העין ויועיל מעפוש השינים וחפירתם (Southernwood (*Artemisia abrotanum*): It is cold [and] used as part of eye remedies; it is beneficial for putrefaction of the teeth and for cavities).

חפץ מאכל :חפץ (*Hanhagat ha-Beri'ut le-Abu 'Ali Ben Zuhr*) = 'appetite' (cf. Honofredi: 'appetitus'); cf. ch. 10: ואמר אריסטו: בלקיחת המרקחות מן הליגנא

---

191 Instead of this loan word, Nathan also uses the regular Hebrew term שפוי כובע (see entry).

192 Ms החנגרה emend. ed.: החנגרי.

אלובין וריברברי ד׳ דרה׳ בכל יום ברקות האצטו׳ יחזק החם אשר בה העוזר לעכול ויתיך הבלגם מפיה ויתן חפץ מאכל ויסיר הרוח אשר בה (Aristotle said: If one takes every day on an empty stomach an electuary prepared from four *dirhams*[193] of aloeswood and rhabarber it strengthens the heat [in the stomach] which is good for the digestion, dissolves the phlegm from the cardia [of the stomach], whets the appetite, and removes wind [from the stomach]). Hebrew חפץ מאכל does not feature in the current dictionaries.

חציי (*Sefer ha-Qanun*, Nathan) = Arabic سهمي 'sagittal' (cf. FAL 131, no. 2860); cf. bk. 1 (fol. 29a): ושלב מחלק לאורך הראש ישר יאמר לו לבדו חציי וכשיחקר מצד חבורו עם הכלילי אז יאמר לו שפודיי (A suture that divides the head longitudinally [and that is] straight is called 'sagittal' when considered on its own, but when it is considered in relation to its connection with the coronal [suture], it is called 'shaped like a spit'). Hebrew חציי features in BM 1707 with the same attestation from the *Sefer ha-Qanun*; see also SRP 39 (285).

חצץ: See entry **חוצץ**.

חרטום: החרטום הנק׳ מנקאר (*Sefer ha-Qanun*, Nathan) = Arabic منقار 'the [coracoid] process'; cf. DKT 550–1, 829, s.v. منقار الغراب; FAL 94, no. 2075 (Greek κορακοειδής; cf. LSG 980)[194]; cf. bk. 1 (fol. 49b): ולמקבצים יש זוג שאחד נפרדין והוא היותר גדול מקבץ עם נטיה לפנים וזה כי צמיחתו מן הזר התחתון מן הכתף ומן החרטום הנק׳ מנקאר (The muscles that flex the forearm are one pair; one of these, the largest, flexes it with an inward rotation, because it arises from the lower (lateral) border and [coracoid] process, called [in Arabic] *minqār*). As an anatomical term, Hebrew חרטום features in BM 1758 in an attestation from the *Sefer ha-Qanun* (trans. Zeraḥyah Ḥen, see next entry): ולו שתי תוספות האחת מהן למעלה ומאחור ונקרא אגרס וחרטום ופי העורב ובהם קשרי הכתף עם השכם and is defined by Ben Yehuda as שם לחלק מעצם ההכתף (a name for a part of the scapula); see also SRP 21 (112–3). Zeraḥyah Ḥen transcribes the Arabic منقار as מינקאר, Joseph Lorki as גומא.

חרטום העורב (*Sefer ha-Qanun*, Nathan) = Arabic منقار الغراب (lit., 'crow's beak'); i.e., 'coracoid process' (cf. DKT 550–1, 829; FAL 94, no. 2075); cf. bk. 1 (fol. 37a): ויש לה שתי תוספות אחת מהן למעלה ומאחור ונקרא אלגזם ופי העורב ובה קשורי הכתף עם התרקוה (It (i.e., scapula) has two processes, one above and [one] behind which is called ʾLGZM (i.e., Arabic الأخرم)[195] and 'crow's beak'; through which the scapula is connected to the clavicle). For Hebrew חרטום

193 The standard *dirham* is 3.125 grams; see Hinz, *Islamische Maße und Gewichte*, 3.

194 In modern terminology it is the 'anchor-shaped' or 'sigmoid process'; cf. Galen, *On the Usefulness of the Parts of the Body*, 2 vols., trans by M. Tallmadge May (Ithaca 1968), 2:615, n. 55; see also DKT 493, n. 12.

195 For an extensive explanation of this term, cf. SRP 21 (113), s.v. ALZEGEM (אלזגם) ḤARṬUM.

העורב, as featuring in the *Sefer ha-Qanun*, cf. SRP 21 (112–3). Zeraḥyah Ḥen renders the Arabic منقار الغراب as פי העורב (see entry), and Joseph Lorki as חרטום ופי העורב.

חרס (*Sefer ha-Shimmush*) = Arabic إبرية 'dandruff' (cf. FL 1:116: 'furfures capitis'); cf. fol. 134b, col. b: ומסגולתה עוד כי הלוקח מסחיטתה ורוחץ בה הראש תנקה החרס וביצי הכנים ממנו ותאריך השער (Another specific property of [beet] is that if someone takes its juice and washes the head with it, it will get rid of the dandruff and eggs of headlice; and [it is good for] the hair growth). In the sense of 'an eruption of the skin, itch', Hebrew חרס features in the Bible (cf. BDB 360) and in Rabbinic literature in an attestation from tb*Bekhorot* 41a, where it is stated to be identical with גרב (itch, scab, scabies, psoriasis)[196]; cf. JD 504.[197] In his *Sefer Almansur*, Shem Tov Ben Isaac translates Arabic إبرية as ילפת (cf. NM 2:12–3).

חשל (*Sefer ha-Qanun*, Nathan) = Arabic ضعف 'feebleness, weakness'; cf. bk. 1 (fol. 39a): ונסתפק בעצמות שלשה כי אם היה נוסף מספרם והיה מקנה זה תוספת מספר תנועות היה בלי ספק מוריש[198] חולשה[199] וחשל באחיזת מה שיהיה צריך לאחוז אל תוספת החזקה בחוזק ([The fingers] only have three bones. If there had been more [than three], more movements would have been possible, but this would without any doubt have caused a weakness and feebleness to hold something that for holding it well would have required extra firmness). In the sense of 'weakness', Hebrew חשל is attested in BM 1805 in liturgical literature only. Zeraḥyah Ḥen renders Arabic ضعف as חולשה, and Joseph Lorki as רפיון.

חִתּוּךְ (*Sefer ha-Qanun*, Zeraḥyah) = Arabic بَطْح 'supination'; cf. bk. 1 (fol. 27a): ואלו הקובצים והפושטים הם בעצמם יפעלו הקיבוב והחיתוך (The same muscles that flex and extend [the wrist] produce [its] pronation and supination). Hebrew חתוך does not feature in this sense in the current dictionaries. For the other translator(s), see entry שטיחה על העורף.

חתך: See entry **סם**.

(חתל) חותל (*Sefer ha-Shimmush*) = Arabic ضُمِّدَ 'to be applied as a poultice'; cf. fol. 124b, col. a: וכשיבושלו ביין ומים ויחותלו בהם השדים אשר נקפא בהם החלב יתיכוהו (And when it is boiled with wine and water and applied as a poultice to the breasts it liquefies the congealed milk in them). Hebrew חתל feature in BM 1824–5 in the Pi'el and is explained by Ben Yehuda as עשה חתול (to apply a bandage). Both, Nathan ha-Me'ati and Zeraḥyah Ḥen, translate

---

196 For the term גרב, cf. NM 3:47.

197 Katzenelsohn (KTM 389) translates חרס as 'Eczema crustosum'.

198 Ms²: מוריש.

199 a وهن Ms חלושה emend. ed.: חולשה.

the same Arabic term as חבש in their translations of Maimonides, *Medical Aphorisms* 9.77, 126. The same holds good for Moses Ibn Tibbon's *Sefer Ṣedat ha-Derakhim* (cf. IJZ 228).

הטיח (טוח) (*Sefer ha-Shimmush*)[200] = Arabic لطخ 'to rub, to smear, to foil, dirty, stain' (cf. WKAS 2.2: 684a–6a); cf. fol. 144a, col. a: המוח חם לח מוליד דם קר חלוק רע אל האסטומ׳ מטיח אותה בלחותו קשה להתעכל וגורם אסטניסות ומסיר תאות המאכל ([Meat] from the brain is hot and moist; it produces cold viscous blood, it is bad for the stomach, it befouls it with its moisture, it is hard to digest, causes nausea and spoils the appetite). In the sense of 'to befoul', Hebrew הטיח is a non-attested semantic borrowing from Arabic لطخ. In the current dictionaries it only features in the sense of 'to plaster, to polish' (JD 522); 'to daub' (BM 1858).

מטיח: See entry **סם**.

טחינה (*Sefer ha-Shimmush*) = Arabic استمراء 'digestion'[201]; cf. fol. 123b, col. 2: ולמי שחלשה טחינתו מן הזקנים והנמלטים מן החליים (... and for the elderly and reconvalescents whose digestion is weak); see also *Sefer Hanhagat ha-Beri'ut* 8.1 (145): והיא הצואה שהיא המותר הטחינה הראשונה ההוה באצטומכא (and these are the excrements which are the remnant of the first digestion in the stomach). Hebrew טחינה features in the current dictionaries in the sense of 'grinding' (BDB 377; JD 528; BM 1866).

טוחן (טחן): See entry **כח**.

טיול (*Sefer ha-Shimmush*) = Arabic رياضة 'physical exercise'; cf. fol. 123b, col. 2: הרביכות: הרביכה זנה מועט וממהרת להתעכל ולרדת מן האסטומ׳ יותר מן הלחם הטבול במרק ולפי כך ראוי להנזר מן הרביכות בעלי היגיעה והטיול והרוצה להנעים גופו (RBYKWT: RBYKH[202] has less nutrition, is quicker digested and descends quicker than bread dipped in soup; therefore, those who strain themselves and do physical exercise and want to fatten their body should refrain from it). Hebrew טיול features in the current dictionaries as a Rabbinic term in the sense of 'walking, going on errands' (JD 530) and as a modern term in the sense of 'trek, hike, trip' (cf. EM 620); see also SHS 1:244 (Ṭet 9). Hebrew טיול

---

200 See also entry הטחה.

201 Arabic *istimrā'* features in al-Zahrāwī's *Taṣrīf* as a synonym for *inhiḍām*; i.e., digestion, although the current dictionaries only register *istimrā'* in the sense of 'quick, easy digestibility' (cf. FL 4:165; L 2702). The explanation of the term in SHS 1:245 (Ṭet 12): 'Arabic *ist mar'* means 'podex or anus of a human being' (L 56, 2702f.)' is faulty and should be corrected as explained above.

202 'RBYKH': I.e., a dish consisting of broken pieces of bread sopped in broth with meat and/or vegetables, cf. entry רביכה.

is also used for Arabic رياضة by the anonymous translator of Maimonides, *Regimen of Health* 1.5–7, 3.12, 4.15 (forthcoming ed. and trans. Bos).

טיחה (*Sammim Libbiyim*) = Arabic تغريّة 'agglutination'; cf. fol. 128a: טין מכתום: הוא שוה המזג בחום והקור מתדמה למזג האדם אלא שיבשו יותר רב מלחותו ויש בו לחות חזק המזג ביובש ולזה יש בו דבקות וטיחה (Sigillate earth: Its temperament in heat and cold is similar to that of a human being, except that its dryness is greater than its moisture. Its moisture is thoroughly mixed with its dryness, thus it has viscosity and agglutination). Hebrew טיחה features in BM 1868 in the sense of 'plastering' and as a medical term in the sense of 'salve' or 'poultice'; cf. NM 1:58, 95. The anonymous author of *Sefer ha-Refu'ot ha-Libbiyot* renders Latin 'confortatio' as חזוק.

טיט: הטיט הנאכל (*Sammim Libbiyim*) = Arabic الطين المأكول 'edible earth' (according to Maimonides (M 172)), the earth of Nishapur is called 'edible earth'; it is a white argil that is transported [through the streets]); cf. fol. 221a: והסותם הוא הסם אשר כאשר עבר במעברם התגבר על הכח המניע לדחותו ועמד[203] נגד כל מציק ומלא את החלל כמו הטיט הנאכל (A blocking (obstruent) [remedy] is a remedy that when it streams through the passages, overcomes their power to expel it, stops at every narrow place and fills the gap. An example is edible earth). Hebrew הטיט הנאכל does not feature in the current dictionaries. The term טיט can be found in the Bible, Rabbinic and modern literature in the sense of 'mud, mire clay, plaster' (cf. BDB 376, JD 530; BM 1868–9; EM 621). The anonymous author of *Sefer ha-Refu'ot ha-Libbiyot* has the same Hebrew term for Latin 'lutum comestibile'.

טרגאאלי (*Sefer ha-Qanun*, Nathan)[204] = Arabic طرجهالي; read طرجهاري (emend. De Koning, DKT 537, n. 2; see also FAL 65, no. 1427) 'arytenoid [cartilage of the larynx]' (from Greek ἀρυταινοειδής; cf. LSG 250); cf. bk. 1 (fols. 46b–47a): והשפוי כובע צריך אל עצלים יאחזו[205] הציניי אל אותו שאין שם לו ועצלים יאחזו[206] הטרגאאלי בו ויקיפוהו[207] ועצלים ירחיקו הטרגאאלי מן האחרים ויפתחו השפוי כובע (The larynx needs muscles to join the thyroid [cartilage] to [the cartilage] that has no name and muscles that join the arytenoid [cartilage] to the [first]) and also muscles that separate the arytenoid [cartilage] from the [two] others for opening the larynx). Hebrew טרגאאלי is a non-attested loan word from the Arabic طرجهالي, which is a corruption of طرجهاري. Zeraḥyah Ḥen transcribes the Arabic طرجهالي as טרגהאלי.

---

203 ועמד נגד כל מציק: فوقف عند كلّ مضيق a.
204 variant reading (fol. 58a) טרגאאלי: טרגאלי.
205 a تضمّ Ms יאחזוקו emend. ed.: יאחזו.
206 יאחזו הטרגאאלי בו: تضمّ الطرجهاري وتطبقه a.
207 a وتطبقه Ms ויקיפהו emend. ed.: ויקיפוהו.

טרוחמטרא (Aramaic) (*Sefer ha-Qanun*, Nathan) = Arabic [208] طروخانطير (emend. De Koning, DKT 569, n. 4; see also ibid. 821; FAL 132, no. 3278) (= Greek τροχαντῆρ; 'trochanter'; cf. LSG 1828); cf. bk. 1 (fol. 53a): ומהם עצל צמיחתו מכל חיצוני עצמות הכסל ומתחבר בעליוני התוספת הגדול הנקרא טרוחמטרא הגדול (Another [muscle of the thigh] that originates from the whole outer side of the ilium and is inserted in the top of the large process (apophyse) which is called 'the large trochanter'). Aramaic טרוחמטרא is a non-attested loan word from Arabic طروخانطير. Joseph Lorki translates the Arabic term as עצם העמוד (see entry).

טריאקי: See entry **סם**.

טריאקיות (*Sammim Libbiyim*) = Arabic ترياقيّة 'having theriacal (antidotal) property'; cf. fol. 124a: הסמים המחזקים אשר להם טריאקיות יכנסו כלם ברפואות הלב לפי שהם נאותים בטבע האדם בסגולה (All the tonic remedies that have theriacal (antidotal) property are part (fall under the category) of cardiacs because they are suited to human nature by their specific property). Hebrew טריאקיות is a non-attested loan word from the Arabic ترياقيّة. The anonymous translator of *Sefer ha-Refu'ot ha-Libbiyot* (fol. 246b) renders Latin 'tiriacalitas' as צריות (see entry).

טריות (*Sefer ha-Shimmush*) = Arabic طراوة 'freshness'; cf. fol. 147a, col. b: ומולידה החצץ בכליות אע"פ שתשתנה כפי מיניה וסוגי בעלי חיים שלה וטרייתה וישנותה ומצועה (And it (i.e., cheese) produces stones in the kidneys, although it differs according to its varieties, kinds of animals [it comes from], freshness, dryness and moderateness). Hebrew טריות features in BM 1927 in an attestation subsequent to Shem Tov Ben Isaac, namely from the *Sefer ha-Qanun*.

יבלת (*Sefer Ṣedat ha-Derakhim*) = Arabic ثألول 'wart' (Greek ἀκροχορδών: 'wart with a thin neck', cf. LSG 58)[209]; cf. bk. 7, ch. 16.1 (IJZ 151, l. 22): היבלת הוא בשר יצמח עגול חזק קשה יצא בכל הגוף וכל שכן בידין והרגלים (Warts are fleshy protrudings of the [skin] that are round, firm and hard. They can appear on the whole body, but especially on the hands and feet). Hebrew יבלת features in the Bible in the sense of 'a running sore or ulcer' (BDB 385); in Rabbinic literature as 'withered excrescense; 1) wart on the skin; 2) parasitic excrescenses on trees, or withered twigs' (JD 561); 'tumor, wart; verruca, porrum; acne' (LOW LIV). Subsequently, Nathan ha-Me'ati renders Plur. Arabic ثآليل as יבלת in his translation of Maimonides, *Medical Aphorisms* 22.25. Ben Yehuda (BM 1946) refers to its occurrence in medieval medical literature as well, i.e., in

208 a(*K. al-Qānūn*, 1:51) طروخابطير : طروخانطير.

209 Cf. IJZ 102, n. 164.

the *Sefer ha-Qanun* and translates the term as 'Auswuchs, excroissance'. Cf. entry מסמר below.

יין: יין הדבש השרוי (*Sefer ha-Shimmush*) = Arabic شراب العسل النقيع 'wine prepared from dried macerated grapes sweetened with honey'; cf. fol. 131b, col. a: יין הדבש השרוי חמומו ונגובו יותר מעטים מן המבושל ולפיכך הוא יותר נאות אל בעלי החמימות ובזמן הסתו (Wine prepared from dried macerated grapes sweetened with honey is less hot and less dry than [the wine] prepared by boiling; for this reason it is more suitable for people with [a hot temperament] and for [consumption during] the winter). Hebrew יין הדבש השרוי does not feature in the current dictionaries.

יין מבושל עד ששב כדבש (*Sefer Ṣedat ha-Derakhim*) = Arabic ربّ العنب 'grape juice (must) boiled down to a syrup'; cf. bk. 2, ch. 17 (fol. 58a): ואם תהיה המורסה קשה יעשה גרגור בחלב שנחלב מיד או בחלב אתון או ביין מבושל עד ששב כדבש (If the tumor [on the tongue] is hard [the patient] should gargle with fresh milk or milk of a donkey or grape juice boiled down to a syrup (lit., 'to the consistency of honey')). Hebrew יין מבושל עד ששב כדבש does not feature in the current dictionaries.

ירידה: ירידת המים בעין (*Hanhagat ha-Beri'ut le-Abu 'Ali Ben Zuhr*) = 'cataract' (cf. Honfredi (recension 1): 'descensus aque ad oculos'; (recension 2): 'fluxum reumatis ad oculos'; cf. ch. 28: ונאמר שכאב הראש כאשר התמיד והתחזק והשקיקה גם כן כאשר התמיד יקרה ממנו ירידת המים בעין ונשירת שער העפעפים (It is said that when a headache, and likewise a migraine, lasts for a long time and becomes more severe it causes a cataract and loss of the hair of the eyelids). Hebrew ירידת המים בעין does not feature in the current dictionaries. The parallel Arabic term نزول الماء, featuring in Maimonides, *Medical Aphorisms* 7.69, is translated by Zeraḥyah Ḥen as ירידת המים בעין as well (cf. NM 1:155–6).

יריעה: היריעה הלבנה (*Sefer Ṣedat ha-Derakhim*)[210] = Arabic الحجاب الملتحم 'conjunctiva' (cf. MMT 687); cf. bk. 2, ch. 1 (fol. 40b): ואולם הסבה מבפנים הוא מותר יטה אל היריעה הלבנה וינפחה כמו שיקרה לשאר האברים (However, the internal cause (of ophthalmia) is a superfluity that streams to the conjunctiva and makes it swell as happens with the other organs). Hebrew היריעה הלבנה (lit., 'the white membrane') does not feature in the current dictionaries. The term יריעה for 'membrane' (of the eye) is, according to David Kaufmann (KDS 86, n. 3), common in the Hebrew translation of Averroes, *K. al-kulliyāt fī 'l-ṭibb*, and also features in Gershon Ben Solomon, *Sha'ar ha-Shamayim*, and Meir Aldabi, *Shevilei Emunah*.

---

210 In addition to היריעה הלבנה, Moses Ibn Tibbon renders Arabic الحجاب الملتحم as המחיצה הלבנה (see entry), while the abbreviated Arabic synonym ملتحم is rendered by him as לֹבֶן (see entry).

ירק: הירק החמוץ (*Sefer ha-Shimmush*) = Arabic البقلة الحامضة (lit., 'the sour plant'), probably a kind of 'sorrel'; cf. Arabic حماض (cf. IBF 323); cf. fol. 136a, col. b: ירקי שדה מיניה רבים והם כלם בכלל ובפרט מולידים מרה שחורה והם רחוקים ממזג האדם ואין ראוי לזון בהם אלא בעת הצורך כירק הססי והירק החמוץ (There are many kinds of wild plants; all of them in general and in particular produce black bile and are very much unlike the human temperament. One should not feed oneself with them unless it cannot be avoided. Examples [of such plants] are field mustard and 'the sour plant' (sorrel)). Hebrew הירק החמוץ does not feature in the current dictionaries.

הירק הססי (*Sefer ha-Shimmush*)[211] = Arabic البقلة الحرشا 'field mustard' (*Sinapis arvensis* L.) (cf. MIG 387); cf. fol. 136a, col. b: ירקי שדה מיניה רבים והם כלם בכלל ובפרט מולידים מרה שחורה והם רחוקים ממזג האדם ואין ראוי לזון בהם אלא בעת הצורך כירק הססי והירק החמוץ. Hebrew הירק הססי does not feature in the current dictionaries. In Rabbinic literature we find ססין, which is explained by Rashi and the *Arukh* as 'poley' (cf. JD 983, s.v. סיסין) and which is, following a Geonic tradition, identical with באבונג 'camomile' (cf. SDA 807; FL 1:376).

יתדי (*Sefer ha-Qanun*, Nathan) = Arabic وتدي 'sphenoid [bone]' (cf. FAL 156, no. 3355); cf. bk. 1 (fol. 29b): אמנם מושב וכן המוח הוא העצם אשר יסבול וישא שאר העצמות ויאמר לו היתדי (The base of the brain is the bone that carries and supports the other bones and that is called 'the sphenoid [bone]'). For Hebrew יתדי, featuring in the *Sefer ha-Qanun*, cf. SRP 32 (218), MD 110.

כאב: כאב המוח (*Sefer Issur ha-Qevurah le-Galienus*)[212] = Arabic إغماء 'swoon, faint, unconsciousness, coma'; cf. par. 1: אני הנחתי ספר בד׳ מאמרים. הראשון מי שיקבר ועודנו חי מפני כאב המוח ([Says Galen:] I composed a book in four parts: The first on someone who is buried due to a coma while he is still alive). Hebrew כאב המוח does not feature in the current dictionaries. Arabic إغماء also features in Maimonides, *Medical Aphorisms* 24.45 (ed. and trans. Bos, 5: 95–6) where it reflects the Greek κάρος (cf. LSG 879: 'heavy sleep, torpor'), and is translated by Zeraḥyah Ḥen as אמשטא, and in ibid., 9.12, where it is translated by Nathan ha-Me'ati as יגונים.

(כוה) כווה: See entry **סם**.

כופרא: כופרי (Aramaic) (*Sefer ha-Shimmush*) = Arabic جفرّى or كفرّى 'envelope, spathe of the palm-flower' (cf. WKAS 1:265b–266a); cf. fol. 140a, col. a: הכופרי והוא לולבי הדקל הרך הנקרא בלשונם אלג׳פרי קודם יביא פריו קרוב מטבע הקור של דקל (KWPRY, i.e., spathes of the young palm tree—called [in Arabic]

211 See also entry ססי.

212 In addition to כאב המוח, Judah al-Ḥarizi translates Arabic إغماء as שעמום (see entry).

ʾLĞPRY, before it bears fruit—are close in coldness to the nature of the palm). Aramaic כופרא, Plur. כופרי features in SDA 565, s.v. כּוּפְּרָא as: 'spadix or inflorescense of palms, spathe, palm pollen'. See also entry לולבי הדקל.

כח: הכח הטוחן (*Sefer Hanhagat ha-Beri'ut*) = 'the digestive faculty'; cf. 8.1 (143): והשלישי הכח הטוחן והוא אשר יבשל המאכלים הנמשכים ויטחון אותם (The third [faculty] (of the four natural faculties of the body) is the digestive faculty that cooks and digests the foods that are attracted to it). Hebrew הכח הטוחן does not feature in the current dictionaries. The standard Hebrew term for 'digestive faculty' is הכח המבשל. Hebrew טחן features in the sense of 'to digest' in BM 1867 in an attestation from Judah Ibn Tibbon's *Ḥovot ha-Levavot*, i.e., his translation of Baḥya Ibn Pakuda's *Duties of the Heart*.

הכח המשליך (*Sefer Hanhagat ha-Beri'ut*) = 'the expulsive faculty'; cf. 8.1 (143–4): והרביעי הכח המשליך והוא אשר ישליך הפסולת הנותר מן המאכלים אחר קחת האברים מהם כל צרכם (The fourth [faculty] (of the four natural facultues of the body) is the expulsive faculty that expels the waste materials that remained from the food once the organs took from them all they needed). Hebrew הכח המשליך does not feature in the current dictionaries. The standard Hebrew term for 'expulsive faculty' is כח דוחה (cf. BM 2317; KTP 2:75).

הכח העוצר (*Sefer Hanhagat ha-Beri'ut*) = 'the retentive faculty'; cf. 8.1 (143): והשני הכח העוצר והוא המעכב אותם ומונע יציאתם עד שתפעל בם התולדה מפעלה (The second [faculty] (of the four natural faculties of the body) is the retentive faculty that retains [the foods] and prevents them from leaving [the body] until nature does its work on them). Hebrew הכח העוצר does not feature in the current dictionaries.[213] In the sense of 'to bind, i.e., retain [the food]', Hebrew עצר features in BM 4660 in an attestation from the *Sod ha-Sodot*, the Hebrew translation of the Arabic *Sirr al-asrār*, known in the Latin version as *Secretum secretorum* (cf. ed. Gaster, 3:273 (112) (Hebrew); 2:805 (translation)).[214] The regular Hebrew term for 'retentive faculty is הכח המחזיק (cf. BM 2317; KTP 2:74).

כחל (*Sefer Ṣedat ha-Derakhim*) = Arabic اكتحل 'to apply as a collyrium'; cf. bk. 2, ch. 4 (fol 45a): ויעשה ממנו גרגרים קטנים ויקח ממנו אחת וישרה אותה במי מטר ויטיף ממנו בעין או תחכך אותה על המשחזת ויכחול בו (Prepare small pills from this, take one pill, steep it in rain water and drip some of it in the eye, or make it fine on a whetstone and apply it as a collyrium [to the eye]). As a medical term, Hebrew כחל features in BM 2322–3 in attestations, a.o., from

213 The term also features as a translation of Arabic القوة الماسكة in Zeraḥyah Ḥen's translation of Maimonides, *Medical Aphorisms* 5.13; 6.74, 88; 23.80 (forthcoming ed. by G. Bos).

214 *Studies and Texts in Folklore, Magic, Mediaeval Romance, Hebrew Apocrypha and Samaritan Archaeology*, coll. and repr. by M. Gaster, 3 vols (New York 1971).

Rabbinic literature and from Joseph Ibn Zabara, *Sefer Sha'ashu'im*, without any further explanation.

הוכחל (*Sammim Libbiyim*) = Arabic اكّتحل 'to be used as a collyrium'; cf. fol. 125a: ולא יופשט חזקו ברוח זולת רוח אבל הוא נאות לעצם הרוח כלו עד שהוא יועיל לרוח אשר במוח למה שנתפרסם ממנו מחזוק הראות כאשר יוכחל בו (Its (i.e., silk) strengthening power is not limited to one specific pneuma, but it is suitable for the substance of any pneuma. Thus it is useful for the pneuma in the brain as was mentioned that it strengthens eyesight when it is used as a collyrium). Hebrew כחל features in BM 2322–3 only in the Qal and Pi'el, and in EM in the Hof'al as a modern term in the sense of 'to be painted with the colour blue'. The anonymous translator renders Latin 'si oculi ex ipso collirientur' as אם יוכחלו ממנו העינים.

כיס: כיס הלב (*Sefer ha-Qanun*, Nathan) = Arabic غلاف القلب 'pericardium' (cf. DKT 842; FAL 62, no. 1389); cf. bk. 1 (fol. 64a): ואחד מנכח כיס הלב ומשלח אליו שריגים רבים מתחלקים כשער וזנין אותו (One branch (i.e., of the vena cava) passes in front of the pericardium and sends many hair-like branches to it that provide it with nutrition). Hebrew כיס הלב features in MD 558, s.v. 'pericardium'. The same term features in Nathan's translation of Maimonides, *Medical Aphorisms* 4.27, 28; 25.72. Zeraḥyah Ḥen renders the Arabic غلاف القلب as קרומות הלב (see entry קרום הלב), and Joseph Lorki as מכסה הלב (see entry).

כיס המים (*Sefer Hanhagat ha-Beri'ut*) = 'urinary bladder'; cf. 8.1 (145): והכליות מושכות המים הרעים אשר בדם ומתפרנסות ממעט האדמימות הנשאר בו ושולחות המותר אל כיס המים והוא מזומן לקבלו ולהוציאו לחוץ על פי האבר הקטן והוא השתן (The kidneys attract the bad watery part of the blood and feed themselves with the small amount of the remaining red part and send the residue to the urinary bladder which is ready to receive it and to expel it through the penis (lit., 'small member'), and this (i.e., what is expelled) is the urine). Hebrew כיס המים does not feature in the current dictionaries. Synonyms featuring in medieval medical literature are כיס מקוה המים (cf. entry חֲלֵב: חלב החטה), מקוה, and כיס הגדול; cf. *Sefer ha-Qanun*: ומנהג הרופאים הקדמונים שיקראו הממרה הכיס הקטן כמו שהוא מנהגם לקרא המקוה הכיס הגדול (as quoted in BM 2347). Hebrew כיס המים features in the sense of 'hydrocele' in Zeraḥyah Ḥen's translation of Maimonides, *Medical Aphorisms* 23.57 (cf. NM 1:158–9).

כיס המרה (*Sefer Hanhagat ha-Beri'ut*) = 'gallbladder'; cf. 8.1 (145): כי הטחול הוכן למשוך ממנה המרה השחורה וכיס המרה לטהר הדם ולנקותו (For the spleen is prepared for drawing the black bile from it (i.e., from the liver) and the gallbladder for cleansing and purifying the blood). Hebrew כיס המרה features in MD 313, s.v. 'gallbladder'. For a variant reading מררה and a synonym הכיס

הקטן, featuring in the *Sefer ha-Qanun* as quoted by Ben Yehuda, cf. previous entry.

ככים :כך (*Sefer Ṣedat ha-Derakhim*) = Arabic لثة 'gums'; cf. bk. 2, ch. 18 (fol. 59a): ומהם מקרים נסתרים כמו שירגיש החולה בתוך שניו דפיקה וכאב חזק ויראה גלויה כאלו אין בה חולי ואולם יקרה להם זה מפני רבוי המותרות והגרתם בהם מן הראש או מן האצטו' או מחדוד מותרות נפסדות נוטות[215] אשר הם נמשכות אל הככים ר"ל מושבי השנים (Some illnesses [affecting the teeth] are hidden, as when the patient feels throbbing in the teeth and a severe pain, while there is no illness to be seen. This happens to him because of a surplus of superfluities that stream from the head or stomach or because of sharp, corrupt, biting[216] superfluities that stream to the gums, i.e., the seat of the teeth). Hebrew ככים is an unattested Hebraisation of Aramaic ככא, Plur. ככין, meaning 'molars' (JD 638, SDA 580). The regular term for 'gums' is חניכים. Hebrew ככים also features, in addition to the regular term חניכים, in the *Hanhagat ha-Beri'ut le-Abu ʿAli Ben Zuhr*, ch. 6: וכן כל אילן עפיץ חריף מן האגוז ומה שדומה לו ינקה השנים ויתיך הבלגם ויתיך הלשון ויזכך הדבור ויעיר תאות המאכל. אמנם בלא חכוך חזק על הככים[217] כמו שזכרתי קודם (Likewise every acrid, sharp [smelling] tree such as hazelnut tree and the like cleanses the teeth and dissolves the phlegm and softens the tongue, cleanses the speech [organs] and wakes up the appetite. But one should not rub the gums in a hard way, as I mentioned before). In his translation of Hippocrates' *Aphorisms* 3.25, Hillel of Verona renders the Latin equivalent 'gingivae' as בשר השנים (cf. NM 3:41).

מוכלח (כלח) (*Sefer ha-Shimmush*) = Arabic هرم 'old'; cf. fol. 142b, col. b: בשר הכבש המוכלח יותר רע מכל מיני בשר הצאן (Meat of an old sheep is worse than that of any other kind of small cattle). Hebrew כלח features in BM 2387 only in the sense of 'to become weak and powerless because of old age' in the Nifʿal, Puʿal and Nitpaʿel conjugations.

כַּלָחוּת (*Sefer ha-Shimmush*) = Arabic هرم 'old age'; cf. fol. 143a, col. a: ולאכול מבשר הצלעות ולבשלו אספידבאג'ה מתובלת בשווי או לבשלו בדבש וכל שכן הקרוב אל הכלחות ([To improve the quality of goats' meat and prevent possible harm] one should eat from the meat of the ribs and cook it [in a dish called] 'SPYDB'ǦH[218], moderately spiced, or cook it with honey, especially [the meat of a goat] that is approaching old age). Hebrew כַּלָחוּת does not feature in the current dictionaries.

---

215 Ms Oxford, Bodleian, Poc. 353, Uri Heb. 314 עוקצות :נוטות.

216 'biting': Trans. after Ms Oxford, Bodleian, Poc. 353, Uri Heb. 314.

217 Mss הכבים emend. ed. :הככים.

218 "SPYDB'ǦH': A kind of dish prepared from meat, onions, butter, oil, parsley, and coriander; cf. entries אספידבאג'ה and הבשר השלוק.

כלי: כלי שעושים <בו> מי ורדים (*Sefer Ṣedat ha-Derakhim*) = Arabic أنبيق 'alembic'; cf. bk. 1, ch. 4 (fol. 9b): וישים האלקנה בכלי שעושים מי ורדים (And he shall put the henna in an alembic). Hebrew כלי שעושים <בו> מי ורדים (lit., 'a vessel for making rose water') does not feature in the current dictionaries.

כלי המציצה (*Sefer Ṣedat ha-Derakhim*) = Arabic محجمة 'cupping glass'; cf. bk. 1, ch. 10 (fol. 14b): ואולם כשיתחמם מחום השמש והאויר הנה הראש יתחמם וימשוך אליו המותרות מכל הגוף כמו שימשוך כלי המציצה (But when [the head] becomes hot because of the heat of the sun and the weather, it attracts the superfluities from the whole body like a cupping glass that attracts [the blood]). Hebrew כלי המציצה features without any further explanation in BM 3251, a.o., in an attestation from Meir Aldabi, *Shevilei Emunah*. For its occurrence in an anonymous translation of Hippocrates' *Aphorisms* 5.50, cf. NM 3:117.

כלילי (*Sefer ha-Qanun*, Nathan) = Arabic إكليلي 'coronal'; cf. bk. 1 (fol. 29a): ומן הראשונים שלב משותף עם המצח קשתי כן)[219] ונקרא הכלילי (To the first sutures belongs one that is common with the frontal bone [and] shaped as a bow like)[220] and called the 'coronal [suture]'). In the sense of 'coronal', Hebrew כלילי features in MD 185 without any reference, and in the sense of 'coronary' it features as a modern term in EM 743. For its occurrence in the Sefer ha-Qanun cf. SRP 38 (279). Zeraḥyah Ḥen translates Arabic إكليلي as עטרי (see entry). Joseph Lorki has הכליל.

כלל: כלל העין (*Sefer ha-Qanun*, Nathan)[221] = Arabic مقلة 'eyeball' (cf. DKT 518–9, 829; FAL 96, no. 2127); cf. bk. 1 (fol. 43a): הפרק הרביעי בנתוח עצלי כלל העין ואמנם העצלים המניעים לכלל[222] העין הם עצלים ששה ארבעה מהם בצד הם הארבעה למעלה ולמטה בשתי קצוות העין הנקרא מאקים (Chapter four: The anatomy of the muscles of the eyeball. There are six muscles that move the eyeball. Four of them are situated at the four sides, above, below, and in the two canthi that are called M'QYM). Hebrew כלל העין does not feature in the current dictionaries. Zeraḥyah Ḥen translates the Arabic مقلة as בת עין (see entry), Joseph Lorki as בת העין.

כמוני: הכמוני (*Sammim Libbiyim*) = Arabic الكموني 'the cumin [stomachic]'[223]; cf. fol. 133a: עוד החולקים מן הרופאים יחשבו שיש מן הטריאק והמטרידיטוס חום עובר

219 I.e., the drawing of a bow : (

220): I.e., the drawing of a bow.

221 In addition to כלל העין, Nathan translates Arabic مقلة as תחתית העין (see entry).

222 a للمقلة Ms לעצלי emend. ed.: לכלל.

223 'the cumin [stomachic]' (جوارشن الكموني): For this compound remedy, cf. Ibn Sīnā, *K. al-Qānūn*, 3:347–9. One variety described by Ibn Sīnā is, a.o., good for intestinal pains caused by cold and for elderly people whose temperament is dominated by phlegm.

הגבול ויעמדו מלהשתמש בשעור חצי משקל ממנו ולא יעמדו מלהשתמש בארבעה משקלים הכמוני ומן הפלפליי (The physicians that have a different opinion think that the theriac and the Mithridates[224] are exceedingly hot and therefore refrain from prescribing [even] half a *mithqāl*[225] of it, but they do not hesitate to prescribe four *mithqāls* of the cumin and pepper [stomachics]). Hebrew הכמוני does not feature in the current dictionaries. The anonymous author of *Sefer ha-Refu'ot ha-Libbiyot* (fol. 252a) transcribes Latin 'dyaciminum'[226] as דיאסימינום.

כמך (*Sefer ha-Shimmush*) = Arabic صير 'fish brine' (cf. D 1:856; FL 2:536: 'Pisciculi sale conditi, e quibus cibus صحناء paratur'); cf. fol. 150, col. b: ואמנם הכמך העשוי ממנו חם יבש גורם צמא ולוטש האסטומכא מהליחה הלבנה העבה והתמדתו מפסדת הדם (But fish brine prepared from it (from salted fish) is hot [and] dry; it causes thirst, cleanses the stomach from the thick phlegm; its frequent use corrupts the blood). Hebrew כמך features in Rabbinic literature; cf. JD 646: '(Pers. Kâmakh, Arabic Kâmah, Fl. to Levy Talm. Dict. II, 4522) *Kamakh, A Persian sauce* of milk, curdled milk &c.'; for the Aram. counterpart cf. SDA 586 s.v. כמכא: '< MIr *kāmak [cf. MP *kāmag*, no. 1 gruel or soup CPD 48]: a type of dish containing milk'; for the Persian term, cf. FL 783 s.v. كامه: '… lac cum oxygala ebullitum, opsonium celebre, quo Ispahanenses frui solent' (milk cooked with sour milk, a famous [appetizer] which the inhabitants of Isfahan used to enjoy); for the Arabic parallel, cf. WKAS 1:351 s.v. كامخ: 'savoury piquant appetizer; vinegar dressing; fruit etc. laid in vinegar'. Subsequent to Ibn Tibbon, כמך features in Nathan ha-Me'ati's glossary to the *Sefer ha-Qanun*, and is explained by him as כמך: אמרתי כמכים מיני רותחים מלשון רבותינו (KMK. I employed (lit., 'said') [the term] KMKYM [for different] kinds of spicy appetizers; [the term is] derived from the language of the Rabbis) (cf. NM 2:115 (Kaf 8), 143).

כֵּן (1) (*Sefer ha-Qanun*, Nathan)[227] = Arabic قاعدة 'basis'; cf. bk. 1 (fol. 39b): ונבראו העצמות שהכנים שלהם יותר רחבים וראשיהם יותר דקים (The bones (of the fingers) have been formed with wider bases and narrower heads). In the sense of 'basis', Hebrew כֵּן is attested for in the Bible, Rabbinic literature (cf. BM 2432), and for modern literature (cf. EM 749–50); for its occurrence in

224 'Mithridates': An antidote ascribed to Mithridates VI. Eupator, king of Pontus (reg. 120–63 BC); see Ullmann, *Medizin im Islam*, 321; for its composition, see Ibn Ḥayyān, *Buch der Gifte* (trans. Siggel, 217); cf. entry זהוב.

225 One *mithqāl* is 4.46 grams; cf. Hinz, *Islamische Maße und Gewichte*, 7.

226 'dyaciminum': cf. BAN 38–9.

227 In addition to כֵּן, Nathan renders the Arabic قاعدة as מכונה (see entry).

the *Sefer ha-Qanun*, cf. SRP 32 (218). Zeraḥyah Ḥen renders the Arabic قاعدة as יסוד, and Joseph Lorki as אדן (quoted by Ben Yehuda; cf. BM 70).

כֵּן (2): כני הפיל (*Sefer Ṣedat ha-Derakhim*) = Arabic بلاذر 'marking nut (*Semecarpus anacardium*)'[228]; cf. bk. 1, ch. 14 (fol. 21b): והיותר מיוחד להועיל בו הרפואה העשויה בכיני[229] הפיל הוא בלאדור כשישתה ממנו בכל יום מדרהם עד שקל במים חמים על צום הנפש (The best remedy for [forgetfulness] is the one prepared from marking nut, i.e., BL'DWR (= Arabic *balāḏur*) when one takes it every day in a dose from one *dirham*[230] to one *mithqāl*[231] with hot water on an empty stomach). Hebrew כני הפיל does not feature in the current dictionaries, it is possibly a calque from Romance in the sense of 'elephant's lice'; cf. Simon Online, s.v. 'Anacardus': 'Anacardus puto grecum est fructus arboris qui et pediculus elephantis a quibusdam vocatur arabice dicitur beladhar' ('Anacardus' is, I believe, Greek; it is the fruit of a tree, which is also called by some 'elephant louse'; in Arabic it is called *beladhar*).[232] The vernacular variant פאדול אורפיאן (read פאזול אורפיאן), featuring in Ms Oxford, Bodleian, Poc. 353, is Old Occitan 'pezol orfian', a loan translation of M. Lat. 'pediculus elefantis'. For Mod. Occ. (Tarn) 'pezoul' (louse), cf. FEW 8:149a; the second element shows a metathesis of the O. Occ. 'orifan/aurifan' (elephant), (FEW 3:213a).[233]

כנף (*Sefer ha-Qanun*, Nathan) = Arabic جناح (lit. 'wing'), i.e., 'transverse process' (Greek: ἀπόφυσις ἐγκάρσια) (cf. DKT 816; FAL 73, no. 1623); cf. bk. 1 (fol. 32a): ומה שיהיה מאלו מונחים לאחור נקרא קוץ וסנסן ומה שיהיה מונח ימין ושמאל נקרא כנף ([The processes] that lie at the back (i.e., of the vertebrae) are called 'spinous[234] processes' and those that lie at the right and left side (i.e., of the vertebrae) are called 'transverse processes'). In the sense of 'transverse process', Hebrew כנף is a non-attested semantic borrowing from the Arabic جناح. In the glossary to the *Sefer ha-Qanun*, Nathan defines the term כנפים as: עצמות בולטים בעצמות השדרה (cf. NM 2:115, 142 (Kaf 6)). Zeraḥyah Ḥen renders the Arabic جناح as כנף as well.

---

228 Cf. G. Bos, 'Baladhur (Marking-nut): A Popular Medieval Drug for Strengthening Memory', *Bulletin of the School of Oriental and African Studies* 59.2 (1996): 229–36.

229 Ms Oxford, Bodleian, Poc. 353, Uri Heb. 314, fol. 6b בכיני הפיל: בפאדול אורפיאן.

230 The standard *dirham* is 3.125 grams; see Hinz, *Islamische Maße und Gewichte*, 3.

231 One *mithqāl* is 4.46 grams; cf. ibid., 7.

232 Cf. commentary ibid.: 'The name pediculus elephantis, lit., 'elephant's louse', is given to the fruit of the tree because of some perceived similarity between the insect Haematomyzus elephantis or 'elephant louse', and the fruit of this tree'; see also *Alphita*, ed. by A. García González (Florence 2007), 148, 346.

233 I thank Julia Zwink for this reference to the Old Occitan.

234 'spinous processes': Cf. entries סנסן and קוץ.

כסלים: כסל (*Sefer ha-Shimmush*) = Arabic حشا, Plur. أحشاء 'inward parts' (D 1:292; UW 629–30); cf. fol. 148b, col. a: איברי העופות: כסלי העוף מיוחסים אל בשרו כיחס כסלי כל בעלי חיים <מיוחסים> אל בשרו (The organs of birds: the inward parts of a bird relate to its flesh in the same way as the intestines of all [other] animals relate to their flesh). Hebrew כסל, Plur. כסלים, only features in the current dictionaries and secondary literature in the sense of 'groin, loin' (cf. JD 654, BM 2464–5); 'pelvis, pelvic girdle, ileum' (read: ilium; LOW LVI). The standard Hebrew term for 'inward parts' is מעים or קרבים.

הלחות הכפורית: כפורי (*Sefer Ṣedat ha-Derakhim*) = Arabic الرطوبة الجلدية 'the crystalline humour'; cf. bk. 2, ch. 2 (Ms Oxford, Bodleian, Poc. 353, Uri Heb. 314, fol. 12a): והלחות הכפורית אם היה דק הנה מי רושילש יסירהו ואם היה עב יצטרך אל מה שהוא יותר חזק (If the crystalline humour is thin it will be cleansed by the juice of poppy[235] anemone (*Anemone coronaria* L.), but if it is thick, it needs something stronger). Hebrew הלחות הכפורית features in BM 2488 in an attestation from Abraham Ibn Daud, *Ha-Emunah ha-Ramah*; however the term is not explained by Ben Yehuda. The same Hebrew term features in Zeraḥyah Ḥen's translation of Maimonides, *Medical Aphorisms* 3.52, while Nathan ha-Me'ati has הלחות הגלדית (cf. NM 2:34). For a detailed discussion of the term as it features in medieval literature, cf. KDS 96–9.

כפיון (*Sefer ha-Shimmush*) = Arabic صرع 'epilepsy'; cf. fol. 132a, col. a: והכווץ והמשיכה המביאים אל הכפיון ([And further harm caused by excessive drinking of wine consists of] spasms and tetanus which lead to epilepsy). In the sense of 'epilepsy', Hebrew כפיון features as a medieval term in EM 762 without attestation. Subsequent to Shem Tov Ben Isaac, the same Hebrew term is used by Nathan ha-Me'ati in his translation of Hippocrates' *Aphorisms* 2.45 (cf. NM 3:119).

כפיפת הארכובה: כפיפה (*Sefer ha-Qanun*, Nathan) = Arabic مثنى الركبة 'the knee pit (popliteal fossa)' (cf. DKT 642–3, n. 3; FAL 90, no. 1978); cf. bk. 1, fol. 67a: והאמצעי נמתח בכפיפת הארכובה יורד (The medial branch [of the vena cava] spreads over the knee pit [and] descends ...). Hebrew כפיפת הארכובה does not feature in the current dictionaries. Masie (MD 306, s.v. 'fossa, popliteal') mentions מרבץ הארכובה as a synonym featuring in the *Sefer ha-Qanun*. Zeraḥyah Ḥen renders the Arabic مثنى الركبة as כפל הארכובה (see entry).

כפיפת המרפק (*Sefer ha-Qanun*, Nathan) = Arabic معطف المرفق 'the elbow pit (cubital fossa)'; cf. bk. 1 (fols. 65b–66a): והשני פונה אל מקום כפיפת המרפק[236] בחיצוני הקנה ומתערב בעומק בשריג גם כן מן האצ<י>לי (The second [branch of

235 'poppy anemone' (RWŠYLŠ): The term is a transcription of Old Cat. Plur. 'rosellas' (cf. BMZ 97).

236 Ms המפרק emend. ed.: המרפק.

the branches of the cephalic vein] proceeds to the elbow pit (cubital fossa) at the outer part of the forearm and joins inside with a branch of the axillary vein). Hebrew כפיפת המרפק is not attested in the current dictionaries. Zeraḥyah Ḥen renders the Arabic معطف المرفق as כפל הקובדי (see entry), and Joseph Lorki as שטח המרפק (?).

יותר נכפל (כפל) (*Sefer ha-Qanun*, Nathan) = Arabic أكثر تكررا 'more frequent'; cf. bk. 1 (fol. 44b): כי תנועות איברי הרקה והשפה יותר רבי המספר ויותר נכפלים ושוקדים (… because the movements of the [different] parts of the cheeks and lips are more numerous and more frequent and last longer). Hebrew נכפל features in the current dictionaries in the sense of 'doubled' and 'multiplied' (cf. BM 2494). Zeraḥyah Ḥen translates the Arabic أكثر تكررا as יותר שניות (see entry), and Joseph Lorki as יותר החזרה.

כפל הארכובה: כֶּפֶל (*Sefer ha-Qanun*, Zeraḥyah) = Arabic مثنى الركبة 'the knee pit (popliteal fossa)' (cf. DKT 642–3, n. 3; FAL 90, no. 1978); cf. bk. 1 (fol. 35a): והאמצעי יתפשט במקום כפל הארכובה ויורד (The medial branch [of the vena cava] spreads over the knee pit and descends …). Hebrew כפל הארכובה does not feature in the current dictionaries. For the other translator(s), see entry כפיפת הארכובה.

כפל הקובדי (*Sefer ha-Qanun*, Zeraḥyah) = Arabic معطف المرفق 'the elbow pit (cubital fossa)'; cf. bk. 1 (fol. 34b): והשני ישתלח אל כפל הקובדי בנראה של הזרוע ויתערבו בו שעיפים מן השחיי (The second [branch of the branches of the cephalic vein] proceeds to the elbow pit (cubital fossa) at the outer part of the forearm and joins inside with branches of the axillary vein). Hebrew-Romance כפל הקובדי[237] is not attested in the current dictionaries. For the other translator(s), see entry כפיפת המרפק.

הכריתה בברזל: כריתה (*Pirqei Arnauṭ de Vilanova*) = Latin 'sectio' (cutting, surgery); cf. 3.7 (44): כמו שהכויה והכריתה בברזל קשה לסבלם כן הרפואות החזקות יקשה ענינם אל הגופים או אל האיברים קלי בהפעלות (Just as cauterization and cutting (surgery) is hard to endure, strong medications are hard [to endure] for bodies and organs that are easily affected). Hebrew הכריתה בברזל does not feature in the current dictionaries. כריתה alone, in the sense of 'cutting', features in BM 2516 in attestations from, a.o., the *Sefer ha-Qanun*. In his translation of Maimonides, *Medical Aphorisms* 15.20, Nathan ha-Me'ati has החתך בברזל and לחתך בברזל for Arabic (ال)قطع بالحديد 'surgery'. Zeraḥyah Ḥen renders the Arabic in both cases as לחתוך בברזל.

---

237 The term קובדי is old Occitan 'covede' or 'copde' for 'elbow' (cf. FEW 2:1447a). I thank Julia Zwink for this reference.

כרמל: הכרמל המהובהב באש (*Sefer ha-Shimmush*) = Arabic فريك (cf. NA 559): 'wheat harvested when it it is still green then toasted in stone pans to get rid of moisture in the grains. To get rid of hull, it is rubbed between the fingers (*yufrak*), and hence the name *farīk*'; see also L 2388: 'wheat that is rubbed and picked, or cleared'; cf. fol. 124a, col. 1: הכרמל המהובהב באש העשוי מן השבלים אשר יש בהם מותר לחות ולא יגמר בשולם (KRML (green toasted wheat) made from the ears that still have some moisture left in them and that are not completely ripened ...). Hebrew הכרמל המהובהב באש does not feature in the current dictionaries. The term כרמל features in the Bible in the sense of '1. garden-land. 2. (fresh), fruit, garden-growth' (BDB 502), and in Rabbinic literature as 'a well-cultivated plot; whence (sub. גרש) (grist of) early ripened and tender barley' (JD 671) (cf. BM 2524: 'fresh early grains'), and in an attestation from Maimonides, *Mishneh Torah, Hilkhot Naḥalot*: 'grain that has not developed into ears' (התבואה קדם שנעשה שבלים) (ibid.).

כת (*Sefer ha-Qanun*, Nathan) = Arabic طائفة 'a detached, or distinct, part or portion, a piece, or bit; [or somewhat] of a thing and of men [i.e., a party, portion, division, or class thereof' (L 1893); cf. bk. 1 (fol. 64b): ויצא לחוץ מהם כת אל העצל היוצא מן החזה (A part (some) of them (i.e., of the branches of the vena cava) emerge [and spread] in the outer muscle of the chest). Hebrew כת features in the current dictionaries in the sense of 'band, party, class, division' (cf. JD 678; BM 2545–7).

כתף (*Sefer ha-Qanun*, Nathan) = Arabic كَتِف 'shoulder, shoulder blade (scapula)'; cf. bk. 1 (fol. 37a): ונוטה אל הצד החיצוני ומחוברת בראש הכתף ונקשרת בה הכתף ובהם יחדו נקשר הזרוע (Then it (i.e., clavicle) goes to the outside and articulates with the acromion process so that the scapula is connected to it, and the humerus to both of them). In addition to the general sense of 'shoulder', Hebrew כתף features in the specific sense of 'shoulder blade' (scapula) as a Biblical term in BDB 509 (cf. SRP 41 (305)). LOW LVII also mentions it as meaning 'Articulatio humeri'.

כתפי: הכתפי (*Sefer ha-Qanun*, Nathan) = Arabic الكتفي 'vein of the shoulder, cephalic vein' (cf. DKT 826; FAL 79, no. 1764); cf. bk. 1 (fol. 65b): אמנם הכתפיי והוא הקיפאל הנה בתחלת מה שיתענף[238] ממנו שריג מתפרק בעור בחלקים הנראים החיצונים מן העצלים[239] (As to the vein of the shoulder, i.e., the cephalic vein, the branch that emerges first out of it spreads out in the skin [and] in the outer parts of the muscle[240]). Hebrew כתפי features in BM 2560 in an attestation from the *Sefer ha-Qanun*.

238 a يتفرع Ms שיתעפף emend. ed.: שיתענף.

239 a העצלים: العضد.

240 'muscle': 'humerus' a.

כתר: כתר מלכות (*Sefer Ṣedat ha-Derakhim*, Ms Munich, Bayerische Staatsbibliothek, Cod. hebr. 19)[241] = Arabic إكليل الملك 'melilot, king's clover' (*Melilotus officinalis*)[242]; cf. bk. 1, ch. 17 (fol. 19a): ואם היתה התעורה מיובש המרה השחורה נצוה החולה לשפוך על ראשו מים שנתבשלו בהם קממילא וכתר[243] מלכות ואניט וקליפת פאפויר וזרע מלוישקלי ומה שדומה להם (And if the sleeplessness is caused by the dryness of the black bile we order the patient to pour over his head water in which camomile, melilot, aneth, poppy [seed] skin and marshmellow seed, or similar ingredients have been cooked). Hebrew כתר מלכות, a variant featuring in Ms Munich, Bayerische Staatsbibliothek, Cod. hebr. 19, fol. 19a,[244] is possibly a non-attested calque of Arabic إكليل الملك (reading الملك as المُلك). In his glossary to the *Sefer ha-Shimmush*, Shem Tov Ben Isaac translates the Arabic as כליל המלך (cf. SHS 1:282 (Kaf 34)). Zeraḥyah Ḥen renders the Arabic إكليل الملك as עטרת המלך (see entry below).

לבוש (*Sefer Ṣedat ha-Derakhim*) = Arabic لباس ('membrane'; cf. WKAS 2.1:142); cf. bk. 2, ch. 6 (fol. 46a): ויכחול ברפואות שיכנס בהם מי המררות וזה כי כל המררות יועילו מקבוץ המים בעין ויטהרו הראות ויסירו מותרי הלחות אשר יתקבץ בלבוש העין (One should apply collyria to the eye that consist of remedies with [different sorts] of bile for all these are good for the accumulation of water in the eye; they give a clear eyesight and remove the superfluous moistures that accumulate in the membranes of the eye). In the sense of 'membrane', Hebrew לבוש is a non-attested semantic borrowing from Arabic لباس; cf. BM 2607 and KDS 85–6 (for other terms used in medieval literature).

לֹבֶן (*Sefer Ṣedat ha-Derakhim*) = Arabic ملتحم 'conjunctiva'; cf. bk. 2, ch. 3 (fol. 43b): הטרפא הוא דם ישפך בלובן מבקיעת הורידים אשר בה (*Ṭarfa* (i.e., a bloodspot in the eye)[245] is the blood that streams in the conjunctiva because of a rupture in its veins). As a medical term Hebrew, לֹבֶן features in BM 2613 in the sense of 'the white of the eye' (i.e., sclera; cf. LOW LVII; JD 694), and 'leucoma, macula cornae'. The Arabic term ملتحم is actually a shortened form for الحجاب الملتحم, which is rendered by Moses Ibn Tibbon as היריעה הלבנה or המחיצה הלבנה (see entries).

241 Cf. entry עטרת המלך.

242 The Arabic term can also stand for other species of *Leguminosae*, e.g., crown vetch (*Coronilla emerus* L.), or scorpion vetch (*Coronilla scorpioides* Koch); cf. DT 3.40 (388).

243 Ms London, British Library, Ar. Or. 26 וכתר מלכות: וקורונא ריאל.

244 The same Hebrew term features in bk. 2, ch. 14 (fol. 41b).

245 The Hebrew term used by Ibn Tibbon for this affliction is אֹדֶם (cf. entry).

לובן הצפורנים (*Sefer Ṣedat ha-Derakhim*) = Arabic بياض الأظفار 'whiteness of the nails'[246]; cf. bk. 7, ch. 27.1 (IJZ 169, ll. 1–3): השער העשרים ושבעה בלובן הצפרנים ורפואת מוגלתם[247] הנקרא גלאיי פעמים יקרה בצפרנים לובן וכאשר נרצה לרפאתו נבוא אליו באחת מאלו הרפואות הנזכרות לזה (Chapter twenty-seven: On whiteness of the nails and the treatment of paronychia[248] (whitlow). The nails are sometimes affected by whiteness, and if we want to treat this, we do so by one of the remedies prescribed [for this disease]). Hebrew לובן הצפורנים does not feature in the current dictionaries.

לבוני: לבני (*Sefer ha-Shimmush*) = Arabic لباني 'pertaining to frankincense'; cf. fol. 138b, col. a: וראוי להנזר ממנו מי שירבו בו הרוחות וימהר אליו הגעש החמוץ ואם יגבר עליו יצרו ויאכל ממנו ראוי לשתות אחריו מיד מן היין החי או לאכול ממרקחת הכמון הלבן[249] או מרקחת הלבוניי (Someone who suffers from many winds and immediate sour eructations should refrain from [eating] them (i.e., apricots). But if he likes them too much and eats them, he should immediately drink unmixed wine or eat the white[250] cumin stomachic or the frankincense stomachic). Hebrew לבני does not feature in the current dictionaries.

ליהב (להב) (*Sefer ha-Shimmush*) = Arabic ألهب 'to make something inflamed, to cause an inflammation' (cf. WKAS 2.3:1454, col. b); cf. fol. 143b, col. a: בשר הגמל חזק החמימות מלהב עם עובי רב ומוליד מרה שחורה (Meat of a camel is very hot and thick, it causes an inflammation and produces black bile). Hebrew ליהב does not feature in a medical context in the current dictionaries; cf. BM 2626 (Ben Yehuda explains the term as דלק ושרף (to burn)).

לולב הדקל: לולב (*Sefer ha-Shimmush*)[251] = Arabic جفرّى or كفرّى 'envelope, spathe of the palm-flower' (cf. WKAS 1:265b–266a); cf. fol. 140a, col. a: הכופרי והוא לולבי הדקל הרך הנקרא בלשונם אלג׳פרי קודם יביא פריו קרוב מטבע הקור של דקל (KWPRY, i.e., spathes of the young palm tree—called [in Arabic] ʾLǦPRY, before it bears fruit—are close in coldness to the nature of the palm). Hebrew לולב הדקל, Plur. לולבים, only features in the current dictionaries in the general sense of 'sprout' (of a plant), and especially as the 'lulav', i.e., the branch of the palm tree used for the festival of Sukkot; cf. JD 698–9; BM 2644; EM 803; LF 2:328).

לֶחֶם: See entry **אח**.

---

246 For Ibn al-Jazzār's discussion, cf. IJZ 67–8 (Arabic text), 129–31 (English translation), 169–70 (Hebrew translation).

247 a الداحس :מוגלתם הנקרא גלאיי.

248 'paronychia (whitlow)': Translated after the Arabic *dāḥis*; cf. IJZ 129, n. 307.

249 om. a :הלבן.

250 'white': om. a. For the composition of this stomachic, cf. QA 58, 69.

251 See also entry כופרא: כופרי.

הלחם האפוי באלפס (*Sefer ha-Shimmush*) = Arabic خبز الماء 'water bread'[252]; cf. fol. 125a, col. a: הלחם האפוי באלפס יותר עב ויותר חזק הכח מלחם הפורני (Water bread (lit., 'bread baked in a stew-pot') is thicker and stronger than bread [baked] in a *furni*[253] (brick oven)). Hebrew הלחם האפוי באלפס does not feature in the current dictionaries. The term אלפס, variant לפס (from Greek λοπάς, λέβης, or from a Semitic root לפס/לפף (cf. HM 126–7)) features as a Rabbinic term in JD 73 in the sense of 'a tightly covered pot, stew-pot', and in BM 258 in the sense of 'pan' or 'saucepan' (modern).

הלחם הרחוץ (*Sefer ha-Shimmush*) = Arabic الخبز المغسول 'washed bread'[254]; cf. fol. 125a, col. 2: הלחם הרחוץ קר לח יאות לחליים החדים ויזיק לבעלי הלחה הלבנה והקרירות וכבר זכרתי רחיצתו במאמר מטעמי החולים ('Washed bread' is cold and moist and good for [those suffering from] acute diseases. It is harmful for patients [with a cold, phlegmatic disease]. I have already mentioned the [washed variety of bread] in the [chapter on] dishes for sick people). Hebrew הלחם הרחוץ does not feature in the current dictionaries. Subsequent to Shem Tov Ben Isaac, the same Hebrew term for Arabic الخبز المغسول features in both Nathan ha-Me'ati's and Zeraḥyah Ḥen's Hebrew translation of Maimonides, *Medical Aphorisms* 20.17.

הלחם השרוי במים עד שיחמיץ (*Sefer ha-Shimmush*) = Arabic البريد 'bread soaked in water'[255]; cf. fol. 125a, col. b: הלחם השרוי במים עד שיחמיץ הנקרא בל־שונם אלבריד הוא רב הרוחות והנפח ומזיק אל האסטומ׳ בלתי[256] מרפה המעים (Bread soaked in water until it turns sour called [in Arabic] *al-barīd* causes many winds and much flatulency, harms the stomach, [and] does[257] not relieve the bowels). Hebrew הלחם השרוי במים עד שיחמיץ does not feature in the current dictionaries.

לטישה (*Sefer ha-Shimmush*) = Arabic جلاء 'a cleansing effect'; cf. fol. 124b, col. a: סובין של חטה חמים יבשים מעטי המזון מאד ומנגבים ולוטשים לטישה רבה יותר מלטישת קמח החטה (Wheat bran is hot [and] dry, only a little bit nutritious

---

252 'water bread': Cf. NA 566: 'called so because a generous amount of water is used in making its dough soft'.

253 *'furni'*: Cf. entry פורני.

254 Cf. NA 566, s.v. *'khubz maghsūl'*: 'literally 'washed bread', used mostly as food for the sick because it is light and easy to digest. Ibn Sīnā describes how to make it: pith is removed from stale bread and soaked in hot water. Next, the water is drained and discarded, and replaced with hot water. The bread is kept in it until it puffs (387). Ibn al-Bayṭār thinks it has no nutritious value (227)'; see also Maimonides, *Medical Aphorisms* 20.17 (ed. and trans. Bos, 4:67; 157, n. 34): Greek πλυτός ἄρτος (cf. LSG 1423: 'a light form of bread').

255 Cf. VL 1:106: 'panis cui superfusa est aqua'; Dozy (D 1:67) translates the term as 'soupe à la semoule'.

256 a مطلق للبطن :בלתי מרפה המעים.

257 'does not relief the bowels': Cf. a: 'relieves the bowels'.

and has a strong drying and cleansing effect, [even] more than wheat flour). In the sense of 'cleansing effect', Hebrew לטישה is a non-attested semantic borrowing from the Arabic جلاء.

לטש (*Sefer ha-Shimmush*) = Arabic جلا 'to cleanse'; cf. fol. 124b, col. a: סובין של חטה חמים יבשים מעטי המזון מאד ומנגבים ולוטשים לטישה רבה יותר מלטישת קמח החטה. In the sense of 'to cleanse', Hebrew לטש is a non-attested semantic borrowing from Arabic جلا. The same Hebrew term is used by Shem Tov Ben Isaac in the *Sefer Almansur*; cf. NM 2:13–4.

ליחה: See entry (**חטא**) **מחטיא**.

לילית (*Sefer Ṣedat ha-Derakhim*) = Arabic عشاء 'nightblindness' (Greek νυκταλωπίασις)[258]; cf. bk. 2, ch. 5 (Ms Oxford, Bodleian, Poc. 353, Uri Heb. 314, fol. 12b: השער הה׳ בלילית הוא בערבי עשא כאשר יקרה לאחד החולי הזה ואות שלו כי בעליו לא יראה בלילה ראוי להקיזו בגיד העליון ולשלשל טבעו בגירא פיגרא או בגרגרי אצטמטיקון (Chapter five: On nightblindness, i.e., Arabic *ʿašā*. If someone is affected by this illness—and its symptom is that he cannot see at night—one should bleed him from the cephalic vein and purge him with *hiera*[259] *picra* and stomachic[260] pills). Hebrew לילית, adj. fem. of לילי, does not feature as a medical term in the current dictionaries. Masie (MD 508, s.v. 'nightblindness') has עורון לילה.

לָמֶד (*Sefer ha-Qanun*, Zeraḥyah) = Arabic لامي '1. shaped like the letter *Lām*; lamdoid [bone]; 2. hyoid [bone]'; h.l., 'hyoid [bone]' (cf. DKT 540–1, 823; FAL 28, no. 544, s.v. العظم اللامي) (Greek λαμβδοειδής 'formed like a Λ'); cf. bk. 1 (fol. 25b): הפרק הי״ג בניתוח המושקלו של הלמד (Chapter thirteen: The anatomy of the muscles of the hyoid [bone]). In the sense of 'hyoid [bone]', Hebrew למד does not feature in the current dictionaries. For the other translator(s), see entry למדי (II.).

למדי (*Sefer ha-Qanun*, Nathan) I. = Arabic لامي 'shaped like the letter *Lām*; lamdoid' (= Greek λαμβδοειδής 'formed like a Λ') (cf. DKT 458–9); cf. bk. 1 (fol. 29a): והשלב השלישי הוא משותף בין הראש מאחור ובין תחתיתו והוא על תבנית זוית מתחברת בנקודתו קצה החציי ונקרא שלב הלמדי להתדמותו לאות למד יונית (The third suture is the one that is common to the occiput and the base of the head. It has the form of an angle that with its top touches the end of the sagittal [suture]. It is called 'lamdoid suture' because it resembles the Greek letter Λ). For Hebrew למדי as featuring in the *Sefer ha-Qanun*, cf. SRP 38;

---

258 Cf. MMT 253; LSG 1183; UW 438–9.

259 '*hiera picra*': For the composition of this compound with aloe as main component, see ʿAlī b. Rabban al-Ṭabarī, *Firdaws al-ḥikma* (ed. Siddiqi, 458); BAN 182–3. It is good, amongst others, for all dyscrasies of the head and for cold humours in eyes and ears.

260 'stomachic pills': Cf. MIG 102.

see also NM 2:144 (Lamed 3); II. = Arabic لامي '1. shaped like the letter *Lām*; lamdoid [bone]; 2. hyoid [bone]'; (cf. DKT 540–1, 823; FAL 28, no. 544, s.v. العظم اللامي)[261]; cf. bk. 1 (fol. 47b): הפרק שלשה עשר בנתוח עצלי הלמדי (Chapter thirteen: The anatomy of the muscles of the hyoid [bone]). Zeraḥyah Ḥen translates the Arabic لامي as למד (cf. entry), and Joseph Lorki as עצם הלאמי (see entry).

ליעוק: לעוק (*Hanhagat ha-Beri'ut le-Abu 'Ali Ben Zuhr*) = 'linctus'; cf. ch. 28: והלעיקה בכל יום מימי הסתו ג׳ ליעוקים דבש או ג׳ ליעוקים מן נופת[262] ירחיק הברסאם (If, in winter, one takes three honey or honeycomb linctuses every day it protects against phrenitis). In the sense of 'linctus', Hebrew ליעוק is a non-attested calque[263] from Arabic لعوق 'linctus, a medicine to be licked with the tongue' (WKAS 2.2:844b).

לפלוף (*Sefer Ṣedat ha-Derakhim*) = Arabic رمص 'pus'; cf. bk. 2, ch. 1 (fol. 41a): והמופת אשר תכיר בו המותר אשר נגר אל המחיצה הלבנה עד שיעשה מורסא הוא כי מי שקרה לו זה מפני מותר דמי ימצא בעיניו כבדות חזק ותראה העין אדומה נפוחה משלכת לפלוף ויכבד מצחו וירבו הדמעות (And the symptom by which one can recognize [the kind of] the superfluity that streams to the conjunctiva and thus causes it to swell is that if someone suffers from it because of a bloody superfluity, his eyes will feel very heavy and will look red and swollen and will excrete pus; his forehead will feel heavy and he will shed many tears). Hebrew לפלוף only features in the current dictionaries for Rabbinic and modern literature (cf. JD 715; BM 2719; EM 821; LOW LVIII).

לקח (*Sefer Ṣedat ha-Derakhim*) = Arabic أخذ 'to start, to begin', cf. bk, 2, ch. 13 (fol. 52b): ואם לא נראה בנחירים דבר ממה שזכרנו ידענו כי הוא מפני ליחה יורדת מוסרחת מלוחה ואז ראוי שנקח להריק הראש בגירש הגדולות (But if we do not observe in the nose anything of the things we mentioned we know that it (i.e., a bad smell in the nose) is caused by a descending putrid, salt fluid. In that case we should begin to cleanse the head with [one of] the great *hieras*[264]). In the sense of 'to begin', Hebrew לקח is a non-attested semantic borrowing from Arabic أخذ. The same Hebrew term is used by Nathan ha-Me'ati to render Arabic اتّخذ 'to prepare' in his translation of Maimonides, *Medical Aphorisms* 23.106 (cf. NM 2:56).

261 See also entries למד, העצם הדומה ללמד בכתיבת היוונים and העצם הלמדי.

262 Mss זפת emend. ed.: נופת.

263 Read as לעוק, it is possibly a loan word.

264 '*hiera*' (from Greek ἱερά): Name used for a number of compound medicines; see Ullmann, *Medizin im Islam*, 296; the main ingredient of many of these was colocynth pulp (cf. Kahl, *Sābūr ibn Sahl's Dispensatory*, 176–9).

לשון: לשון הים, Plur. **לשוני הים** (*Sefer ha-Shimmush*) = Arabic بحيرة, Plur. بحيرات 'lake'; cf. fol. 129a, col. b: המים החמים מן השמש וזולתו וכל שכן כשיהיו מן המים העומדים בברכות ובלשוני הים הנחים מעפשים הדם (Water heated by the sun and the like, especially stagnant water in ponds and lakes putrefy the blood …). Hebrew לשון הים is attested for in the Bible (cf. BDB 546: '(tongue-shaped) bay of sea'), and Rabbinic literature (cf. JD 720: 'small inlet, creek').

לשון הצפרים (Anonymous glossary; Ms Oxford, Bodleian, Mich. Add. 22); cf. fol. 11b: לשון הצפרים לינגא פשארינאש ([Hebrew LSWN HẒPRYM; [Latin] LYNG' PŠ'RYN'Š). The Hebrew term, which is possibly a calque of the Arabic لسان العصافير (cf. M 212), refers to the 'European ash' (*Fraxinus excelsior* L.); cf. LF 2:286.[265] The term features in Zeraḥyah Ḥen's translation of Maimonides, *On Coitus* 8 (forthcoming ed. by G. Bos) and in Judah ben Solomon (fourteenth century), *Kelal Qaṣar min ha-Sammim ha-nifradim*, i.e., his translation of Abū Ṣalt, *K. al-adwiya al-mufrada* (JNK 48 (no. 133)). For Latin 'lingua passerina[s]', cf. SLN 3:91: '1. *Capsella Bursa pastoris* L.; 2. *Thymelaea passerina* L.; 3. *Polygonum aviculare* L.'

לתת (*Sefer Ṣedat ha-Derakhim*) = Arabic لتّ 'to stir, to mix' (WKAS 2.1:184); cf. bk. 1, ch. 23 (fol. 36b): יודקו הסמים וינופו ויחתך הסרפי לחלקים קטנים ויערב הכל וילתות אותו בשמן שקדים מתוקים (Pound the ingredients and strain them, cut the sagapenum into small pieces, mix all this and stir it with sweet almond oil). Hebrew לתת features in the current dictionaries with attestations from Rabbinic literature only (JD 720–1; BM 2747; EM 829).

מאירה: מאירות (*Sefer ha-Shimmush*) = Arabic ذرارح 'cantharides (Spanish flies)' (L. 960); cf. fol. 146b, col. a: חלב הנשים יותר שוה מכל החלבים … ולפיכך הוא מועיל מן העקיצה אשר תקרה באסטומ' ומשחין הריאה והמעים ומשתיית הארנבת הימית ומשתית הסם הנודע בהורג הזאב ומשתית המאירות ועוד יועיל מאדמימות זנב[266] העין (Women's milk is the most balanced of all milks … and for this reason it is good against a burning [sensation] in the stomach, against a tumor in the lung and intestines, against the consumption of sea-hare, of the poison known as 'aconite', and of cantharides (Spanish flies); it is also useful for pterygium in the[267] canthi of the eyes). Hebrew מאירה, Plur. מאירות, means 'curse' and features in the Bible and Rabbinic literature (KB 541; JD 724; BM 2766). The term also features in an agricultural context in a prayer by a farmer: 'May blessings come unto the provisions and may curses stay away from them.' (KT 2:193). Perhaps the Hebrew term מאירות was used for this

265 See also AEY 274, s.v. לשון צפור: '*Delphinium* L. (Larkspur)'.
266 זנב העין: العين a.
267 'the canthi of the eyes': 'the eyes' a.

insect in reference to its potentially devastating effect on the wheat harvest; according to ad-Damīrī, one of its species breeds in wheat (JAD 1:833–4); cf. SHS 1:311 (Mem 16).

מבדיל (*Sefer ha-Qanun*, Zeraḥyah) = Arabic حاجز 'spine of the scapula' (cf. DKT 548–9, 816; FAL 67, no. 1500); cf. bk. 1 (fol. 26b): וחמשה מושקולים צומחים מעצם הכתף ויעסוק[268] מה שבין המבדיל והצלע העליון מן הכתף (There are five [other] muscles [of the arm] which arise from the scapula. One of them arises from the scapula] and[269] occupies the [space] between the spine and the superior border of the scapula). Hebrew מבדיל does not feature in this sense the current dictionaries. For the other translator(s), see entry חוצץ.

מבושים (*Sefer ha-Shimmush*) = Arabic أُنْثَيان 'pudenda'; cf. fol. 126b, col. a: ומתועלות הפולים על דרך הסם כי המערב אותם בורדים ולבונה וחלבוני בצים יועילו מבליטת בת העין והמבשלם ונותנן על המבושים יתיכו נפחם (As remedies, broad beans are good for prolapse of the pupil (i.e., iris) if they are mixed with roses, frankincense and egg yolk; and if they are cooked and put on the pudenda they reduce their swelling). Hebrew מבושים features as a hapax legomenon in the Bible in Deut 25:11 (cf. BDB 102).

מגלא: המוגלא הבלויה (*Sefer Ṣedat ha-Derakhim*) = Arabic قيح 'pus, sputum'; cf. introduction (fol. 3a): השער הי' ברקיקת המוגלא הבלויה (Chapter ten: On vomiting pus). Hebrew מוגלא בלויה does not feature in the current dictionaries. Common however is מוגלא; it features for instance in the translation of Hippocrates' *Aphorisms* 4.75 by Ibn Tibbon, Nathan ha-Me'ati and the anonymous translator.[270]

מגן: מגן הארכובה (*Sefer ha-Qanun*, Nathan)[271] = Arabic عين الركبة 'patella' (cf. DKT 510–1, 818; FAL 126, no. 2777); cf. bk. 1 (fol. 41a): והוכן[272] בצמצום מקודם שלה ברצפה והוא מגן הארכובה (The front of it (i.e., the knee joint) has been craftily prepared with the *raṣfa*; i.e., the patella). Hebrew מגן הארכובה features in MD 552, s.v. 'patella'; see also SRP 26 (159, 164). Zeraḥyah Ḥen and Joseph Lorki render the Arabic عين الركبة as עין הארכובה (see entry).

מדוה: מדוה הגלגולת (*Sefer Ṣedat ha-Derakhim*) = Arabic داء البيضة lit., 'helmet disease', i.e., 'a headache that afflicts the whole head'[273]; cf. bk. 1, ch. 12 (fol.

268 a وتشغل: ויעסוק.

269 'and occupies': Translated after a.

270 Cf. NM 3:172, s.v. עב טיט.

271 In addition to מגן הארכובה, Nathan translates Arabic رصفة, a synonym of عين الركبة, as עגול הארכובה (see entry).

272 a وتهندم: והוכן בְצמצום.

273 Cf. MIG 269: داء البيضة هو الصداع المشتمل على ‹جملة› الراس (*Dā' al-bayḍa* (lit., 'helmet disease') is a headache (*ṣudā'*) which afflicts the head as a whole); see also Maimonides'

השער הי״ב בחולי הנקרא מדוה הגלגלת. פעמים יקרה בגלגלת כאב חזק מזיק קשה :(19a להרפא עד שהחולה ירגיש ממנו כמו שיוכה ראשו במהלומות ולא יוכל לסבול שישמע דבור חזק ולא קול הברה מדבר שיכה בדבר ולא יוכל להביט האורה (Chapter 12: On the illness called MDWH HGLGWLT: Sometimes the head is affected by such a severe harmful and hard-to-cure pain that the patient feels as if he suffers from blows on the head and that he cannot bear to hear loud voices or hard hitting sounds, nor can he look into the light). Hebrew מדוה הגלגולת does not feature in the current dictionaries. Nathan ha-Me'ati translates Arabic بيضة, as it features in Maimonides, *Medical Aphorisms* 23.66 as הכאב הכולל הנקרא כובע, and Zeraḥyah Ḥen transcribes the Arabic بيضة as ביצה.

מדור (*Sefer Ṣedat ha-Derakhim*) = Arabic وعى 'ventricle' (cf. MMT 264–5); h.l., 'hemisphere'; cf. bk. 1, ch. 11 (fol. 18b): המוח יחלק תחלה[274] באורך לשני חלקים: ימין ושמאל וביניהם חוט נמשך באמצע המוח מבדיל בין מדוריו (The brain is first[275] of all divided lengthwise in two halves: right and left, and between these [halves] is a fissure that divides between its ventricles (h.l., hemispheres?)). As an anatomical term, Hebrew מדור features in Rabbinic literature as מדור תחתון in the sense of 'the lowest compartment of the womb' (cf. JD 733).

מדרגה: על מדרגות (*Sefer Ṣedat ha-Derakhim*) = Arabic على تدريج 'gradually'; cf. bk. 1, ch. 22 (fol. 32b): ונתחיל בכל מה שזכרנו מן הרפואה ביותר קל ואחר כך נעלה אל תכליתו והיותר חזק על מדרגות (We begin [the treatment of the epileptic person] with the lightest remedy of all those we mentioned and then we gradually administer stronger ones until the strongest last of all). Hebrew על מדרגות does not feature in the current dictionaries. Moses Ibn Tibbon uses the same Hebrew term to render Arabic على تدريج in his translation of Hippocrates' *Aphorisms* 2.50: אמר המפרש: הקדים הקדמה אמתית וחייב ממנה מה שיתחייב בהתמדת הבריאות בכל הענינים שירגיל האדם עצמו להעתק ממנהג אל מנהג ועל מדרגות (Says the commentator: He has laid down a correct premise and has drawn conclusions from it. [This premise] also implies that regarding the preservation of health in all circumstances one should accustom oneself to change from habit to habit, but only gradually so).

מוקץ: See entry **קיץ**.

Medical Aphorisms 23.66 (trans. Bos, 5:): 'The illness which the physicians call *bayḍa* and *khūdha* (helmet) is an illness affecting the head; it is a chronic headache which is difficult to eliminate whereby minor causes produce attacks that are so severe that the patient does not tolerate the sound of speaking nor a bright light nor any movement. The thing he likes most is to lie down in darkness because of the severity of the pain. *De usu partium* 3.'

274 om. a :תחלה.

275 'first of all': om. a.

מושב (*Sefer ha-Qanun*, Nathan)[276] = Arabic قاعدة 'basis'; cf. bk. 1 (fol. 2b): הנה יש לראש אחר זה גם כן חמשה עצמות כגדרות ואחד כמושב (Then the skull also has five bones that are like walls and one that is like a basis). For Hebrew מושב in the sense of 'basis', featuring in the *Sefer ha-Qanun*, cf. SRP 31–2 (214, 218). Zeraḥyah Ḥen translates the Arabic قاعدة as יסוד. In bk. 1, ch. 4, Zeraḥyah renders the same Arabic term as מכונה (see entry).

ממית (מות): See entry **סם**.

מזג (*Pirqei Arnauṭ de Vilanova*) = Latin 'contempero' (to moderate); cf. 4.34 (58): כאשר יהיה הדם עב יש לחוש שאם נקיז בעת הקור הגובר יורק הדם הרקיק וישאר העב, ולזה אם יביאנו ההכרח להקיז בעת ההיא ראוי למזוג קור האיברים ולהשוותם, לא עם חום האש אך עם תנועה שוה (If one applies venesection when the weather is very cold and the blood is thick, it is to be feared that the thin blood will be expelled and the thick blood will stay [in the organ]. If one has to bleed during that time one should moderate and temper the cold of the organs, not with the heat of the fire but with moderate exercise). Hebrew מזג features in BM 2875 as מזג חמו של דבר and is explained by Ben Yehuda as 'to cool it a little bit' (צינן אותו קצת) (cf. KTP 2:170: 'mischen, zusammensetzen, mildern, mäßigen'). Ben Yehuda also brings an attestation from Gershom Ben Solomon, *Sha'ar ha-Shamayim*: למזוג קרירותו.

מיזג (מזג) (*Sefer ha-Refu'ot ha-Libbiyot*) = Latin 'tempero' (to moderate); cf. fol. 281b: תמר אינדיש: קרים ויבשים בשלישית[277] וחשבו בהם שהם מחזקים הלב אמנם נראה שזה בסגולה לאותם שיש להם רוע מזג נוטה לאדומה כי הוא ממזג בקורו ומנקה מהאדומה בכח המתיך שבו (Tamarind (*Tamarindus indica* L.): It is cold and dry in the third[278] [degree]. It is supposed to strengthen the heart. It seems that this is especially the case for those whose bad temperament tends to be bilious, because [tamarind] moderates by its coldness and cleanses the yellow bile by its dissolving strength). Hebrew מיזג features as a Rabbinic term in JD 752 in the sense of 'to clarify, to make clear', and in EM 888 in the sense of 'to mix'. The anonymous author of *Sammim Libbiyim* renders the Arabic parallel term عدّل as השוה.

מזרקים: מזרק (*Sefer ha-Shimmush*) = Arabic مجار 'passages, i.e., blood vessels'; cf. fol. 130a, col. a: ומי שלא יוכל למצוא דרך לסננם מרוב טרדתו אם יהיה בדרך או בים צריך לקחת אחריהם דברים פותחים הסתומים ומנקים מזרקי[279] הכבד והכליות וכיס מקוה המים (And if someone is too busy to filter it (i.e., thick, turbid water),

---

276 In addition to מושב, Nathan translates the same Arabic term as מושב הכן (cf. bk. 1, ch. 17 (fol. 37a)), and as כֵּן (see entry).

277 בשלישית: in secundo L.

278 'third': 'second' L.

279 מזרקי: סמפוני א^1^ב.

whether he is travelling by land or by sea, he should after drinking it take ingredients that open the blockages and cleanse the blood vessels of the liver, intestines and urinary bladder). Hebrew מזרק, Plur. מזרקים, features in BM 2891 in a quotation from Maimonides, *Mishneh Torah, Hilkhot Shekhitah* 6.8: קני הכבד והם המזרקים שבו (the blood vessels, i.e., *mizraqim*, in which the blood concocts). Ms Oxford, Bodleian, Hunt. Donat 2 (and a marginal gloss in Ms Paris, BN 1163) read סמפונין (see entry).

מחיצה: המחיצה הלבנה (*Sefer Ṣedat ha-Derakhim*)[280] = Arabic الحجاب الملتحم 'conjunctiva'; cf. bk. 2, ch. 1 (fol. 41a): והמופת אשר תכיר בו המותר אשר נגר אל המחיצה הלבנה עד שיעשה מורסא הוא כי מי שקרה לו זה מפני מותר דמי ימצא בעיניו כבדות חזק ותראה העין אדומה נפוחה משלכת לפלוף ויכבד מצחו וירבו הדמעות (And the symptom by which one can recognize [the kind of] the superfluity that streams to the conjunctiva and thus causes it to swell is that if someone suffers from this because of a bloody superfluity, his eyes will feel very heavy and will look red and swollen and will excrete pus; his forehead will feel heavy and he will shed many tears). Hebrew המחיצה הלבנה does not feature in the current dictionaries.

נמחק (מחק) (*Hanhagat ha-Beri'ut le-Abu 'Ali Ben Zuhr*) = 'to be blended, to be steeped' (cf. Latin 'distemperor'; LRM 152); cf. ch. 3: תשמר בריאות העין בעזוב האכילה בלילה והשינה על המלוי והתמדת הכחול אצל השינה באבק אנטימוני הנמחק במי הכמהין שמועיל בקיץ ובחורף (The health of the eyes is preserved if one does not eat at night and does not sleep with a full stomach, and if one regularly powders the eyes when one goes to bed with antimony powder blended with truffle juice; this is benefical in summer and winter). Hebrew נמחק only features in the current dictionaries as a Rabbinic term in the sense of 'to be rubbed out, to be blotted out' (cf. JD 763; EM 908; BM 2929), and as a modern term in the sense of 'to be cancelled, to be waved, to be withdrawn' (cf. EM 908).

מים: המים הגפריתיים והבורקיים (*Pirqei Arnauṭ de Vilanova*) = Latin 'aquae terminales' (thermal waters); cf. 4.104: החלאים הנושנים הוא יעקר שרשם עם הכויות או עם המים הגפריתיים והבורקיים (Chronic diseases can be eradicated by cauterisation or thermal waters). Hebrew המים הגפריתיים והבורקיים (lit., 'sulphurous, nitrous[281] water') does not feature in the current dictionaries.

---

280 In addition to המחיצה הלבנה, Moses Ibn Tibbon renders the Arabic الحجاب الملتحم as היריעה הלבנה (see entry); while the abbreviated form الملتحم is rendered by him as לֹבֶן (see entry).

281 Cf. entry בורקי.

המים השורפים (*Pirqei Arnauṭ de Vilanova*) = Latin 'aqua ardens' (lit., 'burning water'); i.e., 'alcohol'[282]; cf. 4.70 (70): כאשר יהיו החמרים מימיים או נגרים ראוי שנזהר מעשיית המבשלים בהם לחים בפועל, אם לא שיהיה להם כח להריק הליחה המחטיאה, כמו מי חלב העז לבעלי השקוי, או יהיה להם כח להתיך הליחה ולכלותה, כמו המים השורפים בבעלי הפלג (When the matters are watery or fluid one should be wary of the application of ingredients that are actually moist in order to concoct [those matters], unless [these ingredients] have the power to evacuate the peccant humour, such as whey for dropsy patients, or have the power to dissolve and annihilate [those matters], such as alcohol in the case of those who suffer from hemiplegia). Hebrew המים השורפים features, without further explication, as המים השרופים in BM 2970, a.o., in an attestation from the *Teshuvot* composed by Simeon Ben Zemah Duran (1361–1444).

מיץ: מיץ החלב (*Sefer ha-Shimmush*)[283] = Arabic مخيض 'buttermilk' (cf. NA 588: 'sourish buttermilk left after churning the soured milk and extracting its butter')[284]; cf. fol. 146b, col. b–147a, col. a: מיץ החלב אמנם כשתוסר שפותו[285] והתחיל להחמיץ הוא טוב לשלשול[286] המתהוה מן המרה הכרכומית עם כחשות הגוף וחולשתו (Buttermilk: When the butter has been removed and it has begun to turn sour it is good for diarrhea[287] originating from yellow bile which comes with meagerness and weakness of the body). Hebrew מיץ החלב features in the Bible in Prov 30:33: כי מיץ החלב יוציא חמאה 'the squeezing of milk produceth curd' (BDB 568), a passage quoted by Saʿadya Gaon in the introduction to his *Book of Beliefs and Opinions*.[288] In his translation of Maimonides, *Medical Aphorisms* 23.107, Nathan ha-Me'ati explains the term مخيض as חלב משוכשך.

מיתה: מת מיתה משונה (*Sefer ha-Shimmush*) = Arabic مات سقيا 'to die during illness'; cf. fol. 132b, col. b: ואני לא ראיתי מימיי מי שהרגיל[289] השכרות ושתיית היין אחריו והתמדתו שלא מת מיתה משונה (I have never seen anyone who was

282 Cf. J. Maxson Stillman, *The Story of Alchemy and Early Chemistry* (New York 1960), 192: 'Albertus Magnus (ca. 1260) refers to the fact that by 'sublimation' of wine there is produced a light inflammable, supernatant liquid. Arnaldus Villanova, physician and chemist, also describes it and its uses in medicine in about 1300. He calls it aqua ardens or aqua vini and says that some call it aqua vitae.'

283 See also entry חָלָב: החלב החמוץ.

284 Cf. Maimonides, *Medical Aphorisms* 23.107 (ed. and trans. Bos, 5:69): 'Among the names of [different] types of milk are the following: if milk is churned and its butter removed, the rest is called 'buttermilk' (مخيض). From the *Ikhtiyarāt al—Ḥāwī by Ibn al-Tilmīdh*'.

285 a زبده :שפותו.

286 a للخلقة الصفراوية الحارة :לשלשול המתהוה מן המרה הכרכומית.

287 'diarrhea originating from yellow bile': 'hot yellow bile' a.

288 Cf. Judeo-Arabic ed. and Hebrew trans. by J. Ḳafih (Jerusalem 1970), 11a.

289 a واما مداومة السكر وشرب الشراب بعد الخمار :שהרגיל השכרות ושתיית היין אחריו.

constantly drunk and drank wine after [every hangover] who did not die[290] from an unnatural death). Hebrew מיתה משונה features in the current dictionaries in the sense of 'an unnatural, sudden, often violent death'; cf. BM 2982, EM 930.

מיתר (*Sefer Ṣedat ha-Derakhim*) = Arabic رباط 'ligament'; cf. bk. 2, ch. 19 (fol. 61b): ומאשר יקרה לשנים גם כן האיכול והנקוב ופעמים יתחדש בהם התולעת ופעמים ישתנו מראיהם ויהיו כרכומיות או ירוקות או שחורות. זה כלו מתחדש בהם מפני לחה מעופשת רעה מתילדת מהפסד המזון באצטו' וימשכו הליחות האלה וילכו בעצבי המיתרים המחזיקים השנים (The teeth can also be affected by caries and cavities, sometimes by a worm and sometimes their colour changes and becomes yellow or green or black. All this happens to them because of a bad, putrid humour that originates from spoiled food in the stomach. Such humours stream through the nerves of the ligaments that hold the teeth). As a medical term Hebrew מיתר features in BM 2982–3 in the sense of גיד (tendon, sinew), a.o., in an attestation from the *Sefer ha-Qanun*; see also EM 930–2 and NM 1:60. Standard medieval terms for 'ligament' are derivatives from the root קשר such as קשר/קשור/קשירה (cf. NM 1:185–6).

מכונה (*Sefer ha-Qanun*, Zeraḥyah)[291] = Arabic قاعدة 'basis'; cf. bk. 1 (fols. 17b–18a): והרכבת עצם משני עצמות כמו שני המשולשים יפגוש מהם שתי זויות והם מלמעלה ושתי המכונות הממששות בזוית ומתפרדות בשני זויות (The [nose] is composed of two triangular bones whose angles meet above and their bases touch each other at one of the angles and separate at two [other] angles). Hebrew מכונה features in the Bible in the sense of 'fixed resting place, base' (cf. BDB 467) and in Rabbinic literature as 'stall, coop' (JD 781). Nathan ha-Me'ati renders the Arabic term as מושב (see entry).

מכחול (*Sefer Ṣedat ha-Derakhim*) = Arabic ميل 'style' (cf. FL 4:225: 'Stilus, quo collyrium oculo inditur'); cf. bk. 2, ch. 2 (fol. 43b): יודק הכל שחיקה מופלגת וינופה ויולש בלובן ביצה ויעשה ממנו גרגרים ויותך אחד במים ויושם במכחול בעין (Pound all these [ingredients] into a very fine substance, sieve this and knead it with egg white, make pills of it, melt one pill in water and put this into the eye by means of a style). Hebrew מכחול features in Rabbinic literature in the sense of 'staff used for painting the eye' (JD 782) or 'kohl pencil' (BM 2990). Ben Yehuda also refers to its use in medieval medical literature as something with which a medicine is dripped into the ear and the like, and brings an attestation from Nathan ha-Me'ati's translation of Maimonides, *Medical Aphorisms* 9.27 (cf. NM 2:60 and correction to vol. 2, featuring below).

290 'die from an unnatural death': 'die during illness' a.

291 Another term used by Zeraḥyah for Arabic قاعدة is מושב (see entry).

מכסה: המכסה הבצלי (*Sefer Ṣedat ha-Derakhim*) = Arabic الغشاء البصلي 'bulbar conjuctiva' (tunica conjunctiva bulbi); cf. bk. 2, ch. 1 (fol. 40b): הקצידא מורסא חמה תתחדש במכסה המלובש על לובן העין הנקראת הבצלי (Ophthalmia (conjunctivitis) is an inflammation occurring in the membrane that lies over the white of the eye and that is called 'bulbar'). Hebrew המכסה הבצלי is a non-attested calque from Arabic الغشاء البصلي.

מכסה הלב (*Sefer ha-Qanun*, Joseph Lorki) = Arabic غلاف القلب 'pericardium' (cf. DKT 842; FAL 62, no. 1389); cf. bk. 1 (fol. 18b): ואחר כך הולכים כנגד מכסה הלב ומשלחים אליו שריגים רבים ישתרגו כמו השער וזנין אותו (Then they (i.e., two shoots of the ascending branch of the vena cava) pass in front of the pericardium and send many hair-like branches to it that provide it with nutrition). Hebrew מכסה הלב is not attested in the current dictionaries. For the other translator(s), see entry כיס הלב.

מלח: מלח סדומי (cf. Anonymous glossary; Ms Leiden, Universiteitsbibliotheek, Cod. Or. 4732/1); = 'salt of Sodom' cf. fol. 2b: ארמונייקום הוא מלח סדומי חם מאד (Armoniacum (i.e., ammoniacum, gum ammoniac); i.e., salt of Sodom, [it is] very hot). Hebrew מלח סדומי features in LW 3:126 and BM 3030 as מלח סדומית in attestations from Rabbinic literature. It was allegedly so caustic that it could blind the eyes, when one would touch them with one's fingers on which it would adhere after the meal. The danger of Sodomite salt is one of the explanations given for the obligation to wash one's hands after meals (מים אחרונים); see KT 1:119; 501, n. 660; and J. Preuss,[292] *Biblical and Talmudic Medicine*, 525.

ממשות (*Sammim Libbiyim*) = Arabic قوام 'consistency'; cf. fol. 120a: המדקדק הוא הסם אשר מדרכו שישים ממשות הליחות יותר רקיק בהתכה חסרה בחום שוה (A refining [drug] is a drug that has the property to make the consistency of the humours thinner by imperfect dissolution through moderate heat). Hebrew ממשות does not feature in a medical context in the current dictionaries. Ben Yehuda (BM 3073) mentions the term as a synonym of ממש 'substance', and Klatzkin (KTP 2:211) translates it as 'Realität', as featuring in Isaac Israeli, *Yesod Olam*. The anonymous translator of *Sefer ha-Refu'ot ha-Libbiyot* (fol. 244a) renders the Latin parallel term 'substantia' as עצם.

מסמר: מסמרים (*Sefer Ṣedat ha-Derakhim*) = Arabic مسامير (lit. 'nails'), i.e., 'corns, calluses' (Greek: ἧλοι; cf. LSG 769, s.v. ἧλος: 'wart, callus'[293]); cf. bk. 7, ch. 16.0 (IJZ 151, l. 21): השער הי"ו ביבלת והמסמרים (Chapter sixteen: On warts with thin necks and calluses). As a medical term, Hebrew מסמר features in BM 3127 in attestations from the *Sefer ha-Qanun*, and from Moses Ibn Tibbon's transla-

292 J. Preuss, *Biblical and Talmudic Medicine*, trans. and ed. by F. Rosner (New York 1978).

293 Cf. IJZ 102, n. 165; MIG 587.

tion of Ibn Sīnā's *ʿUrǧuza fī al-ṭibb*. The term is defined by Ben Yehuda as 'a name for some of the tumors' (כנוי לקצת המורסות). The term also features in Shem Tov Ben Isaac, *Sefer ha-Shimmush* (cf. NM 1:103); in his glossary to the *Sefer ha-Qanun*, Nathan ha-Me'ati defines מסמרים as: מיני יבלות (kinds of warts with thin necks)[294]; cf. NM 2:116, 146 (Mem 10).

מסננת: מסננת האף (*Pirqei Arnauṭ de Vilanova*) = Latin 'calami narium' (lamina cribrosa; i.e., the cribriform plate of the ethmoid bone); cf. 5.22 (88): ההגרה הבלתי טבעית יאות להטותה אל מעבר טבעי, כמו הזלת הנצור אשר יהיה בדמע העין נטה אותו אל מסננת האף אם העצם כבר נתעפש (An unnatural defluction should be diverted to a natural channel (exit), as [in the case of] a fistula[295] lacrimalis it should be diverted to the lamina cribrosa when the organ is putrefied). Hebrew מסננת features in BM 3127 in an attestation from the *Sefer ha-Qanun*.

מסרק (*Sefer ha-Qanun*, Nathan) = Arabic مشط 'metatarsus' (cf. DKT 512–3, 827–8; FAL 99, no. 2163); cf. bk. 1 (fol. 41b): וארבע עצמות הרסג במה שיתחבר במסרק (... and the four bones of the tarsus to which the metatarsus is articulated). Hebrew מסרק features in BM 3139 in an attestation from the *Sefer ha-Qanun*; see also MD 462, s.v. 'metacarpus' and SRP 28 (184). Zeraḥyah Ḥen translates the Arabic مشط as משרק הכף.

מעבר: מעברי השמירה (*Sefer Issur ha-Qevurah le-Galienus*) = Arabic مجاري الحسة 'the sensory channels'; cf. fol. 136b: ואולם אחת מהעלות היא עלה תהיה בקרום המוח מן המותרות העבים הדבקים ירדו במעברים נקראים מעברי השמירה ויהיה מהם השעמום הדומה למות (One of these conditions is an illness in the cerebral membranes due to thick, viscous residues which descend through the so-called sensory channels, causing death-like coma). Hebrew מעברי השמירה does not feature in the current dictionaries. For the term מעבר in the sense of passage, see NM 3:134.

המעיד (מעד) (*Sefer ha-Shimmush*)[296] = Arabic أزلق 'to make smooth, to soften'; cf. fol. 133b, col. b: ואם יפגושו לחה לבנה יולידו שלשול וקיא יחד ויזיקו בעצבי האצטומ' ויחדשו רוחות פגות והברה וימעידו המזון (And if they (i.e., watermelons) come in contact with phlegm, they produce both diarrhea and vomiting, they harm the nerves of the stomach and cause raw winds and stomach rumble and soften the food). Hebrew המעיד features in BM 3146 in the sense of החליק/השמיט.

מעי: המעי האחרון (*Pirqei Arnauṭ de Vilanova*) = Latin 'anus' (anus); cf. 5.60 (98): האבר אשר יצא מהנחתו הטבעית מבלי הפסד בתמונתו, הנה יתוקן ענינו עם דחייה, כמו המעי האחרון אם יצא מחוץ (The organ that has departed from its natural

294 Cf. entry יבלת.

295 'fistula lacrimalis': Cf. entry הנצור אשר יהיה בדמע העין.

296 See also entry הסם הממעיד.

position without harm to its shape, can be returned to its place through pushing, such as the anus when it has protruded). Hebrew המעי האחרון does not feature in this sense in the current dictionaries.

המעי הזקוף (*Sefer ha-Qanun*, Zeraḥyah) = Arabic المعى المستقيم 'rectum' (cf. DKT 828; FAL 93, no. 2069); cf. bk. 1 (fol. 33b): והחלק השלישי מן הששה הראשונים יקח אל הצד השמאלי ויתפרד בתעלות של העורקים אשר סביב המעי הזקוף (The third branch of the first six [branches of the portal vein] goes to the left side and spreads in the mesenteries that surround the rectum). Hebrew המעי הזקוף is not attested in the current dictionaries. For the other translator(s), see entry המעי הישר.

המעי הישר (*Sefer ha-Qanun*, Nathan) = Arabic المعى المستقيم 'rectum' (cf. DKT 828; FAL 93, no. 2069); cf. bk. 1 (fol. 63b): והחלק השלישי מן הששה הראשונה לוקח אל הצד השמאלי ומתפרד בתעלות העורקים אשר סביב המעי הישר. Hebrew המעי הישר features in BM 3165–6 in several attestations, o.a., from the *Sefer ha-Qanun*, without any further explanation. Zeraḥyah Ḥen translates the Arabic المعى المستقيم as המעי הזקוף (see entry).

המעי הנקרא י״ב אצבעות (*Sefer ha-Qanun*, Joseph Lorki) = Arabic المعى الاثنى عشر 'duodenum' (cf. DKT 828); cf. bk. 1 (fol. 18b): והאחד משני חלקים הקטנים ידבק במעי הנקרא י״ב אצבעות וימשך ממנו המזון (One of the two small branches (i.e., of the portal vein) joins the duodenum to draw nutrition from it). Hebrew המעי הנקרא י״ב אצבעות features as מעי ... בעל שתים עשרה אצבעות in BM 3165 in an attestation from Joseph Ibn Aknin, *Sefer ha-Musar*. For the other translator(s), see entry המעי הנקרא שנים עשר.

המעי הנקרא שנים עשר (*Sefer ha-Qanun*, Nathan) = Arabic المعى الاثنى عشر 'duodenum' (cf. DKT 828); cf. bk. 1 (fols. 63a–63b): והנה אחד משני החלקים מתחבר בחלק המעי הנקרא שנים עשר שימשוך ממנו המזון. Hebrew המעי הנקרא שנים עשר features as המעי השנים עשר in *Sefer Asaph ha-Rofe* (cf. MM 139) and in BM 3166 in an attestation from Meir Aldabi, *Sefer Shevilei Emunah*. Joseph Lorki renders the Arabic المعى الاثنى عشر as המעי הנקרא י״ב אצבעות (see entry).

המעי העור (*Sefer ha-Shimmush*) = Arabic المعى العور 'caecum' (cf. DKT 828; FAL 93, no. 2066); cf. fol. 141b, col. a: והם מועילים אל המעי העור ואל המעי הצם (And they (i.e., walnuts) are good for the caecum and the jejunum). Hebrew המעי העור features as המעי הנקרא עיוורת in BM 3165 without further explanation in an attestation from *Sefer Asaph ha-Rofe* (cf. MA 139, no. 165). Masie (MD 121) mentions an Aramaic parallel מעי סומא, featuring in *Sefer Asaph ha-Rofe*.

המעי הצם (*Sefer ha-Shimmush*) = Arabic المعى الصائم 'jejunum' (cf. DKT 828; FAL 93); cf. fol. 141b, col. a: והם מועילים אל המעי העור ואל המעי הצם. Hebrew המעי הצם features in BM 3165 in an attestation from *Sefer Asaph ha-Rofe* (cf.

MM 139). In his glossary to the *Sefer ha-Qanun*, Nathan mentions בנות החלב and הדורא as synonyms for מעי צם (cf. NM 2:110, 128 (Bet 7)).

מְעֻנָּג: See entry (ענג) **מעונג**.

מערה (*Sefer ha-Qanun*, Nathan) = Arabic مغارة (cf. emend. De Koning, DKT 529, n. 6) 'fossa' (depression, hollow (in the bone); h.l., 'pterygopalatine fossa'; cf. bk. 1 (fol. 45a): ושני אלו העצלים הם נעזרים בשני עצלים שיכנים[297] בתוך הפה יורדים אל הלחי התחתון בהמערה (These two muscles (i.e., of the jaw) are assisted by two [other] muscles that pass through the mouth [and] descend in fossae to the lower jaw). In the sense of 'fossa', Hebrew מערה is a non-attested semantic borrowing from Arabic مغارة.

מְעֻתָּד: See entry **עתד**.

מיצא (*Sefer Ṣedat ha-Derakhim*)[298] = Arabic وضع 'to compose'; cf. bk. 1, ch. 20 (Ms Oxford, Bodleian, Poc. 353, Uri Heb. 314, fol. 8b)[299]: וספר יעקב בן יצחק הכנדי כי אראקאוס אשר מצא הנגונים אמר המלכים יביאוני למושבם כדי שיתענגו בי וישמחו ממני (Jacob Ben Isaac al-Kindī says that Orpheus the composer of melodies (singer, musician) said: Kings invite me to their residences so that they may take pleasure and delight in me). Hebrew מצא does not feature in this sense in the current dictionaries.

מיצטער: See entry **תנועה**.

מקבב: See entry **קבב**.

מקום: מקום שדופק (*Sefer Ṣedat ha-Derakhim*) = Arabic يأفوخ 'sinciput, spot of the anterior fontanel, bregma' (DKT 830); cf. bk. 1; ch. 17 (fols. 24b–25a): ויחלוב על הראש במקום שדופק אחר שיעביר שער הראש חלב אשה או חלב אתון או חלב צאן (And pour on the head, on the sinciput (spot of the anterior fontanel) after it has been shaven, breast milk or milk of a donkey or sheep (goat)). Hebrew מקום שדופק (lit., 'the pulsating spot') does not feature in the current dictionaries. Alternative readings, featuring in Ms Oxford, Bodleian, Poc. 353, Uri Heb. 314, fol. 7a, and Ms Munich, Bayerische Staatsbibliothek, Cod. hebr. 19 (no foliation) are מקום שבתינוק דופק and מקום שמוחו של תינוק דופק.

מקום רחב (*Sefer ha-Qanun*, Zeraḥyah) = Arabic لقمة 'convex part of a vertebra, epiphysis' (cf. WKAS 2.2:124b–1225a; DKT 488–9, 827; FAL 84, nos. 1865–6); cf. bk. 1 (fol. 20a): והיו שתי קצוות הגב יטו אל הפגישה לא נוצר להם מקום רחב (And [since, as it were] the two parts of the spine incline to meet each other, they were not provided with convex parts). Hebrew מקום רחב does

297 a داخل Ms[1] שיכנים: עוברים.

298 The anonymous author of *Sefer Issur ha-Qevurah le-Galienus* renders the same Arabic term with the same sense as הניח (see entry).

299 This section is missing in Ms London, British Library, Ar. Or. 26.

not feature as an anatomical term in the current dictionaries. For the other translator(s), see entry בליטה.

מקום השמיעה (*Sefer ha-Qanun*, Zeraḥyah) = Arabic صماخ '1. the inner cavity of the ear, the tympanic cavity, the middle ear; 2. the external acoustic meatus' (cf. DKT 588–9, 821; FAL 139, no. 3005); cf. bk. 1 (fol. 30b): והחלק הראשון מכל זוג ממנו ילך אל[300] הקרום הפנימי שהוא מקום השמיעה (The first part of each pair (i.e., of acoustic nerves) goes to the membrane that covers the inner cavity of the ear). Hebrew מקום השמיעה does not feature in the current dictionaries. For the other translator(s), see entry נקב האזן.

מקור: מקורות (*Pirqei Arnauṭ de Vilanova*) = Latin 'fontinellae' (fontanels); cf. 5.26 (90): הכויות המריקות ראוי שיעשו לעולם במקורות, והוא המקום אשר יפרדו שם העצלים זה מזה הפרד מבואר או המקום אשר אין שם מונע שלא יתחבר חבור נאות (Cauterization with evacuation should always be applied to the fontanels (i.e., the anterior fontanel and the posterior fontanel), namely at the place where the muscles can be clearly distinguished, or where nothing prevents a proper healing). Hebrew מקור, Plur. מקורות, does not feature in this sense in the current dictionaries.

מקלח: מקלחים (*Sefer Ṣedat ha-Derakhim*) = Arabic حقن 'clysters'; cf. bk. 1, ch. 23 (Ms Oxford, Bodleian, Poc. 353, Uri Heb. 314, fol. 10a): ואם יצטרך למקלחים יעשה להם קלוחים בסמים חמים (If he needs a clyster he should prepare one with hot remedies). Ben Yehuda (BM 5945) mentions the verb קילח in the sense of 'to apply a clyster' in an attestation from Meir Aldabi, *Shevilei Emunah*. For a synonym of מקלח, cf. the entry קלוח.

מְקַשֵּׁר: See entry **קשר**.

מרדים (*Sefer Ṣedat ha-Derakhim*) **I.** = Arabic مرقد 'soporific'; cf. bk. 1, ch. 17 (fol. 25a): ואם נתחדשה התעורה מפני מזונות חמים או סמים חמים יתרפא במה שזכרנו לפי מה שיטה אליו מזגו ויעשה מאלו הרפואות. מזה תואר מרדים מחבור אסחק בן עמרן שירדים בהריח אותו (And if the sleeplessness happens because of [the consumption of] hot foods or hot drugs [the patient] should be treated as we mentioned according to his temperament and take of the following remedies. One of these is a soporific that was composed by Ishāq b. 'Imrān which has a narcotic effect when one inhales it). Hebrew מרדים features in EM 1053 as a modern term. Ben Yehudah (BM 6451) mentions the verb הרדים in the sense of 'to benumb, to stupefy', as featuring in the *Sefer ha-Qanun*; **II.** = Arabic مخدّر 'having a narcotic effect, narcotic'; cf. bk. 2, ch. 18 (fol. 61a): ואם לא ינוח הכאב במה שזכרנו ויביא הצורך אל רפואות יותר חזקות נצוה החולה שיתמיד להניח פלוניה או שכאזניא או תריאק על השן הכואבת ואם לא ינוח הכאב עם זה ראוי שיעשה רפואות מרדימות (If the [toothache] does not abate with the remedies

300 a אל הקרום הפנימי שהוא מקום השמיעה: الغشاء المستبطن للصماخ.

that I mentioned and it is necessary to use stronger ones, we order to patient to keep on putting [the electuary called] PLWNYH[301] or ŠK'ZNY'[302] or theriac on the aching tooth. If the pain does not abate he should apply a narcotic). Nathan ha-Me'ati uses the same Hebrew term for Arabic مخدّر in his translation of Maimonides, *Medical Aphorisms* 8.38–9; 13.43; 24.51. The same term features in the anonymous *Sefer ha-Refu'ot ha-Libbiyot* (fol. 245b) for Latin 'stupefactiva medicina', wich in turn is a translation of Arabic المخدّر.

מרחיק: See entry **עיצל**.

מורסה: מורסת המסך (*Sefer Ṣedat ha-Derakhim*) = Arabic شوصة 'pleurisy'; cf. introduction (fol. 3a): השער הי״ב במורסת המסך הנקרא שוצה ומדוה הצד (On pleurisy called [in Arabic] *šawsa* and [called in Hebrew] *madweh ha-ṣad*). Hebrew מורסת המסך does not feature in the current dictionaries. The synonymous מדוה הצד (for Arabic ذات الجنب) is used by Moses Ibn Tibbon in his translation of Hippocrates' *Aphorisms* 3.23.[303]

מורסת הראש (*Sefer Ṣedat ha-Derakhim*) = Persian سرسام 'phrenitis' (cf. VL 2:193: 'inflammatio capitis, phrenitis'; cf. MIG 899); cf. bk. 1, ch.18 (fol. 26a): מורסת הראש במאמר מוחלט היא מורסא חמה תקרה בקצת קרומות המוח ישיגהו תמיד צער[304] ושגעון וערבוב השכל (In an absolute sense phrenitis is an inflammation in one of the meninges of the brain whereby the patient is always affected by sleeplessness[305], raving, and mental confusion (delirium)). Hebrew מורסת הראש does not feature in the current dictionaries.

ממרק (מרק): See entry **סם**.

מָרָק: מרק תרנגולים קטנים (*Sefer Ṣedat ha-Derakhim*) = Arabic زيرباج (cf. FL 2:270: 'species cibi iusculenti' (a kind of broth))[306]; cf. bk. 1, ch. 10 (fol. 16b): מזה תאר גירא וחבר אותה בן מאסויה יועיל מהסבוב הוקרא סדר בערבי ומכאב הראש שיקרה מליחה לבנה ומרה שחורה יטהר האצטומכא ויתחזק הכבד והוא עומד במעמד הגיראש הגדולות והלקיחה ממנו מדרהם עד שקל ויקחנו במים חמים ויאכל אחריו מרק תרנגולים קטנים או פיישאן (One of these is a recipe of a *hiera*[307] composed by Ibn Māsawayh which is good for dizziness called *sadar* in Arabic and for a headache caused by phlegm and by black bile; it [is a remedy that] cleanses the stomach and strengthens the liver and that belongs to the category of the

301 For this electuary, cf. D 1:282.
302 For this electuary, cf. FAQ 315.
303 Cf. NM 3:125, s.v. מדוה הצד.
304 צער: ارق a.
305 'sleeplessness': Translated according to a.
306 Cf. entry זירבאג above.
307 '*hiera* composed by Ibn Māsawayh': See entry גלגול הראש.

great hieras; one should take from one *dirham*[308] to one *shekel*[309] with hot water, and then eat broth with chickens or francolins). Hebrew מרק תרנגולים קטנים does not feature as the name of a specific dish in the current dictionaries. In bk. 7, ch. 18.5 of *Sefer Ṣedat ha-Derakhim*, Ibn Tibbon renders the Arabic الدرّاج زيرباجات (francolin as *zīrbāj*) as פיישאן מבושל במרק (cf. IJZ 157). Ibn Tibbon's contemporary Shem Tov Ben Isaac did not have a Hebrew equivalent for the Arabic term, but transcribed it as זירבאג (see entry above).

מרקח: מרקחים (*Sefer ha-Shimmush*)[310] = Arabic جوارش or جوارشن, Plur. جوارشنات 'stomachic'. Arabic جوارش is from Persian گوارش ; cf. VL 1:267: 'Medicamentum vel alia res, quae digestionem cibi iuvat' (a medicine or other ingredient that stimulates the digestion of the food; i.e., a stomachic)[311]; cf. fol. 124b, col. a: ודחיית נזקו לבשלו היטב עם יועזר הרבה מבלי שתיית מים אחריו כלל עד שיתעכל וירד מן האסטומ׳ ואחר כך להרגיל אחריו מה שידקדק ויגיר השתן מן המרקחים (To undo its harm (i.e., that caused by the consumption of broth prepared from wheat flour),[312] cook it well with a lot of mint but do not drink any water after it until it is digested and descended from the stomach, and then take a stomachic which thins the urine and makes it flow). Hebrew מרקח features in the Bible in the sense of 'spice, perfume' (cf. BDB 955; BM 3347); Ben Yehuda mentions it also as a synonym for מרקחת (see entry מרקחת).

מרקחים חמים (*Sefer ha-Shimmush*) = Arabic جوارشنات 'stomachics' (see previous entry); cf. fol. 123b, cols. a–b: ואמר אסחק בן סלימאן בלחם מצות כי הוא לא יאות לשום אדם אע״פ שרבים מן הקוצרים והאכרים אוכלים אותו ויתעכל באצטומכתם מרוב יגיעתם ועמלם והנהגתם עליו ונזקו גדול לבעלי המנוחה ומי שהוא חלוש העכול. ותקונו ודחיית נזקו יהיה במה שזכרתי מתקון לחם הסלת בדברים המדקדקים והמגירים השתן מן המרקחים החמים ודומיהם (Isaac Ben Solomon (Isaac Israeli) said regarding unleavened bread that it is not good for any one, although many harvesters and farmers eat it and it is digested in their stomach because of their hard work and labor and they are used to it. But it is very harmful for sedentary people (who do not do hard work) and for someone whose digestion is weak. To correct and undo its harm one should [take] that which I mentioned regarding the correction of bread prepared from fine white wheat flour (semolina), namely, stomachics that have a thinning effect and

308 The standard *dirham* is 3.125 grams; see Hinz, *Islamische Maße und Gewichte*, 3.

309 '*shekel*': I.e., Arabic *mithqāl*. One *mithqāl* is 4.46 grams; cf. ibid., 4–7.

310 In addition to מרקחים, Shem Tov translates Arabic جوارشنات as מרקחים חמים (see next entry); for Sing. جوارشن, Shem Tov has מרקחת (see entry).

311 In his glossary to the *Sefer ha-Qanun*, Nathan ha-Me'ati explains גוארש as שם פרסי כולל לכל מרקחת מעכל (a generic Persian term for every remedy that stimulates digestion); cf. NM 2:111, 130 (Gimel 3).

312 Cf. entry שרף קמח החטה.

that make the urine flow, and similar [remedies]). Hebrew מרקח חם, Plur. מרקחים חמים, does not feature in this sense in the current dictionaries.

מרקחת I. (*Sefer ha-Shimmush*) = Arabic جوارشن 'stomachic' (cf. entry מרקח: מרקחים); cf. fol. 138b, col. a: וראוי להנזר ממנו מי שירבו בו הרוחות וימהר אליו הגעש החמוץ ואם יגבר עליו יצרו ויאכל ממנו ראוי לשתות אחריו מיד מן היין החי או לאכול ממרקחת הכמון הלבן[313] או מרקחת הלבוניי (Someone who suffers from many winds and is quickly affected by sour eructations should refrain from [eating] them (i.e., apricots). But if he likes them too much and eats them, he should immediately drink unmixed wine or eat the white[314] cumin stomachic or the frankincense stomachic). Hebrew מרקחת features in BM 3347–8 as 'aromatic oil, ointment, jam'. Ben Yehuda also refers to a possible meaning of 'medicinal drink' (משקה של סמים). Subsequent to Shem Tov Ben Isaac, Nathan ha-Me'ati uses the same Hebrew term for Arabic جوارشن (stomachic) in his translation of Maimonides, *Medical Aphorisms* 9.47; cf. NM 2:62–3; II. (*Sefer Ṣedat ha-Derakhim*) = Arabic معجون 'electuary'; cf. bk. 1, ch. 23 (fol. 36a): תאר מרקחת יועיל בע״ה מן הרוחות העבות ומן[315] הפלג ועקום הפה והרפיון והרעש והגלגול ותרדמת האיברים ורוח הגבנות וקווץ העצבים וכל חולי שיולד מליחה לבנה דבקה (Recipe of an electuary that is, God willing, good for think winds, hemiplegia, paralysis of the facial nerve, feebleness, tremors, dizziness, numbness, wind [causing?] hunchback, spasms [caused by] the nerves and every illness that arises from viscous phlegm). Subsequent to Moses Ibn Tibbon, Nathan ha-Me'ati uses the same Hebrew term for Arabic معجون (electuary) in his translation of Maimonides, *Medical Aphorisms* 10.56; cf. NM 2:62–3; the term also features in *Hanhagat ha-Beri'ut le-Abu 'Ali Ben Zuhr*, ch. 9 (Honofredi: 'electuarii'): ואכילת מרקחת המצטיק והלנגא אלובי יחזק אותה ויתקן המזג הרע אם יהיה בה (An electuary (stomachic) [prepared] from mastic and aloeswood strengthens [the stomach] and if it suffers from a bad temperament it is improved by it).

מרקחת החבושים (*Sefer ha-Shimmush*) = Arabic جوارشن السفرجل 'the quince stomachic' (for its recipe, cf. QA 69, s.v. جوارشن السفرجل المسهل (the purgative quince electuary)); KTD 88–9, 135–6, no. 135); cf. fol 141b, col. b: והמרבה מאכילת השקדים הרטובים החדשים ראוי לקחת עליהם ממרקחת התמרי או ממרקחת החבושים המשלשל (And if someone eats a large quantity of fresh almonds, he should take the date electuary or the purgative quince stomachic after their consumption). Hebrew מרקחת החבושים does not feature in the current dictionaries.

313 om. a :הלבן.
314 'white': om. a. For the composition of this stomachic, cf. QA 58, 69.
315 om. א :ומן הפלג.

מרקחת התמרי (*Sefer ha-Shimmush*) = Arabic جوارشن التمري 'the date stomachic' (for its recipe, cf. QA 65 s.v. جوارشن التمري لحنين (the date stomachic composed by Ḥunayn)); KTD 92, 225–6, no 145); cf. fol 141b, col. b: והמרבה מאכילת השקדים הרטובים החדשים ראוי לקחת עליהם ממרקחת התמרי או ממרקחת החבושים המשלשל. Hebrew מרקחת התמרי does not feature in the current dictionaries.

משח הנחירים: משח (*Sefer Ṣedat ha-Derakhim*)[316] = Arabic سعط 'to apply an errhine'; cf. bk. 1, ch. 10 (fol. 15a): וימשח נחיריו אחרי הרקת הגוף בשחיטת כרוב או בשחיטת בלידש או בשמן קממילא או בקצת השמנים החמים אשר זכרנו (After emptying the body he should apply an errhine with cabbage extract or beet extract or camomile oil or one of the hot oils mentioned before). Hebrew משח הנחירים does not feature in the current dictionaries.

משחזת (*Sefer Ṣedat ha-Derakhim*) = Arabic مسن 'whetstone' (cf. D 2:593): 'pierre a aiguisser'; cf. Bk. 2, ch. 4 (fol 45a): ויעשה ממנו גרגרים קטנים ויקח ממנו אחת וישרה אותה במי מטר ויטיף ממנו בעין או תחכך אותה על המשחזת ויכחול בו (Prepare small pills from this, take one pill, steep it in rain water and drip some of it in the eye, or make it fine on a whetstone and apply it as a collyrium [to the eye]). Hebrew משחזת features as a Rabbinic term in JD 851; EM 1075 and BM 3367.

משוחפין: מְשֻׁחָף (*Sefer ha-Shimmush*) = Arabic مسلول, Plur. مسلولين 'people suffering from phthisis'; cf. fol. 125b, col. b: ומתועלתיו על דרך הסם כי כשיעשה ממנו שרף מבושל היטב ויורגל בשמן שקדים מתוקים או בחמאה יועיל למשוחפין ובעלי השעול היבש (When it is prepared as a well-cooked broth and applied with sweet almond oil or butter it (i.e., rye) is good as a remedy for those suffering from phthisis and dry cough). Hebrew מְשֻׁחָף (coined from שחפת) does not feature in the current dictionaries. Arabic مسلول is translated as מושחת מחולי by Moses Ibn Tibbon in his translation of Hippocrates' *Aphorisms* 3.10, while Zeraḥyah Ḥen renders the same term as נחלא (see NM 3:146).

משיחת הנחירים: משיחה (*Sefer Ṣedat ha-Derakhim*) = Arabic سعوط 'errhine, snuff medicine'; cf. bk. 1, ch. 10 (Ms Oxford, Bodleian, Poc. 353, Uri Heb. 314, fol. 4b): ויזהר החולה שלא יעשה שפיכת המים על הראש ומשיחת הנחירים רק אחר הרקת הגוף (The patient should be careful only to pour water over his head and to take an errhine once the body has been evacuated). Hebrew משיחת הנחירים does not feature in the currrent dictionaries. A synonymous term used by Moses Ibn Tibbon to render Arabic سعوط is נחירה (cf. entry below). A Hebrew synonym featuring in Rabbinic literature is מעטש (cf. BM 4431); while Masie (MD 266) mentions the Hebrew synonym מעטיש featuring in

316 In addition to משח נחיריו, Ibn Tibbon has שם בנחיריו for Arabic سعط; cf. entry שם בנחיריו.

Sefer Asaph ha-Rofe; cf. NM 3:134–5, s.v. מעטיש: דבר מעטיש (featuring in *Sefer Agur*).

משך (*Sefer Ṣedat ha-Derakhim*) = Arabic مدّ 'to supply with [food]' (cf. L 2696); cf. bk. 1, ch. 1 (fol. 5a): השער מתילד מאיד עשני עב מתחדש מן החום האשי בגוף ויצמח השער ויתוסף במה שימשך מן האיד הזה. (Hair arises from coarse smoky vapor which originates from the fiery heat of the body. Hair grows and becomes longer through [the food] with which it is supplied by the vapor). In the sense of 'to supply with food', Hebrew משך is a non-attested semantic borrowing from Arabic مدّ.

מושך: See entry **סם**.

מְשֻׁכָּר: משוכר (*Sefer Ṣedat ha-Derakhim*) = Arabic مخمور 'drunk, intoxicated'; cf. bk. 19, ch. 1 (fol. 29a): וראוי שיתרפא מזה אחר שיעיין שאם היה המשוכר בעל מזג חם נשים על ראשו שמנים קרים (He should be treated for this (i.e., inebriety) once we have looked [carefully]. If the drunken person has a hot temperament we should put cold oils on his head). Hebrew משוכר does not feature in a medical context in the current dictionaries; cf. EM 1828.

מִשְׁפָּט: משפטים (*Sammim Libbiyim*) = Arabic أحكام 'effects, virtues'[317]; cf. fol. 130a: סוסן אראה[318] אותו קרוב הטבע מן הזעפראן קרוב המשפט ממשפטיו (Wild[319] white iris (*Dietes grandiflora*) (cf. D 1:19): It is close to saffron in nature and effects). In the sense of 'effect', Hebrew משפט is a non-attested semantic borrowing from Arabic حكم. The anonymous author of *Sefer ha-Refu'ot ha-Libbiyot* (fol. 250a) does not render the Latin parallel term 'iudicium'.

משפיע: See entry **שפע**.

מַשְׁקֶה: משקה הדבש (Anonymous glossary; Ms Oxford, Bodleian, Mich. Add. 22) = 'honey drink', h.l., 'hydromel'; cf. fol. 6a: אדרומיל משקה הדבש ('DRWMYL (Latin hydromel(i); LS 871); i.e., honey drink, h.l., hydromel). Hebrew משקה הדבש does not feature in the current dictionaries. A current medieval term for 'hydromel' is מי הדבש, which features, e.g., in the Hebrew translations of Maimonides, *Medical Aphorisms*, both by Nathan ha-Me'ati and Zeraḥyah Ḥen, and is also mentioned by Ben Yehuda (BM 884) in an attestation from Meir Aldabi, *Shevilei Emunah*.

משקה סוכרי (*Sefer Ṣedat ha-Derakhim*)[320] = Arabic جلّاب 'julep'; i.e., a syrup made with rose water and sugar or honey[321]; cf. bk. 1, ch. 18 (fol. 27b):

317 For this unusual meaning of Arabic حكم, cf. D 1:310: 'influence'.

318 a أزاد :(= أراه) אראה אותו.

319 'Wild white iris': Translated after the Arabic سوسن أزاد.

320 In addition to משקה סוכרי, Ibn Tibbon renders Arabic جلّاب as משקה עשוי מסוכרי ומים (see next entry).

321 Cf. NA 552.

וישקוהו בערב מי רמונים עם משקה סוכרי (In the evening one should give him (i.e., the patient suffering fom phrenitis) a potion prepared from pomegranate juice and julep). Hebrew משקה סוכרי does not feature in the current dictionaries.

משקע (*Sefer ha-Qanun*, Nathan) = Arabic مغرز 'the place of growth, insertion, base, root, origin'; cf. bk. 1 (fol. 44a): ולפעמים יקרבו מאד משקע האוזן בקצת האנשים ומתחברים בו ויניע<ו> אזניו (In some people they (i.e., fibers of the muscles of the cheek) come very close to the root (origin) of the ear and are attached to it and move the ear). Hebrew משקע features in the Bible (Ez 34:18) as משקע מים 'water that is settled, clarified, i.e., clear' (cf. BDB 1054; BM 3418), and in modern literature in the sense of 'sediment, residue' (cf. EM 1091). Zeraḥyah Ḥen translates the Arabic مغرز as שורש, and Joseph Lorki as עקר.

מתהפך: See entry **הפך**.

מתח: המתיח הרוח (*Sefer ha-Refu'ot ha-Libbiyot*) = Latin 'dilato spiritum' (to dilate the pneuma); cf. fol. 250b: ובו סגולה לחזק הלב ולשמח והיא מתחדשת ממה שקדמנו בו ובזה הוא ממתיח[322] הרוח ומחזקו וממרקו ומזהירו (And it has the specific property to strengthen and gladden the heart and this occurs to it by what was said before. And thereby it dilates the pneuma, strengthens it, makes it bright and shiny). Hebrew המתיח does not feature in this sense in the current dictionaries. The anonymous translator of *Sammim Libbiyim* translates the Arabic parallel as פשט הרוח (see entry).

מתיקה: See entry **מתקה** below.

מתקה (*Sefer ha-Shimmush*) = Arabic حلاوة 'sweetness'; cf. fol. 133a, col. b: ודחיית נזקו תהיה באכילת מיני מתקה (And its harm (i.e., that of vinegar) can be averted by eating sweatmeats). Hebrew מתקה is a defective spelling for מתיקה 'sweetness' (cf. JD 682; BM 3445–6) which is common in Rabbinic literature in the combination מיני מתיקה (cf. JD ibid.).

נֶאֱמָן (*Sefer Hanhagat ha-Beri'ut*) = 'chronic'; cf. 10.1 (166): ומוליד עליו חלאים רבים רעים ונאמנים (and brings over himself (i.e., he who indulges in sexual intercourse) many bad chronic diseases). Hebrew נֶאֱמָן features in a similar sense in the Bible, in Deut 28:59: וחליים רָעים ונאמנים.

נבוב: הנבוב (*Sefer ha-Qanun*, Nathan)[323] = Arabic الأجوف 'vena cava' (cf. DKT 830, s.v. الوريد الأجوف); cf. bk. 1 (fol. 66a): הפרק החמישי בנתוח הנבוב היורד הנה חתמנו הדבור בחלק העולה מן הנבוב והוא הקטן שבחלקיו (Chapter five: On the anatomy of the inferior vena cava. We have finished the discussion of the

322 Ms Munich 373 מרתיח Ms Vienna 59, fol. 148a: ממתיח.

323 In addition to הנבוב, Nathan has הוריד הנבוב (see entry) to indicate the 'vena cava', conform to the Arabic الوريد الأجوف.

ascending vena cava which is the smaller of the two). Hebrew הנבוב is not attested in the current dictionaries; for the *Sefer ha-Qanun*, cf. SRP 6 (37). Zeraḥyah Ḥen renders the Arabic الأجوف as החלול (see entry), and Joseph Lorki as הפמימי (see entry).

הנבוב היורד (*Sefer ha-Qanun*, Nathan) = Arabic الأجوف النازل 'the inferior vena cava'; cf. bk. 1 (fol. 66a): הפרק החמישי בנתוח הנבוב היורד הנה חתמנו הדבור בחלק העולה מן הנבוב והוא הקטון שבחלקיו. Hebrew הנבוב היורד is not attested in the current dictionaries. Zeraḥyah Ḥen renders the Arabic الأجوف النازل as החלול היורד (see entry), and Joseph Lorki as הוריד הפנימי היורד (see entry).

נבוכות (*Sefer Ṣedat ha-Derakhim*) = Arabic تحيّر 'confusion'; cf. bk. 2, ch. 6 (fol. 45b): ואם סר חליו יורה זה כי החולי היה מפני שתוף האצטמ׳ ואם עמד הדמיון והנבוכות והאופל יורה כי החולי ההוא בעין לבד (If the illness (i.e., dullness of sight; amaurosis) leaves him it indicates that it occurred because of the sympathetic affection (interrelationship) between the stomach [and the eye], but if he continues to see imaginary things, to be confused and to suffer from dullness of sight, it is an indication that the illness is in the eye only). Hebrew נבוכות does not feature in the current dictionaries.

(נגר) מגיר השתן: See entry **סם**.

(נוח) הניח (*Sefer Issur ha-Qevurah le-Galienus*)[324] = Arabic وضع 'to compose'; cf. par. 1: אמר גליינוס: אני הנחתי ספר בד׳ מאמרים (Says Galen: I composed a book in four parts). In the sense of 'to compose', Hebrew הניח is a non-attested semantic borrowing from Arabic وضع.

נוטה: נוטה ל- (*Sefer ha-Qanun*, Nathan) = Arabic شبيه ب- 'similar to'; cf. bk. 1 (fol. 35b): ועצמות העגז נוטים לעצמות הקטן (The bones of the sacrum are similar to those of the loins). Hebrew נוטה ל- does not feature in this sense in the current dictionaries. Zeraḥyah Ḥen and and Joseph Lorki render the Arabic شبيه ب- as דומה ל-.

נחור: ניחור הקול (*Sefer Ṣedat ha-Derakhim*) = Arabic خشونة الصوت 'roughness of the voice'; cf. introduction (fol. 3a): השער הה׳ בניחור הקול (Chapter five: On roughness of the voice). Hebrew ניחור הקול features in BM 3599 in an attestation from Meir Aldabi, *Shevilei Emunah*.

נחירה: נחירות (*Sefer Ṣedat ha-Derakhim*) = Arabic سعوط; Plur. سعوطات 'errhines, snuff medicines'; cf. bk. 1, ch. 23 (Ms Oxford, Bodleian, Poc. 353, Uri Heb. 314, fol. 10a): וישים בנחירי החולה הנחירות אשר נזכור אחר זה (And he shall administer to the patient [one of] the errhines that we shall mention further on). Hebrew נחירה does not feature in this sense in the current dictionaries. A synonymous term used by Moses Ibn Tibbon is משיחת הנחירים (see entry).

---

324 Moses Ibn Tibbon renders the same Arabic term in the same sense as מצא (see entry).

נְחִירַיִם: See entries **משׁח** and **שׂים**.

מנחיר (נחר): See entry **סם**.

נחרה (*Sefer ha-Shimmush*) = Arabic خشونة (= Greek τράχυτης; 'roughness'; cf. UW 682–3); cf. fol. 133, col. a: וכחו לרפות המעים ואיננו מנפח כלל ולא מעורר הקיא ועובר בגוף מהרה ומרכך נחרת החזה ומגיר השתן (Its strength (i.e., of the best kind of honey) is to soften the stools without causing any flatulence or vomiting whatsoever, to pass through the body quickly, to soften roughness on the chest, to stimulate micturition). Hebrew נחרה features in the Bible as 'snorting' [of a horse] (cf. BMB 637), and in BM 3612 (quoting KA 7:93, with regard to the breathing noise made by a woman during sexual intercourse). The same quotation features in the variant reading נחירה (cf. BM 3602), quoting A. Harkavy, *Teshuvot ha-Ge'onim*, Siman 252 (Berlin 1887).

נחש: נחשים (*Sefer Ṣedat ha-Derakhim*) = Arabic حيّات 'round worms' (Greek: ἕλμινθες; cf. UW 235); cf. introduction (fol. 3b): השער הי״ח בתולעים והנחשים המתילדים במעים (On worms and round worms that originate in the intestines). In the sense of 'round worms', Hebrew נחשים is a non-attested semantic borrowing from Arabic حيّات. Subsequent to Moses Ibn Tibbon, Nathan ha-Me'ati uses the same Hebrew term for Arabic حيّات in his translation of Hippocrates' *Aphorisms* 3.26 (cf. NM 3:155).

נטה: See entry **נוטה**.

נטיה: נטית הפה (*Sefer ha-Shimmush*) = Arabic لقوة 'paralysis of the facial nerve' (cf. Isaac Todros, המאמר בלאקואה; ed. by G. Bos, 189[325]); cf. fol. 134b, col. b: ואם יושם ממנה בנחירים מעורבים במרירת עגור תועיל מנטית הפה (And if some of it (i.e., beet) is put into the nostrils mixed with the gall of a crane it is good for paralysis of the facial nerve). Hebrew נטית הפה does not feature in the current dictionaries. For synonyms, see entry עקום הפה.

ניצוציות (*Sammim Libbiyim*) = Arabic شعاعيّة 'radiance'; cf. fol. 129a: כהרבא חם בראשונה יבש בשנית וכבר חשבו שהוא קר ויש לו בושמיות כמפוריית ויש לו מעט ניצוציות[326] (Amber: It is hot in the first and dry in the second [degree]; some people think that it is cold; it has fragrance like camphor and a little bit of radiance). Hebrew ניצוציות, coined after Arabic شعاعيّة, is not attested in the current dictionaries. Just as in the Latin translation, an equivalent for شعاعيّة is missing in the anonymous *Sefer ha-Refu'ot ha-Libbiyot*.

נכות (*Sefer ha-Shimmush*) = Arabic زمانة 'disability'; cf. D 1:604: 'langueur' (languor); L 1254: 'a disease of long continuance; or such as cripples, or deprives of the power to move or to stand or to walk; or want of some one or more

---

325 Cf. G. Bos, 'Isaac Todros on Facial Paresis: Edition of the Hebrew Text with Introduction, English Translation and Glossary', *Korot* 20 (2009–10): 181–203.

326 Ms Munich 57, fol. 125b ניצוציות: ניצוצות.

of the limbs, or members; and privation of the powers, or faculties'; UW 526: 'Verstümmelung' (mutilation) (= Greek πήρωσις); cf. LSG 1401–2: 'maiming, disabling in the limbs or senses'; cf. fol. 130a, col. b: ומנזק היין אל הגוף בכלל למי שיתמידו וישתהו על בלי סדר ויבקש בו השכרות כי הוא יוליד חליים ישנים ... ויחדש הרטט הארוך והפדגרא והנכות (In general, if someone drinks wine constantly until inebriety without any fixed pattern it causes chronic illnesses, constant trembling, podagra, and disability). Hebrew נכות features in EM 1155 as a modern term only.

נכרי I. (*Sefer ha-Shimmush*) = Arabic غريب 'strange, unusual, extraordinary, unnatural'; cf. fol. 147b. col. a: כל הקיבות יש בהן חמימות נכרית וחריפות מקרית (All [sorts of] rennet have unnatural heat and incidental sharpness). In the sense of 'unnatural', i.e., not hailing from the body, Hebrew נכרי features in BM 3672 as חום נכרי in an attestation from Meir Aldabi, *Shevilei Emunah*. The latter term also features in Nathan ha-Me'ati's translation of Maimonides, *Medical Aphorisms* 3.49; 6.6, whereas Zeraḥyah Ḥen has חמימות זר (for Arabic حرارة غريبة); II. (*Sefer Ṣedat ha-Derakhim*) = Arabic وحش 'wild, savage'[327]; cf. bk. 7, ch. 19.1 (IJZ 158, ll. 11–3): הקובא שני מינים: ממנו מין שהוא שוה עם שטח הגוף והויתו ממרה שחורה מתילדת מעכירות הדם ופעמים שיהיה עמו חכוך כשיהיה החומר חזק התנועה ואמנם תתחזק כשיהיה החומר מעופש מאד או נלהב מאד. ואולם המין האחר יקרא הנכרי (There are two kinds of eczema. In the case of one kind [the eczema] is even with the surface of the body (skin) and comes from black bile originating from turbid blood. Sometimes it is accompanied by pruritus if the matter is moving heavily. The movement of the matter becomes heavy when the latter is very putrid or has been affected by burning heat. The second kind is called the 'wild' one).

נעיי (*Sefer ha-Shimmush*) = Arabic مخاطي 'mucous'; cf. fol. 143b, cols. a–b: בשר הדוב נעיי חלוק קשה להתעכל ממהר לרדת מן האסטומ' מגונה המזון מאד (Meat of a bear is mucous, viscous, hard to digest, it passes quickly through the stomach and is very bad food). Hebrew נעיי features as ניעי in BM 3650 in an attestation from the *Sefer ha-Qanun*. The term also features in Nathan ha-Me'ati's glossary to the *Sefer ha-Qanun*; cf. NM 2:117, 149 (Nun 12).

327 'wild, savage': Reflects the Greek 'ἀγρία'; cf. Celsus, *De medicina* 5.28, 18b, ed. and trans. by W. G. Spencer (Cambridge 1977), 2:171: 'Of papules there are two kinds. There is one in which the skin is roughened by very small pustules, and is reddened and slightly eroded ... But the other variety is that which the Greeks call agria [that is, savage]; and in this there is a similar but greater roughness of the skin with ulceration, more severe erosion, and redness ...'; cf. Paul of Aegina, *The Seven Books of Paulus Aegineta* 4.3, trans. by F. Adams (London 1846), 2:25–6.

נעם: הנעים (*Sefer ha-Shimmush*) = Arabic خصب 'to fatten'; cf. fol. 124b, col. a: וינעים הגופים הבריאים וכל שכן כשיהיה מן החטה האדומה הכבדה (It (i.e., broth prepared from wheat flour) fattens the healthy bodies, especially that prepared from heavy red wheat). Hebrew הנעים does not feature in this sense in the current dictionaries.

(נפח) נופח: See entry **סם**.

מנפח: See entry **סם**.

נֶפַח (*Sefer ha-Qanun*, Nathan) = Arabic نفخ 'gas, flatulence'; cf. bk. 1 (fol. 36a): וימלאו הקרבים מן המזון והנפח ויצטרך אל מקום רחב לאויר הנמשך (And when the intestines fill with food and gas (flatulence) and when they need more space because of the inhaled air). Hebrew נֶפַח features in BM 3719 in the sense of 'swelling' or 'tumour'. Zeraḥyah Ḥen renders Arabic نفخ as נפיחה. In his translation of Hippocrates' *Aphorisms*, Moses Ibn Tibbon uses נֶפַח to render both Arabic تقيّخ (suppuration) and نفّاخة (watery vesicle), and Judah Shalom has נֶפַח in the sense of 'inflammation'(cf. BM 3:158). The anonymous translator of *Sefer ha-Refu'ot ha-Libbiyot* has נֶפַח for the parallel Latin term 'inflatio' (flatulence); cf. fol. 248a: אבל ההזנה אשר בה מוליד דם עכור ושחוריי והמותר[328] היותר גובר בו מסבב נפח בגידים וכבר נודע כמות היזק שני הענינים האלו (But the nutrient element in it (i.e., in sweet basil (*Ocimum basilicum* L.)) produces turbid melancholic blood and the superfluity it contains that comes on top of it causes flatulence in the vessels. The extent of the harm [inflicted] by these two things is well-known). The anonymous translator of *Sammim Libbiyim* renders the Arabic parallel term نفخة as נפיחה (see next entry).

נפיחה (*Sammim Libbiyim*) = Arabic نفخة 'flatulence'; cf. fol 126b: והעצם המזוני אשר בו יתילד ממנו דם עכור שחוריי והלחות המותרי אשר בו יתחדש ממנו הנפיחה בעורקים וכבר ידעת הזק שני אלו הענינים (The nutrient substance in it (i.e., sweet basil (*Ocimum basilicum* L.)) produces turbid melancholic blood and the superfluous moisture in it produces flatulence in the vessels. You know how harmful these two things are). Hebrew נפיחה features in BM 3720 in the sense of 'blowing, breath,' and 'swelling (of the flesh)' (נפיחת בשר). It also features in Joseph[329] Delmedigo's translation of Hippocrates' *Aphorisms* 3.24 to render Greek φλεγμονή (inflammation); cf. NM 3:159. The anonymous translator of *Sefer ha-Refu'ot ha-Libbiyot* translates the Latin parallel term 'inflatio' as נפח (see previous entry).

---

328 Et alia superfluitas insuper L :והמותר היותר גובר בו.

329 On Joseph ben Solomon Delmedigo (1591–1655) and his translation of Hippocrates' *Aphorisms*, which was based on the Greek text, see NM 3:11 and the secondary literature listed there.

נפל: See entry **חלי**.

נופת: נֹפֶת (*Sefer Ṣedat ha-Derakhim*) = Arabic شهدة (Greek κηρός) 'honeycomb'[330]; cf. bk. 1, ch. 7 (fol. 11b): השער הז׳ בחולי הנקרא הנופת ובלעז׳ ברשקש[331] ובערבי אלשהדה[332]. פעמים יקרה גם כן בעור הראש נגעים שיהיו בהם נקבים קטנים יצא מהם לחות[333] עב דבק דומה בדבש ולכן נקרא החולי הזה נופת והתילדו מלחה לבנה מלוחה (Chapter seven: On the disease called 'honeycomb', Romance BRŠQŠ[334], Arabic *al-šahda*. Sometimes also the skin of the head is affected by ulcers with small openings from which a thick viscous liquid flows that is similar to honey and for this reason this illness is called 'honeycomb'. It originates from salty phlegm). Hebrew נופת features in BM 3753, in which Ben Yehuda quotes this passage. Following Masie (MD 283), Ben Yehuda translates the term נופת as Latin 'favus'. The anonymous translator of al-Rāzī's *On the Treatment of Small Children* renders Latin 'favositas mellis' as צוף הדבש (cf. ROT 31; NM 2:180) and Bonfos translates the same term as עשניות או אדיות הדבש (cf. ROT 40; NM 2:176).

הנצור אשר יהיה בדמע העין: נצור (*Pirqei Arnauṭ de Vilanova*) = Latin 'fistula lacrimalis' (lacrimal fistula); cf. 5.88 (88): ההגרה הבלתי טבעית יאות להטותה אל מעבר טבעי, כמו הזלת הנצור אשר יהיה בדמע העין נטה אותו אל מסננת האף אם העצם כבר נתעפש (An unnatural defluction should be diverted to a natural channel (exit), as [in the case of] a fistula lacrimalis it should be diverted to the lamina cribrosa when the organ is putrefied). Hebrew הנצור אשר יהיה בדמע העין does not feature in the current dictionaries. Masie (MD 294) mentions נצור הדמעות as a synonym. For נצור in the sense of 'fistula', see BM 3760 with attestations from the *Sefer ha-Qanun*.

נִצָּל מִן (נצל) (*Sefer ha-Shimmush*) I. = Arabic معرًّا من 'free from'; cf. fol. 128b, col. a: מצד ריחם להיותם נצלים מן הסרחון (Regarding their smell, they (i.e., waters) should be free from a putrid smell). Hebrew נצל מן does not feature in this sense in the current dictionaries; II. = Arabic سليم من 'free from'; cf. fol. 146a, col. b: החלב החשוב הוא ההולך על מהלך טבע הבעל חיים אשר הוא ממנו כשיהיה הבעל חיים בריא הגוף יפה המראה ממוצע השומן נצל מן הרזון והמחלות ויתר ההוות (Good milk is that that is according to the nature of the animal from which

330 Cf. UW 344. For another extensive description of this illness in a text attributed to al-Rāzī, which is only preserved in the Hebrew and Latin translations, see ROT 21 (Latin); 31, 40 (Hebrew); 49 (English).

331 Ben Yehuda reads: ברשק (Ms Oxford, Bodleian, Poc. 353, Uri Heb. 314).

332 Ben Yehuda reads: אלסינדא.

333 Ben Yehuda reads: לחה עם.

334 'BRŠQŠ': I.e., the plural of O. Occ./ O. Cat. 'bresca' (honeycomb) (LR 1:256b; DECLC 2:212b). I thank Julia Zwink for this reference.

it comes when it is healthy, of good appearance, moderate in fat, free from leanness, illnesses and other faults). Hebrew נצל מן features in BM 3771 as נצול מן in the sense of 'saved, delivered from'.

נקב האזן: נקב I. (*Sefer Ṣedat ha-Derakhim*) = Arabic ثقب (الأذن) 'ear canal'; cf. bk. 2, ch. 7 (fol. 47b): ואם לא נראה דבר מזה וראינו נקב האזן בריא אין בו נזק ידענו כי העצב אשר בו ילך השמע כואב ואם היה כאב העצב השומע מפני מותר עב קר דבק או מפני רוח עבה או מורסא קרה ... אז ראוי לשלשל המותרות ההם (But if we do not see anything of this but see that the ear canal is clean and not damaged we know that the hearing nerve is painful, and if the pain of the hearing nerve is caused by a cold, thick, viscous superfluity or thick wind or cold swelling ... we should evacuate those superfluities). Hebrew נקב האזן is an unattested calque of the Arabic ثقب (الأذن); II. (*Sefer ha-Qanun*, Nathan) = Arabic صماخ '1. the inner cavity of the ear, the tympanic cavity, the middle ear; 2. the external acoustic meatus' (cf. DKT 588–9, 821; FAL 139, no. 3005); cf. bk. 1 (fol. 57a): והחלק הראשון מכל זוג ממנו יכוון אל הקרום המחפה בתוך אלסמך הוא נקב האוזן (The first part of each pair (i.e., of acoustic nerves) goes to the membrane that covers the SMK (i.e., Arabic صماخ); i.e.. the inner cavity of the ear). Zeraḥyah Ḥen translates the Arabic صماخ as מקום השמיעה (see entry), and Joseph Lorki as פתיחת האזן (see entry).

נקבים (*Sammim Libbiyim*) = Arabic مسامّ 'pores'; cf. fol. 120b: והממרק הוא הסם אשר יכלה מן הליחה הנקפאת והדבקה מה שהיה על שטח האבר ופיות הנקבים (A deterging [drug] is a drug that destroys the congealed, viscous humour that is on the surface of the organ and the openings of the pores). Hebrew נקבים features in Rabbinic literature in the general sense of 'openings [of the body]' (cf. BM 3779; JD 930: 'the organs of the extremities'). The same Hebrew term (for Arabic مسامّ) features in the Hebrew translations of Maimonides, *Medical Aphorisms* by Nathan ha-Me'ati and Zeraḥyah Ḥen. The anonymous translator of *Sefer ha-Refu'ot ha-Libbiyot* (fol. 244a) translates the parallel Latin 'pori' as נקבים as well.

נְקוּב (*Sefer Ṣedat ha-Derakhim*) = Arabic تثقّب 'cavity'; cf. bk. 2, ch. 18 (fol. 59a): כאשר יכאבו ויפסדו יחסר פעולתם ויראו בהם חליים מתחלפים ומהם חליים נראה אותם לעין כמו אכול השנים ונקובם ועפושם ותנועתם ולכלוכם אשר יהיה עליהם ומה שדומה לזה (When [the teeth] hurt and decay, they function less well and different illnesses become visible; some of them visible to the eye, such as caries, cavities, and decay, and when they move or become dirty, and the like). Hebrew נְקוּב features in BM 3790 in an attestation from the *Sefer ha-Difteriah* in the sense of 'perforation' (of the throat by a stone) (אבן ניקוב הגרון).

נקודים: לחם ניקודים (*Sefer ha-Shimmush*) = Arabic بشماط 'biscuit' (cf. D 1:90; FL 1: 126: 'panis bis coctus' (twice[335] cooked bread); cf. fol. 123b, col. a: הכעכין ולחם ניקודים יש בהם תוספת נגוב יוצא משווי הלחם והם מולידים חלט שחורי מאמץ המעים ומנגבים לחות האסטומ׳ והמעים ומולידים סתומים וחול בכליות ומזיקים לבעלי ההדרקון נזק מבואר (Pretzels and biscuits are more dry than bread that is moderately dry. They produce black bile, are constipating, dry the moisture of the stomach and intestines, cause obstructions and kidney stones and cause obvious harm to colic patients). Hebrew נקודים alone features the current dictionaries in the sense of 'crumbs', 'a kind of (hard) biscuit or cake' (BDB 665); 'minute loaves, cakes' or 'crumbled pieces [of bread]' (JD 908); 'biscuit, rusk' (BM 3784).

(נקע) נקוע or **נָקֵעַ** (*Sefer ha-Shimmush*) = Arabic نقيع 'macerated, steeped'; cf. fol. 131b, col. a: שכר התאנים: זה השכר יעשה נקע[336] ויעשה מבושל והנקע יותר לח מן המבושל הרבה והוא מוליד רוחות רבות ונפח (Wine made from figs: This wine can be made through macerating [the figs] or boiling [them]. The macerated [wine] is much moister than the boiled one and causes many winds and flatulence). In the sense of 'macerated', Hebrew נקוע or נָקֵעַ is a non-attested calque of Arabic نقيع. Note that a learned copyist explained this unusual term with the common Hebrew שרוי in a marginal gloss.

נקרה (*Sefer ha-Qanun*, Nathan) = Arabic نقرة 'cavity' (cf. FAL 103, no. 2256); cf. bk. 1 (fol. 32b): ולכל כנף מהם יש שתי נקרות ולכל צלע שתי תוספות מגובנים (Each of these transverse processes (i.e., of the vertebrae) has two cavities and each rib has two tubercles (rounded heads)). As an anatomical term, Hebrew נקרה features in BM 3809 as נקרת הקול in the sense of 'glottis'. Zeraḥyah Ḥen renders the Arabic نقرة as קשר (?). Cf. entry עֹמֶק below.

נרדי: See entry **תרדי**.

נֵרְדְּם: See entry **שרין**.

(נתך) מתיך: See entry **סם**.

(נתר) מתיר הזיעה: See entry **סם**.

סִבוּב (*Sefer Ṣedat ha-Derakhim*) = Arabic دوار 'dizziness, vertigo'; cf. introduction (Ms Oxford, Bodleian, Poc. 353, Uri Heb. 314, fol. 1b): השער הי״ג בגלגול והסבוב (Chapter thirteen: on vertigo and dizziness). Hebrew סבוב features as סבוב הראש in BM 3913 in an attestation from the *Sefer ha-Qanun* (cf. EM

335 'twice cooked bread': So named because originally biscuits were cooked in a twofold process: first baked and then dried out in a slow oven so that they would keep.

336 נקע: שרוי א[1].

1209). Moses Ibn Tibbon also uses סבוב to render the synonymous Arabic term سدر (cf. NM 1:63; 3:127). See also entry גלגול above.[337]

סדיקה (*Sefer Ṣedat ha-Derakhim*) = Arabic شقاق 'fissure'; cf. bk. 7, ch. 30.1 (IJZ 171, ll. 11–4): הנה כשיעורב עם דם המזון מרה שחורה עבה או כרכומית מחודדת יוליד ברגלים ובידים סדיקות מפני תגבורת היובש על דם המזון אבל כי המרה השחורה לכבדו־תה ועביה תצלול ואמנם תוליד הסדיקות בשפל הרגלים והמרה הכרכומית לקלותה רוב מה שתוליד הסדיקות בידים (If the blood [resulting] from the [digestion of the] food is mixed with coarse black bile or sharp yellow bile, it produces fissures in the hands and feet because the dryness prevails over the blood from the food, [and] the black bile, because of its thickness and coarseness [always] sinks and produces fissures in the bottom of the feet, while the yellow bile, because of its lightness mostly produces fissures in the hands). In the sense of 'fissure', Hebrew סדיקה features in BM 3966 in an attestation from Meir Aldabi, *Shevilei Emunah*. In the Hebrew translation of Maimonides, *On Hemorrhoids* 5.2, Moses Ibn Tibbon translates the same Arabic term شقاق in the sense of 'anal fissures' as פרק, and an anonymous translator as סדיקות (cf. ed. Bos, 41, l. 6; 72, l. 6).

סדר (*Sefer Ṣedat ha-Derakhim*) = Arabic قانون 'rule'; cf. bk. 1, ch. 10 (fol. 16b): ובמה שזכרנו מרפואת כאב הראש על דרך הסדר[338] הלמודי מחכמת הרפואה די ספוק (And what we have mentioned of the treatment of headache according to the rules that instruct in the medical art (the theoretical rules of the medical art) is sufficient). Hebrew סדר does not feature in this sense in the current dictionaries; cf. BM 3969–72; KTP 3:94–5. The term recurs in Moses Ibn Tibbon's translation of Averroes, *Middle Commentary on Aristotle's De Anima* (ed. by A. Ivry (Jerusalem 2003), 1, l. 18); cf. NM 3:168, n. 505. Zeraḥyah Ḥen renders Plur. قوانين as סדרים in his translation of Hippocrates' *Aphorisms* 1.1 (cf. NM 3:168).

סחוסי (*Sefer ha-Shimmush*) = Arabic غضروفي 'cartilaginous'; cf. fol. 144a, col. a: האף קר יבש סחוסי קשה להתעכל מעט המזון ([Meat from] the nose is cold, dry, cartilaginous, hard to digest, slightly nutritious). Hebrew סחוסי, adjective formed from סחוס or חסחוס 'cartilage' (cf. JD 486–7; LOW 52; BM 4004–5), features in MD 136 without attestations.

סיטני: סטני (*Sefer ha-Shimmush*); cf. fol. 138b, col. a: והוא מנוגב מעט המימות יקרא המתפלח ובלשון רבותינו הסיטני (This variety of peach] is dry, has only a little bit of moisture; it is called 'the one that can be cut open' and [its name] in Rabbinic Hebrew is SYṬNY). Hebrew סיטני does not feature in the current dictionaries. Löw (FL 4:218) remarks that Plur. סטניות (Sing. סטני) should

337 Cf. NM 3:127, s.v. מחוג הראש.

338 a القانون الطبّي العلمي: הסדר הלמודי מחכמת הרפואה.

be read as סתוניות (Sing. סתוני) 'winter-fruits, late fruits (of grapes)'; cf. JD 1030. However, Plur. סטניות can be found in the fourteenth century Hebrew-Persian dictionary entitled *Sefer ha-Melitsah*, composed by Solomon Ben Samuel, under the rubric מלות נעלמות (words that have vanished; i.e., cannot be found in the dictionaries) without any further explication. (cf. Bacher, 65, no. 701).[339] Bacher (ibid.) explains the term as 'acinus s. granum uvae' (berries or seeds of grapes). Perhaps one might suggest that סיטני, read סיטוני, is a transcription of Latin 'citonia'; i.e., 'quince'.

סיג: סיג הזהב (*Sefer Ṣedat ha-Derakhim*) = Arabic إقليميا الذهب 'gold calamine' (cf. MIG 859); cf. bk. 2, ch. 6 (fol 47a): ואם לא ימצא הפלפל הלבן יושם תמורתו סיג הזהב (But if white pepper cannot be found, put instead of it gold calamine). Hebrew סיג הזהב does not feature in the current dictionaries. The faulty translation of Arabic إقليميا; i.e., Greek καδμεία ('cadmia, calamine'; cf. LS 848) as Hebrew סיג; i.e., 'dross' (cf. BM 4015) goes back to an erroneous identification of Arabic إقليميا as خَبَث 'dross' by Ibn Ǧulǧul as mentioned in Marwan Ibn Ǧanāḥ, *Kitāb al-Talḫīṣ* (MIG 30) and then adopted by later authors like al-Zahrāwī and Ibn Maymūn: إقْلِيميا، قال ابن جلجل: قال أرسطاطاليس يُقال إنّ إقليميا هو خَبَث كلّ جسد ذائب (*Iqlīmiyā* (calamine). Ibn Ǧulǧul: Aristotle said that calamine is said to be the dross (*ḫabaṯ*) of all meltable bodies (i.e., metals)).

סיג הכסף (*Sefer Ṣedat ha-Derakhim*) = Arabic إقليميا الفضّة 'silver calamine' or 'silver cadmia' (cf. MIG 30); cf. bk. 1, ch. 7 (fol. 12a): או יקח סיג הכסף ובלנקט ויודקו בחומץ ושמן ורדים ויטוח בו (Or take silver calamine and ceruse, pound this with vinegar and rose oil and smear it on the spot). Hebrew סיג הכסף does not feature in this sense in the current dictionaries. In the Bible, we find סיגים כסף in Ez 22:18, סיגים מכסף in Prov 25:4 (הגו סיגים מכסף) and כסף סיגים in Prov 26:23, which is commonly translated as 'silver dross', cf. BDB 494; KB 750. In the latter sense, סיג הכסף features in Shem Tov Ben Isaac, *Sefer ha-Shimmush*, bk. 29, as an equivalent to Arabic خبث الفضة 'silver dross' (cf. SHS 1:356–7 (Samekh 6)).

סיג הצפרנים (*Sefer Issur ha-Qevurah le-Galienus*) = Arabic قلامة الأظفار 'nail cuttings'; cf. par. 117 (Ms Leeuwarden, Tresoar Fr. 23, no foliation): ורפואת עלות המאמר הג׳ שיתעשנו בדאם[340] ושישון וקלי[341] החטה המשורפ׳ וסיג הצפרנים והם יקומו לשעתם (The treatment of the third kind of these illnesses

339 W. Bacher, *Ein Hebräisches-Persisches Wörterbuch aus dem vierzehnten Jahrhundert*, = XXIII. Jahresbericht der Landes-Rabbinerschule (Budapest 1900), 65, no. 701 (Hebrew).

340 a בדאם ושישון (= בדארשישעאן): بدارشيشعان.

341 a וקלי החטה: وسويق الشعير.

should consist of fumigation with aspalathus, roasted meal of wheat and nail cuttings. These (patients) will stand up in no time). Hebrew סיג הצפרנים does not feature in the current dictionaries.

סימפונא: See entry **סמפונא**.

סיבי (*Sefer ha-Shimmush*) = Arabic ليفي 'fibrous'; cf. fol. 143a, col. b: בשר הבקר המוכלח איננו טוב כלל מפני התחברות הנגוב והכחשות וחולשת החמימות בו ולפיכך יהיה בשרו סיביי (Meat from old cows is not good at all because it combines dryness, leanness and lack of heat; for this reason it is fibrous …). Hebrew סיבי only features as a modern term in EM 1234.

סכבאג׳: See entry **תבשיל**.

סכסוך הרוחות: סכסוך (*Sefer ha-Shimmush*) = Arabic تهييج الرياح 'arousing winds, flatulences'; cf. fol. 125b, col. a: והמצה ממנו עבה וחלוקה ומתאחרת להתעכל וכבדה על האצטומ׳ ומוסיפה בסכסוך הרוחות רבת הנזק לבעלי החליים הקרים (The unleavened bread prepared from it (i.e., from barley) is thick, viscous, slow to digest, heavy on the stomach, and increasingly arouses winds. It is very harmful for those suffering from cold illnesses). Hebrew סכסוך features in BM 4055 in the sense of 'entanglement, confusion, dispute', and of the 'fire attacking something that cannot be burnt'. The verb סכסך features in the Bible in the sense of 'to provoke' (cf. KB 745). See also SHS 1:362 (Samekh 16).

סוכר ויאולש: סֻכָּר (*Sefer Ṣedat ha-Derakhim*) = Arabic بنفسج مربّا 'violet preserve'; cf. bk. 1, ch. 18 (fol. 27b): ויורק אחר כן בבשול תמראינדיש ופרונש וגוגובש ופרחי ויאולש עם קשיא פישטולא ומאנא ומה שדומה להם וישתה בכל יום מה שירכך הטבע ויכבה חום מרה כרכומית כמו שיקח מנא וסוכר ויאולש מ״א עשרה דרהם וקשיא פשטו־לא מנוקה ה׳ דרהם וימרסהו במי קרא צלויה או במי קשואים[342] וישתה אותו בהיותו צם (Then he (i.e., the patient suffering from phrenitis) should be purged with a decoction of tamarind, prunes, jujube, and violet flowers with Indian laburnum and manna and the like; and every day he should be given a potion which softens the stools and extinguishes the heat of the yellow bile, such as a potion of ten *dirhams*[343] each of manna[344] and violet preserve, five *dirhams* of purified Indian laburnum; this should be mixed with juice of roasted gourd or cucumber[345], and [the patient] should drink it on an empty stomach). Hebrew סכר does not feature in this sense in the current dictionaries.

---

342 add. a קשואים: ويصفّى.

343 The standard *dirham* is 3.125 grams; see Hinz, *Islamische Maße und Gewichte*, 3.

344 'manna': 'from Khurāsān' add. a.

345 'cucumber': 'and strained' add. a.

סוכר כנדי (*Sefer Ṣedat ha-Derakhim*)[346] I. = Arabic سكّر الفانيد 'concentrated juice of the sugar cane'(cf. M 289); NA 596, s.v. 'fānīdh': 'pulled taffy, chewy sugar-candy, usually shape into small discs';[347] cf. bk, 2, ch. 2 (Ms Oxford, Bodleian, Poc. 353, Uri Heb. 314, fol. 12a)[348]: ויועיל מן הלובן שיקח סוכר[349] טוב ב׳ חלקים וקצף הים חלק יודק וינופה וירפא בו או יקח אמידום וסוכר כנדי מכל אחד חלק ויודקו ויתרפא בהם ([A recipe] good for leucoma: take two parts of *ṭabarzad*[350] sugar, one part of alkyonion (lit., sea froth); pound and sieve this [substance] and treat [the leucoma] with it. Or take one part of each of starch and concentrated juice of the sugar cane and pound it and treat it with it). The term סוכר כנדי is a non-attested mixed term, consisting of Hebrew סוכר and Romance כנדי ('candi')[351], which derives from Arabic-Persian *qand* (cf. M 289; MIG 836). According to Nasrallah (NA 599), the term *qand* refers to 'crystallized cane sugar produced by straining and boiling down extracted cane juice then draining and filtering it in cone-shaped clay vessels. At this stage, *qand* is raw and unrefined. For a finer and whiter sugar, it is cooked with water mixed with some milk, and the process of draining and filtering is repeated. The products of this process are *quṭāra* molasses and refined white sugar cones of qand (al-Hassan[352] and Hill 222). The solid cone of the white refined sugar is called *sukkar ublūj* and *ṭabarzad* (see next entry); II. (סוכרי קנדי) = Arabic سكّر طبرزد '*ṭabarzad* sugar'; i.e., fine-quality white and refined cane sugar qand (cf. NA 602)[353]; cf. bk. 2, ch. 2 (fol. 43b): ולו ג״כ תאר עגולים מועילים ללובן ולשחין המתהוה בעין והוא נפלא יקח בלנקט ב׳ שקלים סרקאקולא מתוקנת ב׳ דר׳ דרגאן וגומא ארביקא וסוכרי קנדי וכאנפר מ״א חצי דרהם (Another wonderful recipe by him (i.e., Ibn Māsawayh) for collyria that are good for leucoma and pustules in the eye: take two *sheqels*[354] of ceruse; two *dirhams*[355]

---

346 Cf. entry פנים.

347 According to D. Waines (EI^2 9:804b–805a, s.v. 'sukkar'), it is sugar made in elongated moulds which melted quickly in the mouth.

348 Ms London, British Library, Add. 27542 has a variant reading קנדי (QNDY).

349 סוכר טוב: سكّر طبرزد a.

350 '*ṭabarzad* sugar': Translated according to a سكّر طبرزد, cf. next subentry and entry סכר קשה.

351 Cf. Old Occ. or Old Cat. 'sucre candi' (sugar crystallized in pieces) (FEW 19:83b). I thank Julia Zwink for this reference.

352 A. Y. al-Hassan and D. R. Hill, *Islamic Technology. An Illustrated History* (Cambridge 1986).

353 According to D. Waines (EI^2 9:804b–805a, s.v. 'sukkar'), *sukkar ṭabarzad* is probably that, which is set hard in moulds, while *nabāt* is set on palm sticks placed in the recipient where it was being prepared.

354 '*sheqels* (Arabic *miṯqāls*)': One *mithqāl* is 4.46 grams; cf. Hinz, *Islamische Maße und Gewichte*, 4–7.

355 The standard *dirham* is 3.125 grams; see ibid., 3.

of refined sarcocol, half a *dirham* each of gum tragacanth, gum Arabic, *ṭabarzad* sugar and camphor ...).

סוכר קשה (*Sefer Ṣedat ha-Derakhim*)[356] = Arabic سكّر طبرزد '*ṭabarzad* sugar; i.e., 'fine-quality white and refined cane sugar *qand*' (cf. NA 602)[357]; cf. bk. 7, ch. 8.3 (IJZ 137, ll. 10–14): ומזה גם כן רפואה נסינו אותה ושבחנוה ישתה אותה בתחלת השנפיו והויירולא ותמהר ראותם: יקח ורדים ועדשים קלופים מ"א ארבעה דרהם לאכא מנוקה מעיציה שני דרהם זרע שומר רחב וזרע חבושים ודרגאגאן לבן מכל אחד שקל משתיק דרהם יבושל זה בליטר' מים באש רכה עד שיסור החצי וימרסהו ויסננהו וישתה ממנו רביע ליטר' עם שבעה דרהם סוכר קשה (Another remedy which I tried and found to be good which should be taken in the beginning of smallpox and measles so as to accelerate their eruption: Take four *dirhams*[358] each of the leaves of red roses and of peeled lentils, two *dirhams* of shellac cleansed from its stalks, one *mithqāl*[359] each of horse-fennel seed, quince seed and white gum tragacanth, one *dirham* of mastic. Boil this in one *raṭl*[360] of water on a low fire until half of it has dissipated; macerate and strain it and let [the patient] drink one fourth of a *raṭl* with seven *dirhams* of *ṭabarzad* sugar). Hebrew סכר קשה does not feature in the current dictionaries. Shem Tov Ben Isaac (*Sefer ha-Shimmush*, fol. 139b, col. b) renders the Arabic سكّر طبرزد as הסוכר הטברזד.

סכר הרטוב (*Sefer Ṣedat ha-Derakhim*) = Arabic السكّر السليماني '*Sulaimānī* sugar'[361]; cf. bk. 1, ch. 10 (Ms Oxford, Bodleian, Poc. 353, Uri Heb. 314, fol. 4b): או ישתה מיץ שני הרמונים עם סוכר הרטוב (Or drink the juice of the two kinds of pomegranate with *Sulaimānī* sugar). Shem Tov Ben Isaac (*Sefer ha-Shimmush*, fol. 139b, col. b) renders the Arabic السكّر السليماني as הסוכר הסלימאני.

סם: הסם הדק (*Sefer ha-Refu'ot ha-Libbiyot*) = Latin 'subtiliativa medicina' (the attenuant (refining) remedy); cf. fol. 244a: הסם הדק נאמר אותו שמדקדק עצם

356 See also the previous entry, in which we find the term سكّر طبرزد translated as סכר טוב and סוכרי קנדי; perhaps the term טוב is the first part of a faulty, defective transcription of Arabic طبرزد and should be read as טברזד.

357 Cf. previous entry.

358 The standard *dirham* is 3.125 grams; see Hinz, *Islamische Maße und Gewichte*, 3.

359 One *mithqāl* is 4.46 grams; cf. ibid., 7.

360 The weight of the *raṭl* varies according to region and period; in the eleventh and twelfth century its weight in Egypt was 437.5 grams and subsequently 450 grams. See ibid., 28–33, esp. 29.

361 '*Sulaimānī* sugar': According to D. Waines (EI² 9:804b–805a, s.v. 'sukkar'), it is sugar made from hardened red sugar broken into pieces and further cooked to remove any impurities; the name itself is perhaps connected with *Sulaimānīya*, a town and district in northeastern Iraq where sugar cane was cultivated, cf. WA 2:408–9. According to Nasrallah (NA 601–2), it is 'hard sugar-candy made from white cane sugar. However, compared with regular sugar, it is 'hotter and moister due to the way it is made'.

הליחה מתיך בקלות בחום מזוג (The attenuant remedy is that which makes the consistency of the humours thinner by light (incomplete) dissolution through moderate heat). Hebrew הסם הדק does not feature in the current dictionaries. The anonymous author of *Sammim Libbiyim* has הסם המדקדק (see entry).

הסם החותך (*Sefer ha-Refu'ot ha-Libbiyot*) = Latin 'incisiva medicina' (the incisive remedy); cf. fol. 120b: החותך הוא סם דק נוקב בין שטח האבר ושטח הליחה הדבקה עד שיפרידנו ממנו (The incisive [remedy] is the refining drug that can penetrate the area between the surface of the organ and the surface of the viscous humour, until it separates [the humour] from [the surface of the organ]). Hebrew הסם החותך does not feature in the current dictionaries. The anonymous author of *Sammim Libbiyim* has הסם המחתך (see entry).

הסם הטריאקי (*Sammim Libbiyim*) = Arabic ترياق 'theriac'; cf. fol. 122b: והט־ריאקי והבאדזהר הוא הסם אשר ישנה מזג הרוח הקורה מסם ארסיי אל מזגו הטבעי וישמרהו עליו בסגולה שבו (Theriac and antidote[362] are the remedies that change the temperament of the pneuma resulting from a toxic remedy into its natural temperament and preserve it by their specific quality). Hebrew הסם הטריאקי does not feature in the current dictionaries. For a close parallel, see Nathan ha-Me'ati's glossary to the *Sefer ha-Qanun*: באד זהאר הוא שם לכל רפואה פשוטה שיש לה כח תרייאקיי לדחות איזה ארס ואיזו סם ממית (B'D ZH'R (antidote). This is the name for every simple remedy that is effective as a theriac to expel any poison and any fatal drug) (NM 2:110, 128 (Bet 9)). The anonymous translator of *Sefer ha-Refu'ot ha-Libbiyot* renders the Latin 'medicina tyriacalis' as הצורי, cf. entries צרי and הסם הצרי.

הסם הכווה (*Sammim Libbiyim*) = Arabic الدواء الكاوي 'the caustic remedy'; cf. fol. 121b: והכווה הוא הסם אשר ישרוף העור שריפה יכלה לחותו עד שיתקבצו חלקיו ויקשהו וישוב עצם זה העור סתום המעברים <מ>ליחה נוזלת (The caustic [remedy] is that which burns the skin in such a way that it destroys its humidity and its parts are contracted. It hardens the substance of the skin so that its passages are blocked and no humour can flow through them). Hebrew הסם הכווה does not feature in the current dictionaries. The anonymous author of *Sefer ha-Refu'ot ha-Libbiyot* has הסם הכווה as well.

הסם המאדם (*Sammim Libbiyim*) = Arabic الدواء المحمّر 'the reddening (rubefacient) remedy'; cf. fol. 121a:[363] והמאדם הוא הסם אשר יחמם האבר אשר ימשכהו חמום חזק עד שימשוך אליו הדם הרקיק משיכה חזק יגיע לנראה ממנו ויאדמהו (The

362 'antidote' (B'DZHR): I.e., Arabic بادزهر, derived from Persian *pādzahr* (VL 1:315) and *pāzahr* (ibid., 319), which means 'protecting from poison' (SCP 229); see also MIG 158.

363 a יمשכהו: يماسّه.

rubefacient [remedy] is the one that heats the organ it touches[364] upon to a degree that it strongly attracts the fine blood, so that it reaches the surface [of the organ] and makes it red). Hebrew הסם המאדם does not feature in the current dictionaries. The term אידם features in BM 64 in an attestation from the *Sefer ha-Qanun*. The anonymous author of *Sefer ha-Refu'ot ha-Libbiyot* has הסם המאדם as well.

הסם המאכל (*Sammim Libbiyim*) = Arabic الدواء الأكّال 'the erosive (corroding) remedy'; cf. fol. 121a: והמאכל הוא הסם אשר יגיע מהתכתו והתבערותו[365] שיחסר מעצם הבשר (The erosive [remedy] is the one whose dissolving and ulcerating[366] [property] is such that it reduces the flesh [of the organ] itself). Hebrew הסם המאכל does not feature in the current dictionaries. The term איכל features in BM 213 as ליחה עוקצת מאכלת (biting, erosive (corrosive) humour) in an attestation from the *Sefer ha-Qanun*. This entry is missing in *Sefer ha-Refu'ot ha-Libbiyot*.

הסם המביא דם (*Sefer ha-Refu'ot ha-Libbiyot*) = Latin 'medicina sanguinis eductiva' (the hemorrhagic remedy); cf. fol. 245b: הסם המתיר השתן וזיעה וסם משלשל ומביא הדם או העוצר אותו ודומים יש להם ידיעה נגלית ולכן אינן צריכין ביאור (The diuretic, diaphoretic, purgative, hemorrhagic, styptic and similar remedies are well-known and for that reason do not need an explanation). Hebrew הסם המביא דם does not feature in the current dictionaries. The anonymous author of *Sammim Libbiyim* has הסם המגיר הדם (see entry).

הסם המבשל (*Sammim Libbiyim*) = Arabic الدواء المنضج 'the ripening (coctive) remedy'; cf. fol. 121b: והמבשל הוא הסם אשר יתקן ממשות הליחה אם היה עבה ידקדקהו בשווי ואם היה דק יעבהו עד שיתוקן לדחותו (The ripening [remedy] is the one that corrects the consistency of the humour; when it is thick, it makes it moderately thin, and if it is thin, it makes it thick until it can be expelled). Hebrew מבשל features in BM 641 as הרפואות המבשלות in an attestation from the *Sefer ha-Qanun*. The anonymous author of *Sefer ha-Refu'ot ha-Libbiyot* (fol. 244b) has הסם המבשל as well.

הסם המגיר הדם (*Sammim Libbiyim*) = Arabic الدواء مسيّل الدم 'the hemorrhagic remedy'; cf. fol. 122b: הסם המגיר השתן ולזיעה והמשלשל ומגיר הדם ועוצר אותו ומה שנשאר מאלו ענינם ידוע לא נצטרך להגדרתם[367] (The diuretic, diaphoretic, purgative, hemorrhagic, styptic and other remedies are well-known, we do not need to define them). Hebrew הסם המגיר הדם does not feature in the

364 'touches upon': Translated after a.

365 והתבערותו: وتقريحه a.

366 'ulcerating': Translated after a.

367 Ms Munich 87, fol. 124a להגדתם Ms Munich 280 להדרגתם emend. editor :להגדרתם إلى تحديد a.

current dictionaries. The anonymous author of *Sefer ha-Refu'ot ha-Libbiyot* has הסם המביא דם (see entry).

הסם המגיר לזיעה (*Sammim Libbiyim*) = Arabic الدواء المدّر للعرق 'the diaphoretic remedy'; cf. fol. 122b: הסם המגיר השתן ולזיעה והמשלשל ומגיר הדם ועוצר אותו ומה שנשאר מאלו ענינם ידוע לא נצטרך להגדרתם[368]. Hebrew הסם המגיר לזיעה does not feature in the current dictionaries. The anonymous author of *Sefer ha-Refu'ot ha-Libbiyot* has הסם המתיר הזיעה (see entry).

הסם המגיר השתן (*Sammim Libbiyim*) = Arabic الدواء المدّر للبول 'the diuretic remedy'; cf. fol.122b: הסם המגיר השתן ולזיעה והמשלשל ומגיר הדם ועוצר אותו ומה שנשאר מאלו ענינם ידוע לא נצטרך להגדרתם[369]. Hebrew הסם המגיר השתן does not feature in the current dictionaries. The anonymous author of *Sefer ha-Refu'ot ha-Libbiyot* has הסם המתיר השתן (see entry).

הסם המדביק או המחליק (*Sefer ha-Refu'ot ha-Libbiyot*) = Latin 'inviscativa seu lenificativa medicina' (the agglutinant or mollifacient remedy); cf. fol. 245a: המדביק או המחליק הוא אותו שהוא בדבקות ימתח על שטח האבר מתחלף החל־קים כמו האצטומ' או הרחם או הקנה הישר ולזה יתחדש ויסבב בהם שטח זר וחלק (The agglutinant or mollifacient (smoothing) [remedy] is the one that spreads with its viscosity on the surface of the organ whose parts are of different texture, such as [the cardia of] the stomach, uterus and trachea. In this way it produces upon them a foreign smooth surface). Hebrew הסם המדביק או המחליק does not feature in the current dictionaries. Hebrew רפואה מחליקה features in Hillel of Verona's *Sefer ha-Keritut* in the sense of 'detergent remedy' (for Latin 'medicina abstersiva'). In the same text we find דברים מחליקים in the sense of 'mollifacients' for Latin 'lenificantia'; cf. NM 2:26. The anonymous author of *Sammim Libbiyim* has הסם המטיח (see entry).

הסם המדקדק (*Sammim Libbiyim*) = Arabic الدواء الملطّف (cf. MMT 244–5) 'the attenuant (refining) remedy'; cf. fol. 120a: המדקדק הוא הסם אשר מדרכו שישים ממשות הליחות יותר רקיק בהתכה חסרה בחום שוה (The attenuant [remedy] is that which makes the consistency of the humours thinner by incomplete dissolution through moderate heat). Hebrew הסם המדקדק does not feature in the current dictionaries. The verb דקדק features in the sense of 'to make thin' in BM 986 in an attestation from the *Sefer ha-Qanun*. The anonymous author of *Sefer ha-Refu'ot ha-Libbiyot* has הסם הדק (see entry).

הסם המושך (*Sammim Libbiyim*) = Arabic الدواء الجاذب (cf. MMT 244–5) 'the attracting remedy'; cf. fol. 121a: והמושך הוא הסם אשר לו איכות עוברת מאד

368 Ms Munich 87, fol. 124a להגדתם Ms Munich 280 להדרגתם emend. editor :להגדרתם a إلى تحديد.

369 Ms Munich 87, fol. 124a להגדתם Ms Munich 280 להדרגתם emend. editor :להגדרתם a إلى تحديد.

יגיע הליחה לצד השטח אשר ימששהו אם בסגולה אם בחמום (The attracting [remedy] is the one that has a very penetrating quality (property) to move the humour which it touches upon to the surface. [It does so] either through its specific property or through heating).[370] Hebrew הסם המושך does not feature in the current dictionaries. The anonymous author of *Sefer ha-Refu'ot ha-Libbiyot* has הסם המושך as well.

הסם המחזק (*Sammim Libbiyim*) = Arabic الدواء المقوّي 'the tonic (strengthening) remedy'; cf. fol. 122b: והמחזק הוא הסם אשר ישוה מזג האבר עד שימנעהו מקבלת הפגעים אם לסגולה שבו[371] ואם לשווי מזגו ויקרר מה שהוא יותר חם ויחמם מה שהוא יותר קר לפי מה שזכרו גאלינוס בשמן הוורד (The tonic [remedy] is the one that makes the temperament of the organ balanced so that it prevents it from being affected by disorders. [It does so] either by its specific property[372] or by its moderate temperament so that it cools what is too hot and heats what is too cold, as Galen has said about rose oil). Hebrew הסם המחזק does not feature in the current dictionaries. The anonymous author of *Sefer ha-Refu'ot ha-Libbiyot* has הסם המחזק as well.

הסם המחכך (*Sammim Libbiyim*) = Arabic الدواء المحكّك 'the pruritic remedy'; cf. fol. 121a: והמחכך הוא הסם אשר יגיע מחדותו[373] שימשוך אל הנקבים ליחות עוקצות ולא יגיע אל שישחין כמו האלסכבינג[374] (The pruritic [remedy] is the one that has such a strong[375] heating power that it attracts the irritant humours towards the pores, but not to the extent of producing ulcers. An example is ranunculus[376]). Hebrew הסם המחכך does not feature in the current dictionaries. The anonymous author of *Sefer ha-Refu'ot ha-Libbiyot* has הסם המחכך as well.

הסם המחתך (*Sammim Libbiyim*) = Arabic الدواء المقطّع 'the incisive (cutting,[377] biting, pungent) remedy'; cf. fol. 120b: והמחתך הנה הוא הסם הדק אשר אפשר לו שיעבור במה שבין שטח האבר ושטח הליחה הדבקה המדובקת בו עד

370 Cf. Avicenna, *Tract on Cardiac Drugs and Essays on Arab Cardiotherapy* (*Risālah al-adwiyah al-qalbīyah*), trans. by A. Hameed (Karachi 1983), 33: 'The absorbent drug is the one which moves the humour towards the surface either by its characteristic property of coming into contact with it or by calorification'.

371 שבו: مثل الطين المختوم والترياق add. a

372 'property': 'such as sigillate earth and theriac' add. a.

373 מחדותו: من قوّته وجذبه وتسخينه a.

374 האלסכבינג: الكيكج a.

375 'strong heating power': Translated after the Arabic.

376 'ranunculus': Translated after the Arabic الكيكج. The Hebrew text has 'sagapenum' (= Arabic السكبينج); while Avicenna, *Tract on Cardiac Drugs* (trans. Hameed, 34), has 'wild celery'.

377 Cf. MMT 244–5.

שינקה אותה ממנו (The incisive [remedy] is the refining drug that can penetrate the area between the surface of the organ and the surface of the viscous humour which adheres to it, until it cleanses [the area] from it). Hebrew הסם המחתך does not feature in the current dictionaries. The anonymous author of *Sefer ha-Refu'ot ha-Libbiyot* has הסם החותך (see entry).

הסם המטיח (*Sammim Libbiyim*) = Arabic الدواء الملّس 'the smoothing remedy'; cf. fol. 122a: והמטיח הוא המתדבק אשר יתפשט על פני האבר המתחלף החלקים בהנחה ר״ל כל הנחורים כמו האצטומכא והרחם וקנה הריאה ויתדבק בהם ויתחדש עליהם שטח זר חלק (The smoothing [remedy] is the agglutinant one that spreads on the surface of the organ whose parts are of different texture in their locations, that is to say all the rough [organs], such as [the cardia of] the stomach, uterus and trachea. It sticks to them and produces upon them a foreign smooth surface). Hebrew הסם המטיח does not feature in the current dictionaries. The anonymous author of *Sefer ha-Refu'ot ha-Libbiyot*, fol. has הסם המדביק או המחליק (see entry).

הסם הממית (*Sammim Libbiyim*) = Arabic الدواء القاتل 'the lethal remedy'; cf. fol. 122b: והסם הממית הוא הסם אשר יפסיד עצם מזג הרוח והגוף אם מעצמיותו וצורתו אשר הוא מינו כמו הארסים ואם לתגבורת האיכות הפועלת בו כמו האפיון בקרירותו והאפריביון בחמימותו (The lethal [remedy] is the one that corrupts the substance of the temperament of the pneuma and the body either through its substance and specific form, such as the [different kinds of] poisons, or through the domination (strength) of the quality active in it, such as opium by its coldness or resin spurge (*Euphorbia resinifera* O. Berg) by its heat). Hebrew הסם הממית does not feature in the current dictionaries. The same term features in Zeraḥyah Ḥen's translation of Maimonides, *Medical Aphorisms* 31.34 and in the *Sefer ha-Refu'ot ha-Libbiyot*.

הסם הממעיד (Sammim Libbiyim)[378] = Arabic الدواء المزلّق 'the lubricant remedy'; cf. fol. 122a: והממעיד הוא הסם אשר יטפיח שטח גשם נעצר במעברים ויפרידהו[379] ממה שנעצר בו ואחר יתנועע זה הגשם בכבדותו הטבעי ויהיה מניע אותו במקרה והוא כמו אל<אגא>ש[380] ואללעאבאת[381] (The lubricant [remedy] is the one which moistens the surface of a substance which is blocked in a passage and cures[382] [the dryness] through which it is stuck. Then this matter moves due to its natural heaviness, [the remedy] moving it indirectly. Examples are plums and mucilages). Hebrew הסם הממעיד does not feature in the current

378 See also entry (מעד) המעיד.
379 a فيبرئه :ויפרידהו.
380 a اجّاص :ש<אגא>.
381 a اللعابات :ואללעאבאת.
382 'cures': Translated after the Arabic.

dictionaries. The term הממעיד features in BM 3146 in a similar attestation from Joseph Vidal, *Gerem ha-Maʿalot*: והממעיד הוא אשר יטפיח שטח הגשם הנעצר המעבר וירככהו וכו' ואחר יניעהו בכבד הטבע (The lubricant [remedy] is the one which moistens the surface of a substance which is blocked in a passage and softens it etc., and then moves it due to its natural heaviness). Ben Yehuda (ibid.) explains the term המעיד as החליק/השמיט. The anonymous author of *Sefer ha-Refuʾot ha-Libbiyot* has המשמיט נ"א הממעיד.

הסם הממרק (*Sammim Libbiyim*) = Arabic الدواء الجالي 'the detergent, (cleansing,[383] clearing) remedy'; cf. fol. 120b: והממרק הוא הסם אשר יכלה מן הליחה הנקפאת והדבקה מה שהיה על שטח האבר ופיות הנקבים (The detergent [remedy] is the one which annihilates viscous and thick fluids that exist on the surface of the organ and openings of the pores). Hebrew הסם הממרק does not feature in the current dictionaries. Hebrew מירק features in BM 3345 as רפואה ממרקת in an attestation from Jacob Zahalon (second half of the seventeenth century), *Ozar ha-Hayyim*. The anonymous author of *Sefer ha-Refuʾot ha-Libbiyot* has הממרק as well.

הסם המנגע (*Sefer ha-Refuʾot ha-Libbiyot*) = Latin 'ulcerativa' (ulcerative [remedy]); cf. fol. 244b: והמנגע הוא אותו שיש לו כח חזק לאדם עד שתתך הליחות הנדבקות מהחלקים שיגע בהם ומסבב החבורות ומושך להם המותרות שמהם הוות היציאות כמו סם האנקרדי (The ulcerative [remedy] is the one whose rubricating power is so great that it dissolves the humours that are stuck between the parts [of the organ] that it encounters. It causes [skin] afflictions and attracts residues from which ulcers arise. An example [of such a remedy] is marsh-nut (*Semecarpus anacardium*)).[384] Hebrew הסם המנגע does not feature in the current dictionaries. The verb ניגע features in BM 3520 in an attestation המנגעים פני העור derived from השלמת הטבע (Ms Hamburg, 308,6). The anonymous author of *Sammim Libbiyim* has הסם המשחין (see entry).

הסם המנחיר (*Sammim Libbiyim*) = Arabic الدواء المخشّن 'the roughening remedy'; cf. fol. 120b: והמנחיר הוא הסם אשר ימרק מאבר קשה העצם כמו העצמות והשחוסים והעצבים כאשר יהיה הנחת חלקי האבר מתחלפים וכבר עבר עליו לחות החליק אותו ישיבהו אל נחירותו (A roughening [remedy] is one that cleanses an organ of firm consistency such as bones, cartilages, and nerves when the composition of the parts of the organ is different and a liquid moisture has streamed over it and made it slippery and then made it rough again). Hebrew הסם המנחיר does not feature in the current dictionaries. In the sense of 'to make something rough', Hebrew הנחיר features in BM 3612 in an attestation from

383 Cf. MMT 242–3, s.v. دواء جلّاء.

384 Cf. Bos, 'Baladhur (Marking-nut)', 229–36.

the *Sefer ha-Qanun*. The anonymous author of *Sefer ha-Refu'ot ha-Libbiyot* (fol. 244a) has הסם המנחיר as well.

הסם המנפח (*Sefer ha-Refu'ot ha-Libbiyot*) = Latin 'inflativa medicina' (the remedy that produces gas (flatulence)); cf. fol. 245a: המנפח הוא אותו אשר בעצמו לחות גסה זרה מתגברת מעורבת אל היושר וכשיפעל בה החום הטבעי יוליד רוח שאינו נתך כמו הפישולש (The flatulent [remedy] is the one whose substance is dominated by a foreign thick moisture, moderately mixed. When innate heat acts upon it it produces gas that does not dissolve. An example is beans[385]). Hebrew הסם המנפח does not feature in the current dictionaries. The anonymous author of *Sammim Libbiyim* has הסם הנופח (see entry).

הסם המעבה (*Sammim Libbiyim*) = Arabic الدواء المغلّظ 'the thickening remedy'; cf. fol. 122a: הסם המעבה הפך המדקדק (The thickening remedy is the one opposite the attenuant (refining) remedy). Hebrew הסם המעבה does not feature in the current dictionaries. The anonymous author of *Sefer ha-Refu'ot ha-Libbiyot* has הסם המעבה as well.

הסם המעכל (*Sammim Libbiyim*) = Arabic الدواء الهاضم 'the digestive remedy'; cf. fol. 120b: והמעכל הוא הסם אשר ישנה המזון אל הדמות הליחות המשובחות אשר יזונו הגוף והליחות אל הדמות הגוף (The digestive [remedy] is the one that changes the food so that it becomes similar to (assimilated by) the wholesome humours that feed the body and so that these humours become similar to (are assimilated by) the body). Hebrew הסם המעכל does not feature in the current dictionaries. The term מעכל features as הכח המעכל (the digestive faculty) in BM 4471 in some attestations from medieval literature. The anonymous author of *Sefer ha-Refu'ot ha-Libbiyot* has הסם המעכל as well.

הסם המעפש (*Sammim Libbiyim*) = Arabic الدواء المعفّن 'the putrefying remedy'; cf. fol. 121b: והמעפש הוא הסם אשר יפסיד התדבקות האבר בהתכתו מה שבו מן הרוח הטבעי והתכת חומו הטבעי ולא יגיע אל שיאכלהו או יצ<י>להו או ישרפהו אבל ישאר בו לחות יתעצם בו חום בלתי טבעי (The putrefactive [remedy] is the one that corrupts the continuity of the organ through the dissolution of the natural pneuma and of the innate heat, but it does not go to such an extent as to erode, roast or burn it, but lets a moisture remain in it in which an unnatural heat is active). Hebrew הסם המעפש does not feature in the current dictionaries. Ben Yehuda (BM 4625) mentions the verb עיפש in an attestation from the *Sefer ha-Qanun*. The anonymous author of *Sefer ha-Refu'ot ha-Libbiyot* has הסם המעפש as well.

---

385 'beans' (PYŠWLŠ): I.e., Old Occ. 'faizols' or Old Cat. 'fesols'; cf. SHS 1:481 (Resh 4). The term stands for Arabic لوبيا, a sort of bean, presumably the black-eyed pea (*Vigna unguiculata* subsp. *unguiculata* (L.) Walp.) [olim: *Vigna sinensis; Dolichos lubia*]; cf. MIG 249.

הסם המפיג (*Sammim Libbiyim*) = Arabic الدواء المفجّج 'the remedy that makes crude (unripe)'; cf. fol. 122b: והמפיג הוא הסם המונע מהבשול והעכול לקרירותו כמו המים הקרים כאשר ישתו במורסות האצטומכא (The [remedy] that makes crude is the one that, because of its coldness, prevents ripening (concoction) and digestion, such as cold water when it is drunk in case of an inflammation of the stomach [lining]). Hebrew הסם המפיג does not feature in the current dictionaries. The anonymous author of *Sefer ha-Refu'ot ha-Libbiyot* has הסם המפיג as well.

הסם המרדים (*Sammim Libbiyim*) = Arabic الدواء المخدّر 'the benumbing[386] (stupefying, narcotic, soporific) remedy'; cf. fol. 122b: והמרדים הוא הסם הקר אשר יגיע מקרירותו לאבר אל שישנה עצם מה שיעבור בו מן הרוח אל מזג קר יבש יוצא ממזגו אשר בו יקבל הכוחות המרגישות והמניעות וישנה מזג האבר ככה ויבטל החוש (The benumbing [remedy] is the one that, being cold, cools an organ so much that it changes the temperament of the substance of the pneuma that passes through it into a cold and dry one. As a result it does not have the temperament any more through which [the organ] receives the perceptive faculties and those that cause movement. In this way it changes the temperament of the organ and benumbs the senses). Hebrewהסם המרדים does not feature as a medical term in the current dictionaries. Hebrew מרדים, Plur. מרדימים, features in Nathan ha-Me'ati's translation of Maimonides, *Medical Aphorisms* 8.39 (cf. NM 2:62). Ben Yehuda (BM 6451) refers to הרדים in the sense of 'to benumb the power, to benumb the senses, to weaken and paralyze them' in an attestation from the *Sefer ha-Qanun*. In the sense of 'narcotic', Hebrew מרדים features as a modern term in EM 1053. The anonymous author of *Sefer ha-Refu'ot ha-Libbiyot* has הסם המרדים as well.

הסם המרפה (*Sammim Libbiyim*) = Arabic الدواء المرخي 'the relaxant (slackening[387]) remedy'; cf. fol. 120b: והמרפה[388] הוא אשר ישים ממשות האברים קצרי הנקבים יותר רך ללחותו וחומו ויקרה מזה שישים הנקבים רחבים וידחה מה שבהם מן המותרים יותר נקל (The relaxant [remedy] is the one which renders the consistency of the organs that have constricted (hard) pores softer by its fluidity and heat so that the pores become wider and the expulsion of their superfluous contents becomes easier). Hebrew הסם המרפה does not feature in the current dictionaries. The anonymous author of *Sefer ha-Refu'ot ha-Libbiyot* has הסם המרפה as well.

386 Cf. MMT 242–3.
387 Cf. ibid.
388 Ms והמרפא emend. ed.: והמרפה.

הסם המרתיע (*Sammim Libbiyim*)[389] = Arabic الدواء الرادع 'the repellent remedy'; cf. fol. 122b: והמרתיע הוא הסם הקר אשר יחדש באבר קור יעבה אותו וייצר נקביו ויקפיא הנוזל אליו ויעבהו בכבוי חומו וימנעהו ובפרט כאשר היה עב הממשות כמו שמן הורד המקורר וה<ד>בסרקאטונא[390] וזולתה (The repellent [remedy] is the one that being cold produces coldness in an organ, condenses it, constricts its pores, congeals the [matter] that flows to it, and thickens it by extinguishing its heat and stops [its flow], especially when it is thick in consistency. Examples are cooled rose oil and [mucilage of] fleawort and the like). In the sense of 'repellent remedy', Hebrew מרתיע features in BM 6771 in attestations from the *Sefer ha-Qanun*, from Moses Narboni (*c.* 1300–62 CE),[391] *Sefer Oraḥ Ḥayyim*, and from Tuviah ha-Kohen, *Ma'aseh Tuviah*.

הסם המשבר הרוח (*Sammim Libbiyim*) = Arabic الدواء الكاسر الرياح 'the carminative remedy'; cf. fol. 122a: הסם המשבר הרוח הוא הסם אשר ישיג[392] בחומו הדק העובר מה שיקצר בו <החום> החלוש אם ישתנה הלחות אל רוח ולא יותך. ולפעמים יהיה מגיע התכתו להתיך מה שבעורקים מנפח המזונות והסמים כמו זרע רודא ואנג'ילקשטי (The carminative [remedy] is the one which corrects by its penetrating refining heat the weak [bodily] heat when it turns humidity into gaseousness and does not dissolve. Sometimes its dissolution goes to the extent that it dissolves the flatulence produced inside the vessels by foods and drugs. Examples [of carminatives] are rue and chaste tree). Hebrew הסם המשבר הרוח does not feature in the current dictionaries. The anonymous author of *Sefer ha-Refu'ot ha-Libbiyot* has הסם השובר רוח (see entry).

הסם המשחין (*Sammim Libbiyim*) = Arabic الدواء المقرّح 'the ulcerative remedy'; cf. fol. 121a: והמשחין הוא הסם אשר יפליג התאדמותו עד שיתיך הליחות המגיעות בין חלקי מה שיפגשהו ויחדש אליהם חבורות וימשוך אליהם מותרים וישוב כמו נגע וזה כמו הבלאדור (The ulcerative [remedy] is the one whose rubricating power is so great that it dissolves the humours between the parts of the organ that it encounters. It attracts residues and creates ulcers. An example [of such a remedy] is marsh-nut (*Semecarpus anacardium*))[393]. Hebrew הסם משחין does not feature in the current dictionaries. The verb השחין features in BM 7027 in the sense of 'to cause leprosy' (הכהו בשחין) in an attestation from Nathan ha-Me'ati's Hebrew translation of Maimonides, *Medical Aphorisms*.

---

389 See also entry (רתע) הרתיע.

390 a بزرقطونا: בסרקאטונא.

391 On the author and the *Sefer Oraḥ Ḥayyim*, see G. Bos 'R. Moshe Narboni, Philosopher and Physician. A Critical Analysis of *Sefer Orah Hayyim*', *Medieval Encounters* 2.1 (1995): 219–51.

392 a يتدارك Ms Munich 280, fol. 122a יתיך :(Ms Leiden, Or. 4719, fol. 165a) ישיג.

393 Cf. Bos, 'Baladhur (Marking-nut)', 229–36.

The anonymous author of *Sefer ha-Refu'ot ha-Libbiyot* has הסם המנגע (see entry).

הסם המשלשל (*Sammim Libbiyim*) = Arabic الدواء المسهل 'the purgative remedy'; cf. fol. 122b: הסם המגיר השתן ולזיעה והמשלשל ומגיר הדם ועוצר אותו ומה שנשאר מאלו ענינם ידוע לא נצטרך להגדרתם[394] (The diuretic, diaphoretic, purgative, hemorrhagic, styptic and other [remedies] are well-known, we do not need to define them). Hebrew הסם המשלשל features in BM 7199 in Plur. סמים המשלשלים in an attestation from Solomon Ibn Ayyub's Hebrew translation of Ibn Rushd's commentary on Ibn Sīnā's *'Urǧūza*, which he completed in the year 1261.[395] The anonymous author of *Sefer ha-Refu'ot ha-Libbiyot* has סם משלשל.

הסם המתיך (*Sammim Libbiyim*) = Arabic الدواء المحلّل 'the resolvent, (melting,[396] reducing) remedy'; cf. fol. 120a–b: המתיך הוא הסם אשר יתיך הליחה בהפרידו[397] אותה והוציאו אותה מן המקום אשר נסתבכה בו חלק אחר חלק עד יכלה אותו להפלגת חומו (The resolvent [remedy] is the remedy which resolves the humour by vaporizing[398] and expelling it, bit by bit, from the place where it is stuck until it annihilates it through its excessive heat). Hebrew הסם המתיך does not feature in the current dictionaries. The verb התיך features in BM 3872 in the sense of 'to melt'. The anonymous author of *Sefer ha-Refu'ot ha-Libbiyot* (fol. 244a) has הסם המתיך as well.

הסם המתיר הזיעה (*Sefer ha-Refu'ot ha-Libbiyot*) = Latin 'medicina provocativa sudoris' (the diaphoretic remedy); cf. fol. 245b: הסם המתיר השתן וזיעה וסם משלשל ומביא דם או העוצר אותו ודומים יש להם ידיעה נגלית ולכן אינן צריכין ביאור (The diuretic, diaphoretic, purgative, hemorrhagic, styptic and similar [remedies] are well-known and for that reason do not need an explanation). Hebrew הסם המתיר לזיעה does not feature in the current dictionaries. Hebrew התיר את השתן features in BM 3888 in an attestation from the *Sefer Asaph ha-Rofe*. The anonymous author of *Sammim Libbiyim* has הסם המגיר הזיעה (see entry).

הסם המתיר השתן (*Sefer ha-Refu'ot ha-Libbiyot*) = Latin 'medicina provocativa urine' (the diuretic remedy); cf. fol. 245b: הסם המתיר השתן וזיעה וסם משלשל ומביא דם או העוצר אותו ודומים יש להם ידיעה נגלית ולכן אינן צריכין ביאור. Hebrew הסם המתיר השתן does not feature in the current dictionaries. Hebrew התיר

394 Ms Munich 87, fol. 124a להגדתם Ms Munich 280 להדרגתם emend. editor :להגדרתם a إلى تحديد.

395 Cf. Steinschneider, *Hebräische Übersetzungen des Mittelalters*, 700.

396 Cf. MMS 242–3.

397 Ms Paris, BN, Arabe 5966, fol. 72b بتبخيره :בהפרידו.

398 Translated after the Arabic.

את השתן features in BM 3888 in an attestation from the *Sefer Asaph ha-Rofe*. The anonymous author of *Sammim Libbiyim* has הסם המגיר השתן (see entry).

הסם הנופח (*Sammim Libbiyim*) = Arabic الدواء المنفخ 'the remedy that produces gas (flatulence)'; cf. fol. 121b: והנופח הוא הסם בעצמיותו ליחות עבה זרה וכאשר יפעל בו החום הטבעי השוה ישתנה רוח ולא יותך כמו הלוביא (The flatulent [remedy] is the one whose substance has foreign thick moisture. When moderate innate heat acts upon it it changes into gas and does not dissolve. An example is beans[399]). The anonymous author of *Sefer ha-Refu'ot ha-Libbiyot* (fol. 244a) has הסם המנפח (see entry).

הסם הנושך (*Sefer ha-Refu'ot ha-Libbiyot*) = Latin 'mordicativa medicina' (the irritant remedy); cf. fol. 244b: הנושך הוא אותו שיש בו איכות דק נושך עושה בפרוק חבור מרבה המספר מהחלקים הקטנים ומקרובי ההנחה (The irritant [remedy] is one that has a fine irritant quality (property) of producing breaches of continuity [by breaking up] small particles with similar form in large number). Hebrew הסם הנושך does not feature in the current dictionaries. Zeraḥyah Ḥen renders the parallel Arabic term الأدوية اللذّاعة, featuring in Maimonides, *Medical Aphorisms* 21.58 as הרפואות הנושכות. The anonymous author of *Sammim Libbiyim* has הסם העוקץ (see entry).

הסם הסותם (*Sammim Libbiyim*) = Arabic الدواء المسدّد 'the obstruent (clogging[400]; stopping the pores) remedy'; cf. fol. 122a: והסותם הוא הסם אשר כאשר עבר במעברים התגבר על הכח המניע לדחותו ועמד נגד כל מציק ומלא את החלל כמו הטיט הנאכל (The obstruent [remedy] is the one that, when it passes inside the passages overcomes their motive power to expel it, and stops at every narrow and open place and fills it up. An example is edible[401] earth). Hebrew הסם הסותם does not feature in the current dictionaries. The anonymous author of *Sefer ha-Refu'ot ha-Libbiyot* has הסם הסותם as well.

הסם העוצר 1. (*Sefer ha-Refu'ot ha-Libbiyot*) = Latin 'compressiva medicina' (the astringent remedy); cf. fol. 245a: העוצר הוא אותו שהוא יבש מסבב לאבר יובש ומקבץ אותו לעצמו ולזה סותם המעברים (The astringent [remedy] is the desiccant one which produces dryness and constriction in the organ by blocking its passages). Hebrew הסם העוצר does not feature in the current dictionaries. Both, Nathan ha-Me'ati and Zeraḥyah Ḥen, render the Arabic الأدوية الحابسة (the binding remedies), featuring in Maimonides, *Medical Aphorisms* 13.28,

399 'beans' (LWBY'): I.e., Arabic لوبيا, a sort of bean, presumably the black-eyed pea (*Vigna unguiculata* subsp. *unguiculata* (L.) Walp. [olim: *Vigna sinensis; Dolichos lubia*]; cf. MIG 249.

400 Cf. MMT 242–3.

401 'edible earth': The Muslim world knew different types of 'edible earth', the most famous of which was that from Nishapur; cf. M 172.

as הרפואות העוצרות. The latter term also features in an anonymous translation of *On the Treatment of Small Children* that was attributed to al-Rāzī, whereby עוצר stands for Latin 'stipticus' (cf. ROT 33, l. 16; NM 2:180). The anonymous author of *Sammim Libbiyim* renders the parallel Arabic الدواء المقبّض as הסם הקובץ (see entry); II. (*Sammim Libbiyim*) = Arabic الدواء العاصر 'the constrictive remedy'; cf. fol. 125a: והעוצר הוא הסם אשר יגיע מקביצותו וחברו חלקי האבר קצתם אל קצת אל שיוכרחו הלחויות הרקיקים אשר יעמדו בפנימיותו אל שיתלחצו ושיתנועעו התנועה הנבדלת ממנו (The constrictive [remedy] is that whose constrictive action and joining of the parts of the organ reaches such a degree that the thin humours found in its spaces are necessarily compressed and move in a separate (opposite) direction). The anonymous translator of *Sefer ha-Refu'ot ha-Libbiyot* has הסם העוצר as well.

הסם העוצר הדם (*Sammim Libbiyim*) = Arabic الدواء الحابس الدم 'the styptic remedy'; cf. fol.122b: הסם המגיר השתן ולזיעה והמשלשל ומגיר הדם ועוצר אותו ומה שנשאר מאלו ענינם ידוע לא נצטרך להגדרתם[402] (The diuretic, diaphoretic, purgative, hemorrhagic, styptic and other [remedies] are well-known, we do not need to define them). Hebrew הסם העוצר הדם does not feature in the current dictionaries. The anonymous author of *Sefer ha-Refu'ot ha-Libbiyot* has הסם העוצר הדם as well.

הסם העוקץ (*Sammim Libbiyim*) = Arabic الدواء اللاذع 'the irritant (corrosive)[403] remedy'; cf. fol. 121a: והעוקץ הוא הסם אשר לו איכות דקה עוברת תחדש פרוק במחובר רב המספר מתקרב ההנחה קטון השעור (The irritant [remedy] is one that has a fine penetrating quality (property) of breaking up many small continuous particles that have a similar form). Hebrew הסם העוקץ does not feature in the current dictionaries. Nathan ha-Me'ati renders the parallel Arabic term الأدوية اللذّاعة, featuring in Maimonides, *Medical Aphorisms* 21.58, as הסמים העוקצים. The anonymous author of *Sefer ha-Refu'ot ha-Libbiyot* has הסם הנושך (see entry).

הסם הפותח (*Sammim Libbiyim*) = Arabic الدواء المفتّح 'the deobstruent remedy'; cf. fol. 120b: והפותח הוא אשר יגיע[404] החומר הנופל בחללות המעברים ויוציאהו לא בפיותיהם לבד (The deobstruent [remedy] is the one which not only expels the matter from the opening of the pores but also that found in the cavities of the passages by moving[405] it). Hebrew הסם הפותח does not feature in this

402 Ms Munich 87, fol. 124a להגדתם Ms Munich 280 להדרגתם emend. editor :להגדרתם a إلى تحديد.

403 Cf. MMT 242–3.

404 a يحرّك :יגיע.

405 Translated after the Arabic.

sense in the current dictionaries. The anonymous author of *Sefer ha-Refu'ot ha-Libbiyot* (fol. 244a) has הסם הפותח as well.

הסם הצרי (*Sefer ha-Refu'ot ha-Libbiyot*)[406] = Latin 'medicina tyriacalis' (theriac); cf. fol. 251a: פוסתיק: יש לו ריחניות ועפיצות עם דביקות ומפני זה הוא משמח הלב ולזה הוא נמנה בכל הסמים הצריים (Pistachio: It possesses aroma and astringency along with viscosity, and for this reason it exhilarates the heart and is counted among all the theriacs). Hebrew הסם הצרי does not feature in the current dictionaries. The anonymous author of *Sammim Libbiyim* renders Arabic ترياقات as תריאקות.

הסם הקובץ (*Sammim Libbiyim*) = Arabic الدواء المقبّض 'the astringent remedy'; cf. fol. 122a: והקובץ הוא הסם היבש אשר יחדש באבר יובש והתקבצות אל עצמו ויסתים לזה המעברים (The astringent [remedy] is the desiccant one which produces dryness and constriction in the organ by blocking its passages). Hebrew הסם הקובץ does not feature in this sense in the current dictionaries. Hebrew קובץ features in BM 5715 as מאכל קובץ in an attestation from the *Sefer ha-Qanun*. He explains the term as מאכל המקווץ את הבטן ועוצר (cf. NM 2:81). The anonymous author of *Sefer ha-Refu'ot ha-Libbiyot* has הסם העוצר (see entry).

הסם הרוחץ (*Sammim Libbiyim*) = Arabic الدواء الغسّال 'the abluent remedy'; cf. fol. 120b: והרוחץ הוא הסם אשר ימרק לא בכח פועלת בו אבל בכח מתפעלת והוא הלחות כשילך על פיות הנקבים וירכך מה שיש עליהם מן הליחות הדבקות והנקפאות בלחותו והזלתו והתערבו בהם (The abluent [remedy] is the one that cleanses not through its active power but through its passive power, namely the humidity, by flowing over the openings of the pores. Thus it softens the viscous and congealed humours which are on the openings, through its humidity, its flow, and its mixing with them). Hebrew הסם הרוחץ does not feature in the current dictionaries. The anonymous author of *Sefer ha-Refu'ot ha-Libbiyot* has הסם הרוחץ as well.

הסם השובר רוח (*Sefer ha-Refu'ot ha-Libbiyot*) = Latin 'frangitiva ventositatis medicina' (the carminative remedy); cf. fol. 245a: השובר רוח הוא הסם ממלא בחומו הדק העובר חסרון החום החלוש אשר הוא בלתי יכול להתיך הלחות המנפח כשפועל בה והתרת זאת הרפואה הגיע לפעמים להתיך הנפח ההווה בגידים מהמזונות ומהסמים כמו זרע רודא ואנגילקושט (The carminative [remedy] is the one which replenishes by its fine penetrating heat the weak [bodily] heat when this heat is so weak that it cannot dissolve, through its activity, the flatulent moisture. Sometimes dissolution of this remedy goes to the extent that it dissolves the flatulence produced inside the vessels by foods and drugs. Examples [of carminatives] are rue and chaste tree). Hebrew הסם השובר

406 In addition, the author has צרי (see entry).

רוח does not feature in the current dictionaries. The anonymous author of *Sammim Libbiyim* has הסם המשבר הרוח (see entry).

הסם השורף (*Sammim Libbiyim*) = Arabic الدواء المحرق 'the corrosive remedy'; cf. fol. 120b: והשורף הוא הסם אשר ישרוף לחות הליחות וישאיר אפריותם כמו אלפרביון ואלחלתית (The corrosive [remedy] is that which burns (evaporates) the moisture of the humours and lets their residue remain, such as resin spurge (*Euphorbia resinifera* O. Berg) and asafoetida (the gum resin of *Ferula assa-foetida* L.). Hebrew הסם השורף does not feature in the current dictionaries. The anonymous author of *Sefer ha-Refu'ot ha-Libbiyot* has הסם השורף as well.

סַמּוּר (*Sefer ha-Shimmush*) = Arabic سمّور 'sable (martes zibellina)'; cf. L 1426; D 1:683; cf. fol. 150b, col. a: הסמור חשוב וטוב אל החזה והכליות והכבד ([A garment from] sable is good and beneficial for chest, kidneys and liver). Hebrew סמור only features as a modern term in EM 1251 for 'marbled polecat' (*Vormela pergusna*); but cf. Wikipedia, entry סמור (genus *Mustela*).

סמפון: סמפונות (*Sefer Ṣedat ha-Derakhim*) = Arabic خيشوم; Plur. خياشيم '[nasal] arteries' (cf. FL 1:491: 'venae in interiore naso'); cf. bk. 2, ch. 14 (fol. 54a): ואם יקרה הרבמס מפני ליחה חמה חדה נגרת מן המוח אל הנחירים ימצא החולה מזה תגבורת שרפה בחוטם וחום ולהבה ושעירות בגרונו ובשני בסמפונות אשר מן החוטם אל הפה הנקראים כיאשם דומה לעשן (If the rheum (cold) occurs because of a hot, sharp fluid that streams from the brain to the nostrils, the patient will have a sensation of burning heat in his nose and of blazing heat and roughness similar to smoke in his throat and in the two arteries that go from the nose to the mouth and that are called [in Arabic] KY'ŠM). Hebrew סמפון (from Greek σίφων 'tube'; cf. KL 2:389; HM 150), Plur. סמפונות, is attested in Rabbinic literature in JD 982 (s.v. סימפון) in the sense of 'ramified blood-vessel, artery; bronchiae.' See also EM 1253; KTM 394. For the Aramaic parallel סמפונא, see next entry.

סמפונא: סמפונין (Aramaic) (*Sefer ha-Shimmush*) (Ms Oxford, Bodleian, Hunt. Donat 2[407]) = Arabic مجار 'passages, i.e., blood vessels'; cf. fol. 211a, col. a: ומי שלא יוכל למצוא דרך לסנגם מרוב טרדתו אם יהיה בדרך או בים צריך לקחת אחריהם דברים פותחים הסתומים ומנקים סמפוני[408] הכבד והכליות וכיס מקוה המים (And if someone is too busy to filter them (i.e. thick, turbid water), whether he is travelling by land or by sea, he should take ingredients that open the blockages and cleanse the blood vessels of the liver, intestines and urinary bladder). Aramaic סמפונא, Plur. סמפונין, features in JD 982 (s.v. סימפונא) in the sense of 'ramified blood-vessel, artery; bronchiae' with a reference to

407 Ms Paris, BN 1163 reads מזרקים (see entry), and סמפונין in a marginal gloss.

408 סמפוני (= ב): אי¹ מזרקי א.

tb*Hullin* 49a: סימפונא רבא דכבדא (the large blood-vessel of the liver)[409]; see also SDA 806, s.v. סימפונא: 'bronchus, blood vessel'. For the Hebrew parallel term סמפון, Plur. סמפונות, cf. previous entry.

סנון: סינונים (*Sefer Ṣedat ha-Derakhim*) = Arabic سنونات (cf. FL 2:361, s.v. سنون: 'dentifricium') 'dentifrices'; cf. introduction (fol. 2b): השער הכ"א בסינונים[410] אשר ינקו השנים (Chapter twenty-one: On dentifrices for cleaning the teeth). Hebrew סנון, Plur. סינונים, features in BM 4122 in the sense of 'filtering'. A variant reading שינונים, featuring in Ms London, British Library, Add. 27542, is mentioned in BM 7320 in an attestation from the *Sefer ha-Qanun*. Ben Yehuda defines Sing. שִׁנּוּן as a 'paste or powder to clean the teeth' (משחה או אבקה לנקוי השנים).

סנסן: סנסנים (*Sefer ha-Qanun*, Nathan)[411] = Arabic سنسنة, Plur. سناسن 'spinous processes' (Greek ἄκανθα) (cf. DKT 819; FAL 140, no. 3019); cf. bk. 1 (fol. 32a): ובעד השנית שהשדרה מחסה ומגן לאיברים הנכבדים המונחים לפניה ולכן ברא לה קוצים וסנסנים ([The second use] of the spinal cord is that it covers and protects the noble organs that lie in front of it. For this reason He created spines and spinous processes for it). In the sense of 'spinous process', Hebrew סנסן features in BM 4127 in an attestation from the *Sefer ha-Qanun*. Zeraḥyah Ḥen renders the Arabic شوك وسناسن as קוצים.

סְנַפִּיר: סנפירות (*Sefer Ṣedat ha-Derakhim*) I. = Arabic إبرية 'scurf, dandruff' (cf. FL 1:3: 'furfuratio capitis'; Greek: πιτυρίασις (cf. LSG 1409)); cf. introduction (Ms Oxford, Bodleian, Poc. 353, Uri Heb. 314), fol. 1b: השער הה' בסנפירות המתילדות בעור הראש (Chapter five: On scurf (dandruff) which originates on the skin of the head). As a medical term, Hebrew סְנַפִּיר features in BM 4128 in a quotation of the mentioned passage. Ben Yehuda defines the term as מין מרסה מִן המרסות הצומחות בראש, Ichtyosis (cf. MD 374), pityriosiforme(?); II. = Arabic نخالة 'scales'[412]; cf. bk. 7, ch. 19.1 (IJZ 158, ll. 11–3): הקובא שני מינים: ממנו מין שהוא שוה עם שטח הגוף והויתו ממרה שחורה מתילדת מעכירות הדם ופעמים שיהיה עמו חכוך כשיהיה החומר חזק התנועה ואמנם תתחזק כשיהיה החומר מעופש מאד או נלהב מאד. ואולם המין האחר יקרא הנכרי[413] ובו שריפה והוא בולט יוצא משטח הגוף והוא נוטה למראה[414] תכלת והקודם נוטה אל האדמימות ובמין הזה השני סנפירות[415] רב כעין

409 Cf. KTM 394, s.v. סמפון הכבד: 'Ductus hepaticus'.

410 London, British Library, Add. 27542, fol. 2a בסינונים: בשינונים.

411 Cf. entries כנף and קוץ.

412 The Arabic term, usually meaning 'bran', is a semantic borrowing from the Greek 'πίτυρον', meaning both 'bran', and a 'bran-like eruption on the skin, esp. the head, scurf, dandruff' (LSG 1409); UW 530: 'Hautschorf, Kopfkleie'.

413 a הנכרי: الوحشة.

414 a למראה תכלת: إلى الغبرة.

415 a סנפירות רב כעין מורסן: نخالة كثيرة.

מורסן ונגוב ופעמים סדיקות וחכוך (There are two kinds of eczema. In the case of one kind [the eczema] is even with the surface of the body (skin) and comes from black bile originating from turbid blood. Sometimes it is accompanied by pruritus if the matter is moving heavily. The movement of the matter becomes especially heavy when the latter is very putrid or has been affected by burning heat. The second kind is called the 'wild'[416] one. It is burning hot and protrudes and stands out from the surface of the body (skin); its color tends to that of dust, while the color of the first [kind] tends towards red. The second kind is very scaly and very dry and sometimes it has splits and is accompanied by pruritus); cf. IJZ 53 (Arabic), 113 (English), 158 (Hebrew); III. = Arabic خشكريشة 'eschar'; cf. 7.22.1: הנגעים אמנם יתילדו ממשיכת הדם וכל שכן הנגעים האדומים והם נגעים רעים שיש עמהם קדחת ועליהם סנפירות ומראיהם אדום ואדמימותם נוטה למראה אפר (Ulcers, especially red ulcers originate from the attraction of blood [to a certain spot]. These are malignant ulcers which are accompanied by fever and eschars, and their redness tends sowewhat towards ash-grey); cf. IJZ 58 (Arabic), 118 (English), 162 (Hebrew); NM 1:63.

ססי (*Sefer ha-Shimmush*)[417] I. = Arabic ما كان به خشونة 'that which is harsh, rough' (خشن) (Greek αὐστηρός 'harsh, rough, bitter'; cf. LSG 278); cf. Galen, *De alimentorum facultatibus* 2.10 (ed. Helmreich,[418] 280, ll. 17–8): μικταὶ δ' ἔκ τε γλυκείας και αὐστηρᾶς ποιότητος αἱ πλεῖσται (most [raisins] being a mixture of sweet and harsh qualities) (trans. Grant);[419] cf. fol. 137a, cols. a–b: והצמוקים הקובצים והססיים מורכבים משתי כחות כח מבשל ומתיך התכה בינוני וכח קובץ ומחזק (Astringent, harsh raisins have two powers (properties), the ripening, moderately dissolving power and the astringent, strengthening power). Hebrew ססי does not feature in the current dictionaries. In his glossary to the *Sefer ha-Shimmush*, Shem Tov Ben Isaac identifies the Hebrew term as Arabic أخرش 'rough, harsh, coarse' (cf. SHS 1:361 (Samekh 14; next entry); II. = Arabic أخرش 'rough, hard'; cf. fol. 149a: הדגים הימיים על שני מינים המין האחד האדום הנקרא רויל הנצוד בסלעי הים והדגים הססיים (There are two kinds of sea fish: the red kind that is called RWYL (i.e., mullet), that is caught between the cliffs and the kind with a rough (hard) [skin]).

סער (*Sefer Ṣedat ha-Derakhim*)[420] I. = Arabic أرق 'wakefulness, engendered by anxiety and grief; sleeplessness' (cf. L 50); cf. bk. 1, ch. 17 (fol. 25b): תאר

---

416 'wild': Cf. entry נכרי.

417 See also entry ירק ססי.

418 Galen, *De alimentorum facultatibus*, ed. by G. Helmreich, = Corpus Medicorum Graecorum 5.4.2, (Leipzig 1923).

419 Galen, *On Food and Diet*, trans. by M. Grant (London 2000).

420 See also entry צער.

עוגות ירדימו החולה כשיהיה בו סער חזק וחום חזק מחבור אצחק (A prescription of pastilles that make the patient sleep when he suffers from severe sleeplessness and high fever, composed by Isḥāq[421] [b. ʿImrān]). Hebrew סער features in the current dictionaries in the sense of 'tempest' (BM 4137–8), 'tempest, esp. fig.: of passionate acts of men' (BDB 704), and of רעש/מהומה/צרה 'tumult, disturbance, confusion, trouble, misfortune' (EM 1260); II. = Arabic كرب 'distress'; cf. bk. 1; ch. 18 (fol. 26a): ויקרה לחולה עם עלות החולי וקרוב חזקתו מקרים מפחידים כמו צמא חזק ונגוב פה ושעירות לשון ושחרותה וסער ודפיקת לב (And when the illlness becomes severe and burning hot, the patient suffers from frightening afflictions such as severe thirst, dryness of the mouth, roughness and blackness of the tongue, distress and cardialgia). Subsequently, Arabic كرب is translated as סער by Zeraḥyah Ḥen in his translation of Maimonides, *Medical Aphorisms* 13.47; cf. NM 1:173–4.

ספחת (*Sefer ha-Shimmush*) = Arabic قوباء 'eczema' (cf. IJZ 105); cf. fol. 138b, col. b: ומועיל מן הספחת והנתק כשיוטח נו (And it (i.e., citron) is good for eczema and freckles when it is rubbed on them). Hebrew ספחת features in the Bible as 'eruption, scab' (BDB 705), and in Rabbinic literature as 'rising on the skin, sore' (JD 1012), or as 'a scaly skin-disease, Pityriasis capitis, psoriasis' (LOW LXVII), cf. BM 4155: 'psoriasis' (following MD 606); for the alternative spelling מספחת, cf. SHS 1:321 (Mem 36).

סֻפַּק על (ספק) (*Sefer Issur ha-Qevurah le-Galienus*) = Arabic أشكل على 'to be difficult for'; cf. par. 75: וזה החולי יסופק על הרופאים מאד כי אין לו הוראה מדפיקת עורק ויראה בעליו מת אמתי (This condition is very difficult to handle for physicians, as there is no (reliable) method of diagnosis, [as] from the pulse, and the patient looks really dead). In the sense of 'to be difficult for', Hebrew סֻפַּק עַל is a non-attested semantic borrowing from أشكل على.

סקירה (*Sefer ha-Qanun*, Nathan) = Arabic لحاظ 'external angle of the eye' (cf. DKT 586–7, 826; FAL 82, no. 1806; FL 4:91); cf. bk. 1 (fol. 57a): והחלק השני עובר בנקב הנברא בעת[422] הסקירה[423] (The second part (i.e., of the third branch of the trochlear pair of nerves) penetrates the hole that has been created close[424] to the external[425] angle of the eye). In the sense of 'external angle of the eye', Hebrew סקירה is a non-attested semantic borrowing from Arabic لحاظ,

421 On the physician Isḥāq b. ʿImrān, teacher of Isaac Israeli and active in Qayrawān in the beginning of the tenth century and foremost known for his treatise *On Melancholy*; cf. Ullmann, *Medizin im Islam*, 125–6.

422 a בעת: عند.

423 Ms הסקירא emend. ed.: הסקירה.

424 'close to': Translated after a.

425 'the external angle': Read: 'the internal angle'; cf. DKT 587, n. 3.

read as لِحَاظ. Zeraḥyah Ḥen translates the Arabic لحاظ as עיון (see entry), and Joseph Lorki as קצה העין מצד האזן (see entry).

סתום: סתומים (*Sefer Ṣedat ha-Derakhim*) = Arabic سدّة, Plur. سدد 'obstructions'; cf. introduction (fol. 3b): השער הב׳ בסתומים המתילדים בכבד (Chapter five: On obstructions in the liver). Hebrew סתום features in Rabbinic literature in the sense of 'closing up, pasting over' (JD 1031). In a medical sense, it is mentioned in BM 4231 in an attestation from Shem Tov Ibn Falaquera, *Sefer ha-Mevakkesh* (composed in 1263): סתום הכבד. Ben Yehuda explains the term as having the same meaning as סתימה, which he explains as 'closure', clogging' (סגירה/מלוי של נקב).

(סתם) סותם: See entry **סם**.

(סתר) נסתר מן (*Sefer ha-Qanun*, Nathan) = Arabic محجوب عن 'prevented from'; cf. bk. 1 (fol. 56b): והנה זכר לנפילת החתוך הזה תועלות שלשה אחד מהם שיהיה הרוח הנוזל אל אחת האישונים בלתי נסתר מהזיל אל האחרת[426] ([The physicians] mentioned three advantages of the fact that they (i.e., the optic nerves) cross. One of these is that the pneuma that streams to one of the eyes is not prevented from streaming to the other). In the sense of 'prevented from', Hebrew נסתר מן is a non-attested semantic borrowing from Arabic محجوب عن, which can also mean 'hidden from'. Zeraḥyah Ḥen translates Arabic محجوب عن as נפסק מן, and Joseph Lorki as עצור מן.

(עבד) עִבֵּד (Sefer ha-Shimmush) = Arabic بدغ 'to fortify, to tone' (cf. D 1:423: بدغ المعدة 'fortifier l'estomac'); cf. fol. 137b, col. a: ואחרי כן מחזקים האסטומ׳ ומעבדים אותה מבלי מזיקים לעצביה (And then they (i.e., pomegranates) fortify and strengthen the stomach without causing harm to the nerves). Hebrew עִבֵּד does not feature in this sense in the current dictionaries. For a similar use of עִבֵּד by Shem Tov Ben Isaac in the *Sefer Almansur*, see NM 2:16.

(עבה) מעבה: See entry **סם**.

עבי: עובי (*Sammim Libbiyim*)[427] = Arabic متانة 'compactness, firmness, solidity'; cf. fol. 129a: כמתרי יש בו בשמיות וקביצות ועובי עצמיות (Pear (*Pyrus communis* L.) is aromatic, astringent and firm in its substance). Hebrew עבי features in BM 4274–5 in the sense of 'thickness' and in KTP 3:120 as 'Dichte, Masse, Körperlichkeit, Stofflichkeit'. The anonymous translator of *Sefer ha-Refu'ot ha-Libbiyot* renders Latin 'soliditas substantie' as עצם מקשיי.

426 Ms האחרות emend. ed.: האחרת.

427 In addition to עבי, the anonymous author of *Sammim Libbiyim* renders Arabic متانة as התקשרות (see entry).

עִגּוּל (*Sefer Ṣedat ha-Derakhim*) = Arabic شياف 'eye-salve (collyrium)[428]'; cf. bk. 2, ch. 1 (fol. 42b): ומזה תואר עגולים לבנים כוללים מועילים בע״ה לקצידה החמה והדפיקה (Recipe of white eye-salves (collyria) that are generally, God willing, good for hot ophthalmia[429] and throbbing pain). Hebrew עגול does not feature in this sense in the current dictionaries; cf. BM 4301–3, EM 321. Moses Ibn Tibbon renders the same Arabic term with the Rabbinic Hebrew term קילור (cf. NM 1:112).

עגול הארכובה (*Sefer ha-Qanun*, Nathan)[430] = Arabic رصفة 'patella' (cf. DKT 570–5, 818; FAL 126, no. 2777); cf. bk. 1 (fol. 54a): ויש לו שתי קצוות אחד מהם בשריי ומתחבר בעגול הארכובה קודם שיהיה מיתר והאחר קרומיי מתחבר בקצה הפנימי משתי קצוות פחד הירך ([This muscle] (i.e., of the knee joint) has two ends, one is fleshy and inserted on the patella before becoming a tendon, and the other which is membranous is inserted on the inner end of the thigh bone). Hebrew עגול הארכובה is not attested in the current dictionaries. Zeraḥyah Ḥen transcribes the Arabic رصفة as רצפה (see entry), and Joseph Lorki as חולית הארכובה (see entry).

העגול השחור שבבשר (*Sefer ha-Qanun*, Nathan)[431] = Arabic لَبّة[432] (Greek σφαγή) (cf. DKT 608–9, 826; WKAS 2.1:84b) 'fossa iugularis, jugular fossa'; cf. bk. 1 (fol 61a): אמנם החלק העולה משני חלקי האוריטי הנה הוא מתחלק לשני חלקים הגדול שבהם מתחיל עולה אצל סביב העגול השחור שבבשר הנקרא ליפה (The ascending part of the two parts of the aorta divides into two parts. The largest goes upwards towards the jugular fossa which is called LYPH [in Arabic] ...). Hebrew העגול השחור שבבשר is not attested in the current dictionaries. Zeraḥyah Ḥen transcribes the Arabic لَبّة as לכה (read: לבה); Joseph Lorki translates it as אמצע החזה (see entry).

עגז (*Sefer ha-Qanun*, Nathan)[433] = Arabic عجز 'sacrum' (cf. DKT 486–7, 821; FAL 6, no. 99); cf. bk. 1 (fol. 35b): הפרק אחד עשר בנתוח העגז (Chapter eleven: On the anatomy of the sacrum). Hebrew עגז is a loan word from Arabic عجز (cf. SRP 42 (326): 'buttocks'). In the glossary to the *Sefer ha-Qanun*, Nathan defines the term as שם פרק במקום הפרשות (The name of a limb (bone) that is located in the region of the 'ramifications' (pelvic girdle)); cf. BM 2:117, 153 (Ayin 1).

---

428 For Arabic شياف in the sense of 'suppository', cf. entry פתילה.

429 'ophthalmia' (קצידה): See NM 3:206 and Gerrit Bos, 'Two Notes on A Complete Dictionary of Ancient and Modern Hebrew', *Ha-Lashon* (forthcoming).

430 In addition to עגול הארכובה Nathan translates Arabic عين الركبة, a synonym of رصفة as מגן הארכובה (see entry).

431 The same term features as שחור השר (= הבשר) in fol. 63a.

432 a لثة emend. De Koning (DKT 609, n. 1): لَبّة.

433 A Hebrew term used by Nathan for 'sacrum' is העצם הרחב (see entry), which is a loan translation of Arabic العظم العريض.

Zeraḥyah Ḥen renders the Arabic عجز as זקן (see entry), and Joseph Lorki as עצם הטבעת (see entry).

עגזי: See entry **עצב**.

עדשה[434]: **עדשי הפנים** (*Sefer Ṣedat ha-Derakhim*) = Arabic كلف 'freckles' (cf. WKAS 1: 323); cf. introduction (Ms Oxford, Bodleian, Poc. 353, Uri Heb. 314, fol. 1b): השער הכ״ה בעדשי הפנים והוא אלכלף (Chapter twenty-five: On freckles, i.e., [Arabic] *kalaf*). Hebrew עדשי הפנים features in BM 4350 in an attestation from Pseudo-Ibn Ezra, *Sefer ha-nisyonot*.[435] Instead of עדשי הפנים, Ms London, British Library Ar. Or. 26, fol. 3a, has נתק, a term also featuring in Shem Tov Ben Isaac, *Sefer Almansur* (cf. NM 2:15–6).

עוג (*Sammim Libbiyim*) = Arabic عجن 'to knead'; cf. fol. 134b: וישמר שיושמו הסמים האחרים על ענינם ויועג כמו שזכרנו (And take care to add the other ingredients as they are and knead them in the way that I mentioned). Hebrew עוג features in the Bible in the sense of 'to bake' (cf. KB 794; BM 4351). Ben Yehuda also gives an attestation from *Sefer Refu'ah le-Rambam* (ed. Grossberg): ותעוג בהם שאר הסמנים, but does not give its specific meaning of 'to knead'.

עֲוִוּת I. (*Sefer Ṣedat ha-Derakhim*) = Arabic مغص (Greek στρόφος; cf. UW 644) 'colic'; cf. introduction (fol. 3b): השער הי״ג בעוות והמשברים הוא אל מגת ובלע' טרנקדש (Chapter thirteen: On colic and MŠBRYM (?), i.e., [Arabic] مغص and Romance ṬRNQDŠ[436]). As a medical term, Hebrew עוות features in BM 4361 in an attestation from the commentary by the otherwise unknown Jacob bar Joseph Ibn Zabara on Hippocrates' *Aphorisms*, and is defined by Ben Yehuda as synonymous with עוית 'convulsion'. For the composition of this commentary Ibn Zabara extensively used Moses Ibn Tibbon's Hebrew translation of Maimonides' commentary on the *Aphorisms* (cf. NM 3:11). In the sense of 'colic', Hebrew עוות also features in Hillel of Verona's translation of Hippocrates' *Aphorisms* 5.41 (cf. NM 3:172); II. (*Hanhagat ha-Beri'ut le-Abu 'Ali Ben Zuhr*) = 'twitching' (cf. Honofredi: 'tortura'); cf. ch. 28: עוות הפנים חזק הכח יבשר באלקוה שיקרב חדושה וראוי כאשר ירגיש זה שיעשה שלשול חזק ויחפף הפנים בחומץ יין חזק כבר הורתח בהם פודנג' וימעט המזון וירחיק השתיה בכלל ויעשה גרגרים ועטושים (A severe twitching of the face indicates that facial paresis is about to occur. When one feels this one should use a strong purgative and wash the face with strong wine vinegar in which mint has been

434 'עדשה': Thus EM 1881; according to Ben Yehuda (BM 4349–50), Sing. is עדש.

435 Cf. *Sefer Hanisyonot. The Book of Medical Experiences attributed to Ibn Ezra*, ed. by J. O. Leibowitz and S. Marcus (Jerusalem 1984), 184, l. 5.

436 'ṬRNQDŠ': I.e., 'trencadas', Plur. of Old Occ. 'trencada' (stomach ache) (LR 5:416b; cf. also FEW 13.2:280b, s.v. '*trinicare', modern Occ. 'trincado' (colique très aiguë). I thank Julia Zwink for this reference.

cooked. One should take little food and not drink at all and apply gargles and sternutatories).

אותם שיראו בעוות (*Sefer ha-Qanun*, Zeraḥyah) = Arabic أحول, Plur. حول 'squinting'; cf. bk. 1 (fol. 30a): ועל כן יקרה לאותם שיראו בעוות שיראו הדבר שני דברים בסור אחת משתי הבבות לצד מעלה או לצד מטה (For this reason those who squint see a single object as if it is double when one of the pupils turns upwards or downwards). Hebrew אותו שיראה בעוות, Plur. אותם שיראו בעוות, is not attested in the current dictionaries; see also NM 2:179, 'עוות ההבטה' for Latin 'obliquitas aspectus'. For the other translator(s), see entry (עות) מעוות הראות.

עורק: העורק התרדמיי (*Sefer ha-Qanun*, Nathan) = Arabic العرق السباتي 'carotid artery' (DKT 584–5, 822; FAL 77, no. 1707); cf. bk 1 (fols. 56b–57a): שריג יוצא ממבוא העורק התרדמיי (One branch (i.e., of the third pair of encephalic nerves) passes through the entry of the carotid artery). Hebrew העורק התרדמי is not attested in the current dictionaries. Zeraḥyah Ḥen translates the Arabic العرق السباتي as הגיד הנקר' סובאת ופירושו תרדמה. A translation of this term is missing in Joseph Lorki.

העורקים הנחים (*Sefer ha-Qanun*, Nathan) = Arabic العروق الساكنة 'non-throbbing vessels, veins' (cf. DKT 822; FAL 77, no. 1704); cf. bk. 1 (fol. 63a): אמנם העורקים הנחים הנה צמיחת כלם מן הכבד (All veins emerge from the liver). In the sense of 'non-throbbing vessel, vein', Hebrew העורק הנח is a non-attested loan translation from Arabic العرق الساكن. Zeraḥyah Ḥen renders the Arabic العروق الساكنة as הגידים הנחים (see entry), Joseph Lorki has הגידים הנחים as well.

מעוות הראות (עות) (*Sefer ha-Qanun*, Nathan) = Arabic أحول, Plur. حول 'squinting'; cf. bk. 1 (fol. 56b): לכן יקרה למעוות[437] הראות הנק' נירש שיראה הדבר כשני דברים בעת שתטה אחת האישונים למעלה או למטה (For this reason those who squint (which is called NRYŠ) see a single object as if it is double when one of the pupils turns upwards or downwards). Hebrew מעוות הראות does not feature in the current dictionaries. Zeraḥyah Ḥen translates the Arabic حول as אותם שיראו בעוות (see entry עוות).

עטרה: עטרת המלך (Zeraḥyah Ḥen's translation of Maimonides, *Medical Aphorisms* (forthcoming ed. Bos))[438] = Arabic إكليل الملك 'melilot, king's clover (*Melilotus officinalis*)'[439]; cf. 21.69: הרפואות החמות בראשונה היבשות מאותן שמשמשין אותן שבעה ועשרים והם אורז ואנזרוט אשטוכדוס אסמרינו הנקרא בעברי עטרת המלך (There are twenty-seven drugs that are hot and dry in the

---

437 Ms[1]: למעוות.

438 Cf. entry כתר מלכות.

439 The Arabic term can also stand for other species of *Leguminosae*, e.g. crown vetch (*Coronilla emerus* L.), or scorpion vetch (*Coronilla scorpioides* Koch; cf. DT 3:40 (388)).

first [degree] and which are commonly used: rice, sarcocol, French lavender, ʾSMRYNW (read: RSMRYNW), called in Hebrew ʿṬRT HMLK, i.e., melilot ...). Hebrew עטרת המלך does not feature in the current dictionaries. In his translation of the same aphorism, Nathan ha-Meʾati renders the Arabic as Romance מלילוט; in the *Sefer Ṣedat ha-Derakhim*, Moses Ibn Tibbon renders it as כתר מלכות (see entry).

עטרי (*Sefer ha-Qanun*, Zeraḥyah) = Arabic إكليلي 'coronal'; cf. bk. 1 (fol. 17a): ומן הראשונים חוליה משותפת עם המצח והוא עשוי כקשת וזה צורתו (ונקרא העטרי (To the first sutures belongs one that is common with the frontal bone and shaped like a bow, and this is its shape (, and called the coronal suture). Hebrew עטרי, adjective coined from עטרה does not feature in the current dictionaries. For the other translator(s), cf. entry כלילי.

עיון (*Sefer ha-Qanun*, Zeraḥyah) = Arabic لحاظ 'external angle of the eye'; cf. DKT 586–7, 826; FAL 82, no. 1806); cf. bk. 1 (fol. 30a): והחלק השני יעבור בנקב הנברא במקום[440] העיון (The second part (i.e., of the third branch of the trochlear pair of nerves) penetrates the hole that has been created close to the external[441] angle of the eye). In the sense of 'external angle of the eye', Hebrew עיון is a non-attested semantic borrowing from Arabic لحّاظ, read as لِحَاظ. For the other translator(s), see entry סקירה.

עין הארכובה: עין (*Sefer ha-Qanun*, Zeraḥyah) = Arabic عين الركبة 'patella' (cf. DKT 510–1, 818; FAL 126, no. 2777); cf. bk. 1 (fol. 22b): וראשה נעשה עם תחבולה ברצפה והיא עין הארכובה (The front of it (i.e., the knee joint) has been craftily prepared with the *raṣfa*; i.e., the patella). Hebrew עין הארכובה features in MD 552, s.v. 'patella', referring to the *Sefer ha-Qanun*; see also SRP 26 (164). For the other translator(s), see entry מגן הארכובה.

עין הכתף (*Sefer ha-Qanun*, Nathan) = Arabic عين[442] الكتف 'the process of the scapula that is shaped like the Arabic letter *ʿayin*'; i.e., the spine of the scapula (cf. DKT 494–5, 824) (Greek: σιγμοειδής; cf. LSG 1596: 'of the shape of sigma; crescent shaped, semi-circular')[443]; cf. bk. 1 (fol. 37a): והתוספת הזאת היא כמו הסנסן לחוליות נבראים לשמירה ונקרא עין הכתף (Just like the spinous processes, this process (apophysis) has been created for protection and is called '*ʿayin* of the scapula'). Hebrew עין הכתף, a combination of the

440 a במקום: عند.

441 'the external angle': Read: 'the internal angle'; cf. DKT 586–7.

442 a عير emend. De Koning (DKT 495, n. 1): عين.

443 My translation is based on Singer-Rabin (SRP 22 (118)) who—as the translation 'eye of the scapula' is unintelligible—suggest that the Arabic term عين الكتف does not mean 'eye of the scapula' (cf. FAL 6) but 'the *ʿayin* of the scapula', i.e., the Arabic letter *ʿayin*, as it closely resembles the Greek uncial sigma. For an extensive discussion, see FAL 97, nos. 2276–7.

Hebrew transcription of the Arabic letter عين and Hebrew כתף (i.e., shoulder blade) features in BM 4446 as a Hebrew term without further explanation with an attestation from Joseph Lorki's version of the mentioned quotation: והתוספת הזאת כמו הסנאסן בחוליות נבראת להגן ונקראת עין הכתף. For an extensive discussion of the Hebrew term, see SRP 22 (118). Zeraḥyah Ḥen translates Arabic عين الكتف as עין הכתף as well.

עינים (*Sefer ha-Qanun*, Nathan) = Arabic عين, Dualis عينان (*K. al-Qānūn*, ed. by Bulaq, 1877), but cf. emend. De Koning (DKT 497, n. 4: عتبتان (= Greek βαθμίς, Plur. βαθμίδες) (lit. 'thresholds'); i.e., 'the olecranon and coronoid fossa [of the humerus]' (cf. FAL 27, no. 510); cf. bk. 1 (fol. 38a): ואבוקראט קרא אלו שתי נקרות שני עינים (Hippocrates called these two cavities 'two eyes' (read: two thresholds, i.e., the olecranon and coronoid fossa). Hebrew עינים is based on the corrupt Arabic version عينان which should be read as عتبتان (see above). Zeraḥyah Ḥen renders the Arabic عينان as עינות.

עכוב: עכוב השתן (*Sefer ha-Shimmush*) = Arabic عسر البول 'dysuria'; cf. fol. 136a, col. a: ויש פחד מן הפטריות שאינם ממיתים שלא יקרה מהן חניקה וגנוח ועלוף וקרירות הידים והרגלים ועל הרוב ירדוף אותן שלשול וקיא חזקים (And if someone takes mushrooms that cause non-fatal [poisonings], he has to fear that he will suffer from quinsy, asthma, fainting, cold hands and feet, and in most cases he will be attacked by severe cholera). Hebrew עכוב השתן does not feature in the current dictionaries. Hebrew synonyms, featuring in translations of Hippocrates' *Aphorisms*, are עיצור השתן (*Sefer Agur*); עוצר השתן (Moses Ibn Tibbon and Zeraḥyah Ḥen); קושי השתן (Anonymous); קשי יציאת השתן (Nathan ha-Me'ati); דיסוריאה (Hillel of Verona), and קשי ההשתנה (Joseph Delmedigo) (cf. NM 3:179).

עכול: העכול השני (*Sefer ha-Shimmush*) = Arabic الهضم الثاني 'the second digestion' (i.e., that in the liver)[444]; cf. fol. 135a, col. b: והממעט מאכילתו חי אחר האכילה יתמעטו רוחותיו העת ההיא וירפה המעים ויעבור בקלות המזון בגידים ויחזק העכול השני אשר בכבד (If someone eats a little bit of it (i.e., radish) after the meal while it is fresh he will at that time hardly have any flatulence, his stools will be soft, his food pass easily through the vessels, and his second digestion in the liver will be strong). Hebrew העכול השני does not feature in the current dictionaries. Ben Yehuda (BM 4468–9) mentions the first and third digestion in

444 Following Galen, medieval doctors considered the physiology of nutrition in terms of three orders of digestion: the first in the stomach, the second in the liver—the major nutritive organ where the food is turned into blood—and the third in the rest of the organs which the nutriments reach via the veins; cf. Maimonides, *On Asthma* (ed. Bos, 1:8, and 124, n. 1).

attestations from Tuviah ha-Kohen's *Ma'aseh Tuviah*, and Jacob Ben Joseph Zabara's translation of Hippocrates' *Aphorisms*.

עכירות: עכירות הראות (*Hanhagat ha-Beri'ut le-Abu 'Ali Ben Zuhr*) = 'clouded (blurred) vision' (cf. Honofredi: 'obscuritas oculorum'); cf. 34: הרחיק עצמך מהאכילה מעכירות הראות בלילה (Avoid eating at night so that you are safe from (do not suffer from) clouded (blurred) vision). Hebrew עכירות on its own features in BM 4470, o.a., as עכירות החושים in an attestation from Moses Narboni,[445] *Sefer Oraḥ Ḥayyim*.

(עכל) מעכל: See entry **סם**.

עלה: עלה בשנים (*Sefer Ṣedat ha-Derakhim*) = Arabic مسنّ 'advanced in years, old' (cf. Ms Oxford, Bodleian, Poc. 353, Uri Heb. 314, fol. 10a): ואם עלה בשנים או היה חלוש ראוי שנזהר מהוצאת הדם ויסתפק על מה שזכרנו מהרפואה הכללית והפרטית (If he (i.e., someone suffering from apoplexy) is advanced in years or weak we should be careful not be extract blood but contend ourselves to give him the general and particular treatment that we mentioned). Hebrew עלה בשנים does not feature in the current dictionaries.

עִלָּה: העלה הרוחנית (*Shemot ha-Mashqim*) 'disorder of the spiritual members';[446] cf. 18 (57): דיאה קלמינטום ... בשעת שכיבה עם[447] בשול ריגליסיאה מנוק<ה> כנגד העלה הרוחנית (Dyacalamentum ... When the patient goes to bed, with a[448] decoction of purified licorice for disorders of the spiritual members). Hebrew העלה הרוחנית does not feature in the current dictionaries.

עלקא (Aramaic) (*Sefer ha-Shimmush*) = Arabic علق 'leech'; cf. fol. 126b. col. a: והנותן גריסיהם על מקום העלקא יפסיקו הדם (If their broth (i.e., of broad beans) is put on the spot of the leech it stops the bleeding). Aramaic עלקא is attested for Rabbinic literature only; cf. SDA 869. In the Glossary to the *Sefer ha-Shimmush*, Shem Tov Ben Isaac translates the Arabic علق as Hebrew נימי המים and as Romance (Old Occ.) 'eruges' (cf. SHS 1:343 (Nun 15)). The same Romance term (for the Arabic علق) features in the *Sefer Ṣedat ha-Derakhim*, bk. 2, ch. 6 (fol. 46a).

עמוד: העמוד העליון (*Sefer ha-Qanun*, Joseph Lorki)[449] = Arabic الزَند الأعلى 'radius' (cf. FAL 172, no. 3683); cf. bk. 1 (fol. 12b): ואמנם פרק המרפק מתחבר מפרק העמוד העליון ופרק התחתון עם קנה הזרוע (The elbow is formed by the articulation of

---

445 On the author and the *Sefer Oraḥ Ḥayyim*, see Bos, 'R. Moshe Narboni, Philosopher and Physician', 219–51.

446 'spiritual members': Bodily members involved in breathing (and so in taking in air and spirit), namely the lungs, the trachea, and the epiglottis; cf. entry האברים הישרים.

447 cum decoctione enule et liquiritie munde L: עם בשול ריגליסיאה מנוק<ה>.

448 'a decoction of purified licorice': 'a decoction of elecampagne and prepared licorice' L.

449 Cf. entry זנד.

the radius, ulna and humerus). Hebrew העמוד העליון does not feature in the current dictionaries. For the other translator(s), see entry הזנאד הֶעליון.

העמוד התחתון (*Sefer ha-Qanun*, Joseph Lorki) = Arabic الزند الأسفل 'ulna' (cf. FAL 172, no. 3684); cf. bk. 1 (fol. 12b): ואמנם פרק המרפק מתחבר מפרק העמוד העליון ופרק התחתון עם קנה הזרוע. Hebrew התחתון, read העמוד התחתון, features in MD 747, s.v. 'ulna', with a reference to Saul Tchernichowsky. For the other translator(s), see entry הזנאד התחתון.

שני עמודים (*Sefer ha-Qanun*, Joseph Lorki) = Arabic الزندان 'the two bones of the forearm' (radius and ulna) (cf. DKT 497, n. 6; SRP 24 (142); FAL 172, no. 3682)[450]; cf. bk. 1 (fol. 12b): הזרוע מחובר משתי עצמות דבקות ונקראים שני עמודים (The forearm is composed of two bones that are attached to each other and that are called the two *zand*). In the sense of 'bone of the forearm', Hebrew עמוד features in MD 747, referring to Saul Tchernichowsky. For the other translator(s), see entry זנד.

עמידה (*Sefer ha-Qanun*, Zeraḥyah) = Arabic وقوف 'maturity'; cf. bk. 1 (fol. 18a): וברוב הם צומחות באמצע זמן הגדול והוא אחר היותו רואה קרי עד שיגיע אל העמידה כי העמידה קרובה משלשים שנה ועל כן נקראות שני[451] החלומות (In most cases [wisdom teeth] appear during the time of growth, namely from the time that one has a noctornal pollution until one reaches maturity. For [one reaches] maturity at about thirty years and therefore [these teeth] are called 'wisdom teeth'[452]). Hebrew עמידה does not feature in this sense in the current dictionaries. Nathan ha-Me'ati renders the Arabic وقوف as העמדה (see entry).

עֹמֶק: העומק אשר בעליון אחורי הצואר (*Sefer Ṣedat ha-Derakhim*) = Arabic نقرة 'the nape of the neck (Nackengrube, fovea nuchae)'[453]; cf. bk. 1, ch. 10 (fol. 14b): ואם היה חלוש ולא תהיה בו קדחת נשים לו כוסות המציצה בחיצון כל אחד משוקיו גבוה טפח מן העקב או נשים כוסות המציצה בעומק אשר בעליון אחורי הצואר (If [the patient] is weak but does not suffer from fever one should put a cupping glass on the outside of [one of] his legs, one span above the heel, or on the nape of the neck). Hebrew העומק אשר בעליון אחורי הצואר does not feature in the current dictionaries. Arabic نقرة also features in Maimonides, *Medical Aphorisms* 12.43, and is translated by Nathan ha-Me'ati as הנקרה בעורף (cf. entry נקרה above), and by Zeraḥyah Ḥen as חולית הצואר.

---

450 Arabic *zand* originally means 'one of a pair of sticks used for producing fire' (cf. L 1257).

451 שני החלומות: أسنان الحُلُم (a: أسنان الحِلْم).

452 See entry שן: שני החלומות.

453 Cf. FL 4:321, s.v. نُقْرَةٌ: 'Scrobs in occipitis inferiore parte (ubi desinit pars protuberantior occipitis); HA 188–90.

עמקי (*Sefer ha-Shimmush*) = Arabic سهلي '[growing] in the plains'; cf. fol. 135a, col. b: האספרגוס שני מינים: עמקי והררי (Asparagus (*Asparagus officinalis* L.) consists of two kinds: [one variety that grows] in the plains and [another variety that grows] in the mountains). Hebrew עמקי, adjective coined from עֵמֶק, does not feature in the current dictionaries.

ענב (*Sefer ha-Shimmush*) = Arabic حبّ 'berries'; cf. fol. 139a. col. b: עינבי ההדס הקרירות והיבישות גוברים עליהם (Myrtle berries are dominated by cold and dryness). Hebrew ענב features in the Bible in the sense of 'grape(s)' (cf. BDB 772) and in Rabbinic literature in the sense of 'grapes with the tendrils, also berry' (JD 1091). The term עינבי ההדס features in *Mishnah Sukkah* 3.2. as ענבי הדס and is mentioned in LW 3:666; BM 5574.

הענבית :ענבי (*Sefer Ṣedat ha-Derakhim*) = Arabic العنبية 'the grapelike [tunic]'; Latin 'uveon'; cf. bk. 2, ch. 6 (fol. 45b): ואם יהיה החולי מפני לחות עבה עומדת בין הכפורית והענבית ראוי שנצוה החולה להקיז הגיד העליון ויוציא מן הדם בשעור הצורך והכח (But if the illness (i.e., dullness of sight, amaurosis)[454] is caused by thick moisture between the crystalline and grapelike [tunic] we should order that the patient be bled from the cephalic vein and that as much blood is extracted as is necessary and as the patient can tolerate). In the sense of 'grapelike [tunic]', Hebrew ענבית features in BM 4575, a.o. as ענבי in an attestation from Judah Ben Barzillai's *Commentary on Sefer Yetsirah*, and as המחיצה הענבית in an attestation from Samuel Ibn Tibbon's translation of Maimonides, *Guide of the Perplexed*.[455] Shem Tov Ben Isaac, Moses Ibn Tibbon's contemporary, renders Arabic الطبقة العنبيّة as הגלד הענבי (cf. NM 1:82). According to Masie (MD 756, s.v. 'uvea'), the term ענבית can already be found in the *Sefer Asaph ha-Rofe*.

מעונג (ענג) (*Sefer Ṣedat ha-Derakhim*) = Arabic راهق 'adolescent'; cf. bk. 1, ch. 6 (fol. 11a): ויעשה מאילו הטיחות מהם תאר טיחה מועילה בע"ה מן המוגלא והנגעים שיהיו בראש וכל שכן במעונגים והבחורים והוא מנוסה (The following liniments may be used: One of them is a liniment that is, God willing, beneficial for weeping [spots] and ulcers occurring on the head, especially of adolescents and juveniles—it has been proved). Hebrew מעונג features in BM 4576 in the sense of 'someone who is used to luxury, pleasure'; cf. EM 1002–3. Hillel of Verona uses the term מעונג to render Latin 'delicatus' (soft); cf. NM 1:30.

ענן (*Sefer Ṣedat ha-Derakhim*) = Arabic ضبابة 'cloud in the eye'; 'mist over the eyes' (Greek νεφέλη, cf. UW 434: 'Wolke im Auge' or ἀχλύς, cf. ibid. 154: 'Nebelschleier vor den Augen', LSG 297: 'a mist over the eyes'); cf. bk. 2, ch. 6, fol. 46b): תאר עגולים טובים מועילים מן הענן והדמע והאכול ויובש העפעפים מסבות

454 See entry אפל above.

455 For a detailed discussion of the term הענבית, cf. KDS 90–2.

עשנים כרכומיים (A recipe for collyria that are good and beneficial for a cloud in the eye, persistent flow of tears (epiphora), gangrene, and dryness of the eyelids, caused by bilious vapors). In the sense of an eye disease (מחלה בעין), Hebrew ענן features in BM 4599 in an attestation from the *Sefer ha-Qanun*.

עִסּוּי (*Sefer ha-Qanun*, Nathan) = Arabic عَصْر 'extraction, evacuation'; cf. bk. 1 (fol. 52a): אמנם הבטן הנה עצליו שמנה ישתתפו בתועלות ומהם העזרה[456] על עסוי[457] איזה מה בקרבים מן היציאה והשתן (The abdomen has eight muscles which share a common purpose. One of these is to assist the evacuation of the feces and urine in the bowels). As a medical term, Hebrew עסוי features in BM 4617 and is defined by Ben Yehuda as the name of an illness; cf. NM 3:177–8, with an attestation from Nathan's translation of Hippocrates' *Aphorisms* 7.27, where it stands for Arabic زَحير 'tenesmus'. Zeraḥyah Ḥen translates Arabic عَصْر as לעצור, and Joseph Lorki as סחיטה.

עסיס (*Sefer ha-Shimmush*) = Arabic رُبّ 'rob' (i.e., fruit juice boiled down to syrup); cf. fol. 132, col. b: ואחר להרגיל אחד מן העסיסים החמוצים אם הוא בעל מזג חם (Then he should take (as part of the treatment of inebriety) one of the sour robs if he has a hot temperament). Hebrew עסיס only features in the current dictionaries in the sense of 'pressed out juice' (BDB 779; EM 1350); 'must, young wine' (JD 1098; BM 4607–8).

עפיצות (*Sefer ha-Refu'ot ha-Libbiyot*) I. = Latin 'stipticitas' (astringency); cf. fol. 249a: ועם זה יש בו דקות והנה ניאות ברוח לריחניותו ועפיצותו (Besides, it (i.e., the myrtle) has refining [power] and it is favorable to the pneuma because of its aroma and astringency). Hebrew עפיצות features in BM 4616, a.o., in an attestation from Nathan ha-Me'ati's translation of Maimonides, *Medical Aphorisms*, where it stands for Arabic عفوصة (sharpness, acridity). The term is explained by Ben Yehuda as 'the taste of something that is sharp, sour' (טעם של דבר שהוא עפוץ). The anonymous translator of *Sammim Libbiyim* renders the parallel Arabic قبض as קביצות; II. = Latin 'pontificas' (acridity, bitterness) (cf. LRM 359, s.v. 'ponticiticas'); cf. fol. 250a: מיראבולמש קיבולש ואינדיש קרים בראשונה ויבשים בשניה ולהם עפיצות שמורה על שיש לו קביצות עצמי (Chebulic or Indian myrobalan is cold in the first and dry in the second [degree]. Its acridity indicates that it has a natural astringency). The anonymous translator of *Sammim Libbiyim* (fol. 127a) renders the parallel Arabic عفوصة as עפיצות as well.

עפצי (*Sefer ha-Refu'ot ha-Libbiyot*) = Latin 'stipticus' (astringent); cf. fols. 247a–b: אבל אותם שאומרים שהוא קר מתחלפים ג״כ שקצתם מניחים קרירותו בראשונה וקצתם בשניה אבל ידמה שהוא בסוף הראשונה ויובשו בשנית מפני זה הוא מהרפואות

456 Ms העזר ל? emend. ed.: העזרה על.

457 Ms עסוי איזה עסוי בקרבים emend. ed.: עסוי איזה מה בקרבים.

העפציות (But those who say that it (i.e., emblic myrobalan) is cold also disagree; some say that it is cold in the first [degree] and others [say that it is cold] in the second [degree]. But it seems that it [is cold] in the end of the first [degree] and dry in the second [degree]. On this account it is included in the astringent remedies). Hebrew עפצי features in BM 4619 in attestations from Tuviah ha-Kohen's *Ma'aseh Tuviah* and from Isaac Satanow's commentary on Aristotle's *Nicomachean Ethics*. Ben Yehuda (BM 4619) explains the term as עפוץ (sharp, sour). The anonymous translator of *Sammim Libbiyim* renders the parallel Arabic قابض (astringent) as קובץ (cf. NM 1:81).

מעפש (עפש): See entry **סם**.

עץ (*Sefer ha-Shimmush*) = Arabic عود 'stalk, stem'; cf. fol. 127a, col. b: ולתבל הבשר בכוסבר הלח ובצלים ועץ של שבת ושרשי כרשין וכשיצטמקו העדשים לשפוך מימיהם ולרחצם במים אחרים חמים (And season them (i.e., the lentils) with fresh coriander, onions, aneth stems, and leek root. When the lentils are boiled down, pour the [remaining] water out, and wash them with new hot water).[458] Hebrew עץ features in the current dictionaries in the general sense of 'tree' or 'wood' (cf. BM 4627–30). In the Bible, we find the term in the sense of 'stalk' or 'stem' in Js 2:6: עצי פשתן (stalks, stems of flax) (KB 864).

עצב: העצב אשר בו ילך השמע (*Sefer Ṣedat ha-Derakhim*) = Arabic العصب الذي يجري فيه السمع 'the acoustic (auditory) nerve'; cf. bk. 2, ch. 7 (fol. 47b): ואם לא נראה דבר מזה וראינו נקב האזן בריא אין בו נזק ידענו כי העצב אשר בו ילך השמע כואב ואם היה כאב העצב השומע מפני מותר עב קר דבק או מפני רוח עבה או מורסא קרה ... אז ראוי לשלשל המותרות ההם (But if we do not see anything of this but see that the ear canal is clean and not damaged we know that the acoustic (auditory) nerve is painful, and if the pain of the acoustic nerve is caused by a cold, thick, viscous superfluity or thick wind or cold swelling ... we should evacuate those superfluities). Hebrew העצב אשר בו ילך השמע is an unattested calque of Arabic العصب الذي يجري فيه السمع. In addition to this term, Ibn Tibbon has העצב השומע (see entry).

העצב החוזר (*Sefer ha-Qanun*, Zeraḥyah) = Arabic العصب الراجع 'recurrent laryngeal nerve' (cf. DKT 590–1, 822; FAL 24, no. 455); cf. bk. 1 (fol. 30b): ועל כן נקרא[459] העצב החוזר (For this reason they are called 'recurrent laryngeal nerves'). Hebrew העצב החוזר features in MD 502, s.v. 'nervus recurrens', referring to the *Sefer ha-Qanun*. For the other translator(s), see entry העצב החוזר למפרע.

---

458 Cf. entry צמק: הצטמק.

459 Ms נקרב emend. ed.: נקרא.

העצב החוזר למפרע (*Sefer ha-Qanun*, Nathan)[460] = Arabic العصب الراجع 're-current laryngeal nerve' (cf. DKT 590–1, 822; FAL 24, no. 455); cf. bk. 1 (fol. 58a): ולכן נקר' העצב החוזר למפרע. Hebrew העצב החוזר למפרע features as העצב החוזר in MD 502, s.v. 'nervus recurrens', referring to the Hebrew translation of the *K. al-Qānūn*. Zeraḥyah Ḥen and Joseph Lorki translate the Arabic العصب الراجع as העצב החוזר (see entry).

העצב השומע (*Sefer Ṣedat ha-Derakhim*) = Arabic العصبة السامعة 'the acoustic (auditory) nerve' (cf. FAL 25, no. 468); cf. bk. 2, ch. 7 (fol. 47b): ואם לא נראה דבר מזה וראינו נקב האזן בריא אין בו נזק ידענו כי העצב אשר בו ילך השמע כואב ואם היה כאב העצב השומע מפני מותר עב קר דבק או מפני רוח עבה או מורסא קרה ... אז ראוי לשלשל המותרות ההם (But if we do not see anything of this but see that the ear canal is clean and not damaged we know that the acoustic (auditory) nerve is painful, and if the pain of the acoustic nerve is caused by a cold, thick, viscous superfluity or thick wind or cold swelling ... we should evacuate those superfluities). Hebrew העצב השומע is an unattested calque from the Arabic العصبة السامعة. In addition to העצב השומע, Ibn Tibbon has העצב אשר בו ילך השמע (cf. entry).

[העצבים] העגזיים (*Sefer ha-Qanun*, Nathan) = Arabic العصب العجزي 'nerves of the sacrum; sacral nerves'; cf. bk. 1 (fol. 60a): הזוג הראשון מן העגזיים מתערב בקטניים כפי האמור[461] (The first pair of the sacral [nerves] mixes with the coccygeal nerves, as has been said (before)). Hebrew עגזי is a non-attested adjective coined from עגז (see entry). Zeraḥyah Ḥen translates the Arabic العصب العجزي as עצבי עצם הזקן (see entry זקן), and Joseph Lorki as עצב פי הטבעת (see entry עגז).

[העצבים] הקטניים (*Sefer ha-Qanun*, Nathan) – Arabic العصب القطني 'nerves of the coccyx'; cf. bk. 1 (fol. 60a): הזוג הראשון מן העגזיים מתערב בקטניים כפי האמור[462]. Hebrew קטני is a non-attested adjective coined from קטן (see entry). Zeraḥyah Ḥen translates the Arabic العصب القطنية as עצבי עצם הקוטן, and Joseph Lorki as עצבי עצם המתנים.

עצביות (*Sefer ha-Qanun*, Nathan) = Arabic عصبانية 'having the property of a nerve, membrane'; cf. bk. 1 (fol. 50a): והאחר יותר קצר ממנו ופתיליו אל ההתרחבות וקצהו יותר חזק העצביות (The other [pronator muscle] is shorter, has broad fibers and is more membranous at the end). Hebrew עצביות is a non-attested loan translation from the Arabic عصبانية. Zeraḥyah Ḥen and Joseph Lorki translate the Arabic عصبانية as עצבי.

460 In addition to העצב החוזר למפרע, Nathan (ibid.) translates Arabic العصب الراجع as העצבים החוזרים לאחור.

461 a قيل Ms האחור emend. ed.: האמור.

462 a قيل Ms האחור emend. ed.: האמור.

עִצּוּר: עצור המעים (*Sefer ha-Shimmush*) = Arabic حبس البطن ‘constipation’; cf. fol. 142a, col. b: ותקונם ודחית נזקם לרוצה לתתם עוזרים לעצור המעים מבלי נזק לקלותם או לצלותם על האפר החם (To improve [their quality] and undo their harm (i.e., of chestnuts), if someone wants to give them as a remedy for constipation without [causing harm], one should roast them or grill them in hot ashes). Hebrew עצור המעים does not feature in the current dictionaries. Ben Yehuda (BM 4641) mentions the occurrence of עִצּוּר in the general sense of ‘closure of the body openings’ in an attestation from Meir Aldabi’s *Shevilei Emunah*; see also NM 2:179, s.v. עִצּוּר. In the *Sefer Agur*, we find the term עיצור הבטן for ‘constipation’ (cf. NM 3:178–9).

עִצּוּם: עיצום (*Sefer ha-Shimmush*) = Arabic زحير ‘tenesmus’ (Greek τεινεσμός; cf. UW 669); cf. fol. 146b, col. a: חלב הבקר יותר עב מכל החלבים ויותר רחוק מן העכול והירידה ויותר כבד על האסטומ׳ ושלשולו הבטן יותר מועט אלא שהוא זן יותר מכל החלבים ועל כן חלבם מועיל מן השלשול המררי והעיצום הכרכומי (Cows’ milk is thicker than all the other [kinds of] milk, it is harder to be digested and to go down, it is heavier on the stomach, and it is not so good for relieving the bowels, but it is more nutritious than all the other [kinds of] milk. For this reason [cow’s] milk is good against bilious diarrhea and tenesmus [and discharge of] yellow bile). Hebrew עצום does not feature as a medical term in the current dictionaries. The same Hebrew term is used by Shem Tov Ben Isaac in the *Sefer Almansur* to render Arabic سحج (Greek κοιλιακός; cf. UWS 1: 567: ‘dysentery’); see NM 2:16. Arabic زحير also features in Hippocrates’ *Aphorisms* 7.27 and is rendered by Moses Ibn Tibbon as Romance פונץ, by Nathan ha-Me’ati as עסוי, by Zeraḥyah Ḥen as שלשול מעיים הנק׳ בערבי זחיר, and by the anonymous translator as שלשול של זחיר עצור. Judah Shalom has טנשמון, *Sefer Agur* עיות הבטן and Joseph Delmedigo עסוי (cf. Nathan) (cf. NM 3:172–3).

העיצום וההפשטה (*Sefer ha-Shimmush*) = Arabic سحوج الأمعاء ‘intestinal abrasion’ (for Arabic سحوج, Greek ἀπόσυρμα, cf. UW 126); cf. fol. 125a, col. b: הארז אמר אסחק כי הארז חם בתחלת המעלה הראשונה ואמר זולתו כי הוא קרוב מן השווי. והלחם העשוי ממנו יזון פחות מלחם החטה ויותר מתאחר להתעכל ועוצר המעים ומועיל מן העיצום וההפשטה ומן השחין המתהוה בהם (Rice: Isaac [Israeli] said that rice is hot in the beginning of the first degree; and someone else said that it is nearly moderate. Bread prepared from [rice] is less nutritious than wheat bread and slower to digest; it binds the bowels, and is good for intestinal abrasion and intestinal ulcers). Hebrew העיצום וההפשטה does not feature in the current dictionaries. For עיצום, used by Shem Tov Ben Isaac in *Sefer Almansur* as a translation of Arabic سحج, see previous entry. A cognate of הפשטה, namely הפשט for Arabic سحج, features in Nathan ha-Me’ati’s translation of Maimonides, *Medical Aphorisms* 21.27 (cf. NM 2:40–1).

עצל: העצל הישר מעצלי הבטן (*Sefer ha-Qanun*, Nathan) = Arabic العضل المستقيم من عضل البطن (the rectus abdominis muscle); cf. bk. 1 (fols. 48b–49a): ומזה זוג אצל קצוותיהם ומתדבק באמצע החזה מה שבין השחוס[463] הנקר' אלחנגרי והתרקוה ומתדבק לעצל הישר מעצלי הבטן (Another pair [of muscles] is situated at the ends of the sides [of the chest] and is attached to the sternum between the xiphoid cartilage and the clavicle and joins the rectus abdominis muscle). Hebrew העצל הישר מעצלי הבטן does not feature in the current dictionaries. Zeraḥyah Ḥen translates the Arabic العضل المستقيم من عضل البطن as המושקלו הישר מן מושקלו של הבטן.

העצל המחזיר לאחור (*Sefer ha-Qanun*, Joseph Lorki) = Arabic العضل المدير 'rotator muscles'; cf. bk. 1 (fol. 16a): היותר גדולים בעצלי הירך הם המותחים אותו אח"כ אשר יקבצנו ... ואחריה העצל המרחיק ואחריו המקרב ואחריו המחזיר לאחור (The largest muscles of the thigh are the ones that extend it; next to them are those that flex it, after these come the abductor muscles, then the adductor muscles, and finally the rotator muscles). Hebrew העצל המחזיר לאחור is not attested in the current dictionaries. For the other translator(s), see entry העצל המסבב.

העצל המסבב (*Sefer ha-Qanun*, Nathan) = Arabic العضل المدير 'rotator muscles'; cf. bk. 1 (fol. 53a): הגדול שבעצלי פחד הירך הוא אותו אשר יפשיטהו ואחריו אותו אשר יקבצהו ... ואחריו העצל המרחיק ואחריו העצל המקרב ואחר העצל המסבב. Hebrew העצל המסבב is not attested in the current dictionaries; the term מסבב on its own features as מסובב in MD 636, s.v. 'rotator'. Zeraḥyah Ḥen translates the Arabic العضل المديرة as המושקלו המסביב, and Joseph Lorki as העצל המחזיר לאחור (see entry).

העצל המקרב (*Sefer ha-Qanun*, Nathan) = Arabic العضل المقرب 'adductor muscles'; cf. bk. 1 (fol. 53a): הגדול שבעצלי פחד הירך הוא אותו אשר יפשיטהו ואחריו אותו אשר יקבצהו ... ואחריו העצל המרחיק ואחריו העצל המקרב ואחר העצל המסבב. Hebrew העצל המקרב is not attested in the current dictionaries; the term מקרב on its own features in MD 12, s.v. 'adductor'. Zeraḥyah Ḥen translates the Arabic العضل المقربة as המושקלו המקרבת.

העצל המרחיק (*Sefer ha-Qanun*, Nathan) = Arabic العضل المبعد 'abductor muscles'; cf. bk. 1 (fol. 53a): גדול שבעצלי פחד הירך הוא אותו אשר יפשיטהו ואחריו אותו אשר יקבצהו ... ואחריו העצל המרחיק ואחריו העצל המקרב ואחר העצל המסבב. Hebrew העצל המרחיק is not attested in the current dictionaries. Zeraḥyah Ḥen translates the Arabic العضل المبعدة as המושקלו המרחק.

עצלה (*Sammim Libbiyim*) 1. = Arabic بلادة 'amentia'; cf. fol. 128b: כנדר: לבונה אליבנום חם בשניה יבש בראשונה מחזק הרוח אשר בלב ואשר במוח ולזה הוא מועיל מן העצלה והשכחה (Frankincense, *levonah* (Hebrew); olibanum (Latin); it is hot

463 Ms השחוסי emend. ed.: השחוס.

in the second and dry in the first [degree]; it strengthens the pneuma in the heart and brain; therefore it is good for amentia and amnesia). Hebrew עצלה features in BM 4645 in the sense of 'indolence, laziness'. The anonymous translator of *Sefer ha-Refu'ot ha-Libbiyot* renders Latin 'ebetudo' as גסי השכל (those who have a coarse brain); II. = Arabic كلال 'weariness, fatigue'; cf. fol. 130a: נינופר: הוא קרוב במשפטו מן הכאמפור אלא שהוא יותר לח ולחותו תחדש ברוח אשר במות עצלה ורפיון (Water lily: In its actions it is close to camphor. However, it is more moist and its moisture produces fatigue and weakness in the pneuma that is in the brain). The anonymous author of *Sefer ha-Refu'ot ha-Libbiyot* has Hebrew עצלה for Latin 'pigrities'.

עצם: עצם אבניי (*Sefer ha-Qanun*, Nathan) = Arabic عظم حجري (lit. 'stony bone'); i.e., 'the petrous part of the temporal bone'; cf. DKT 823; FAL 28, no. 535); cf. bk. 1 (fol. 57b): וגם המוצא אשר יש לו בעצם אבניי קשה סובל נקבים רבים (Their exit (i.e., of the nerves of the temples) in the petrous part of the hard stony bone endures many holes). Hebrew עצם אבניי, a loan translation of the Arabic عظم حجري, is not attested in the current dictionaries. Zeraḥyah Ḥen translates the Arabic عظم حجري صلب as עצם קשה כאבן, and Joseph Lorki as עצם כאבן קשה.

העצם הדומה ללמד בכתיבת היוונים (*Sefer ha-Qanun*, Nathan)[464] = Arabic العظم الشبيه اللام في كتابة اليونانيين 'the bone resembling the letter L in the Greek alphabet'; i.e., the hyoid bone' (cf. DKT 516–7, 823; FAL 28, no. 544); cf. bk. 1 (fol. 42b): הנה כל העצמות אם מנית אותם יהיו רמ"ח לבד השומשמניים ובלעדי העצם הדומה ללמד[465] בכתיבת היוונים[466] (If you count all the bones they number two hundred and forty-eight, except for the sesamoid bones and the hyoid bone). Hebrew העצם הדומה ללמד בכתיבת היוונים does not feature in the current dictionaries or secondary literature. A variant reading של עצם הלמדא features in MD 364, s.v. 'hyoid'. Joseph Lorki translates the Arabic العظم الشبيه اللام في كتابة اليونانيين as העצם הנק' לאמי דומה אל הלמד היונית.

עצם דומה לעצמות הקוביא (*Sefer ha-Qanun*, Zeraḥyah) = Arabic نردي 'cuboid bone'; cf. DKT 512–3, 823; FAL 29, no. 550); cf. bk. 1 (fol. 23a): ואחד מהם עצם דומה לעצמות הקוביא והוא עשוי בששה פנים מונחים על הצד החיצון (One of these (i.e., of the tarsal bones) is the cuboid bone made of six sides [and] lies on the outer side [of the foot]). For עצם דומה לעצמות הקוביא as featuring in Zeraḥyah's translation, cf. SRP 28 (180). Aramaic קוביא (from Greek κυβεία) is attested for in Rabbinic literature in the sense of 'dice (playing)', cf. JD 1323; HM 188. For the other translator(s), see entry עצם תרדי.

---

464 See also entries למד, למדי, and העצם הלמדי.

465 add. Ms ללמד: הדומה.

466 Ms היוונית emend. ed.: היוונים.

עצם החזה (*Sefer ha-Qanun*, Zeraḥyah) = Arabic قصّ 'sternum' (cf. FAL 123, no. 2697); cf. bk. 1, ch. 15 (fol. 20b): הפרק הט"ו בניתוח עצם האנצולא והוא עצם החזה. זה העצם הוא מחובר משבעה עצמות ולא מעצם אחד כמו שנודע בו בשאר המקומות מן התועלת (Chapter fifteen: On the anatomy of the 'ṢM ha-'NṢWL', i.e., sternum. The sternum is composed of seven bones. Because of its use it was not made from one bone as we know from other places). In the sense of 'sternum', Hebrew עצם החזה features in MD 677, s.v. 'sternum' (cf. SRP 22 (121)). For the other translator(s), see entry אמצע החזה.

עצם החלצים (*Sefer ha-Qanun*, Zeraḥyah) = Arabic عظم الخاصرة 'ilium' (cf. FAL 28, no. 542); DKT 506–7, 823); cf. bk. 1 (fol. 22a): וכל אחד מהם יחלק אל ארבעה חלקים ומה שסמוך לצד החיצון נקרא בער' אלכרקפה ועצם החלצים (Each one of them (i.e., the two hip bones) is divided into four parts. The outer part is called in Arabic *al-ḥarqafa*[467] and [in Hebrew] 'ṢM ha-ḤLṢYM). Hebrew עצם החלצים does not feature in the current dictionaries. For the other translator(s), see entry עצם הכסל.

עצם הטבעת (*Sefer ha-Qanun*, Joseph Lorki)[468] = Arabic عجز 'sacrum' (cf. DKT 486–7, 821; FAL 6, no. 99); cf. bk. 1 (fol. 12a): פרק י"א בנתוח עצם הטבעת (Chapter eleven: On the anatomy of the sacrum). As featured in the *Sefer ha-Qanun*, the term עצם הטבעת is discussed as עצם פי הטבעת in SRP 42 (326). For the other translator(s), see entry עגז.

עצם הכסל (*Sefer ha-Qanun*, Nathan) = Arabic عظم الخاصرة 'ilium' (cf. FAL 28, no. 542; DKT 506–7, 823); cf. bk. 1 (fol. 40a): וכל אחד מהם מתחלק לד' חלקים ואשר יטה לצד החיצונים נקרא אלחרכפא ועצם הכסל (Each one of them (i.e., the two hip bones) is divided into four parts. The outer part is called [in Arabic] *al-ḥarqafa*[469] and [in Hebrew] 'ṢM ha-KSL). Hebrew עצם הכסל features in MD 529, s.v. 'os ilei'; see also SRP 35 (238). Zeraḥyah Ḥen renders Arabic عظم الخاصرة as עצם החלצים (see entry).

עצם הכתף (*Sefer ha-Qanun*, Nathan) = Arabic عظم الكتف 'scapula' (cf. FAL 28, no. 541); cf. bk. 1 (fol. 49a): וחמשה עצלים צמיחתם מעצמות הכתף מהם עצל תולדתו מעצם הכתף ומתחבר[470] מה שבין החוצץ והצלע העליון לכתף (There are five [other] muscles [of the arm] which arise from the scapula. One of them arises from the scapula and[471] occupies the [space] between the spine and

467 '*al-ḥarqafa*' (ilium): Cf. DKT 506–7, 816; FAL nos. 1525–6.

468 In addition to עצם הטבעת, Joseph Lorki translates Arabic عجز as פי הטבעת (cf. entry העצבים העגזיים).

469 '*al-ḥarqafa*' (ilium): Cf. DKT 506–7, 816; FAL nos. 1525–6.

470 a ומתחבר: وتشغل.

471 'and occupies': Translates after Arabic وتشغل.

the superior border of the scapula). Hebrew עצם הכתף does not feature in the current dictionaries.

העצם הלמדי (*Sefer ha-Qanun*, Nathan)[472] = Arabic العظم اللامي 'the hyoid bone' (cf. DKT 540–1, 823; FAL 28, no. 544); cf. bk. 1 (fol. 47b): העצלים המניעים הלשון הם תשעה שנים רחבים באים מהתוספות[473] החיציות ומתחברים בצדדיו ושנים ארוכים צמיחתם מעליוני העצם הלמדי (There are nine muscles which move the tongue. Two transverse [muscles] come from the 'arrow-like' (styloid) processes and are inserted into the sides [of the tongue]. Two longitudinal [muscles] originate from the upper parts of the hyoid bone …). Hebrew העצם הלמדי features in Nathan's glossary to the *Sefer ha-Qanun*. Nathan remarks that he called it thus because of its resemblance to the Greek letter Lambda: למד: באמרי עצם למדי להדמותו לאות למד יונית (cf. NM 2:115 (Lamed 3), 144). Zeraḥyah Ḥen translates the Arabic العظم اللامي as עצם הלמדי, and Joseph Lorki as עצם הלאמי.

עצם מקום שער הרגלים (*Sefer ha-Qanun*, Joseph Lorki) = Arabic عظم العانة '1. hip bone; 2. pubic bone' (cf. DKT 823; FAL 25, nos. 528–9); cf. bk. 1 (fol. 18a): ולפי שאין[474] לעצל הצומח מצד מקום עצם שער הרגלים דרך אל הרגלים מאחורי הגוף ומפנימי הירכים לרוב מה ששם מהעצלים[475] והגידים (And because [the nerves for] the muscles that come from the region of the pubic bone cannot go to the legs through the posterior parts of the body, nor through the inner parts of the thighs, because of the large number of muscles and veins being there …). Hebrew עצם מקום שער הרגלים does not feature in the current dictionaries. For the other translator(s), see entry גב הערוה.

עצם העמוד (*Sefer ha-Qanun*, Joseph Lorki) = Arabic طروخانطير[476] (emend. De Koning, DKT 569, n. 4; see also ibid. 821; FAL 132, no. 3278) (= Greek τροχαντήρ; 'trochanter'; cf. LSG 1828); cf. bk. 1 (fol. 16a): ומהם עצל תולדתו בכל שטח עצם עצמות הכסלים ויתדבק בעליון עצם העמוד הגדול (Another [muscle of the thigh] that originates from the whole outer side of the ilium and is inserted in the top of the large trochanter). Hebrew עצם העמוד is not attested in the current dictionaries. For the other translator(s), see entry טרוחמטרא.

העצם הרחב (*Sefer ha-Qanun*, Nathan)[477] = Arabic العظم العريض 'sacrum' (cf. DKT 570–1; FAL 28, no. 531); cf. bk. 1 (fol. 53b): ואמנם מטים לחוץ הם שני עצלים

472 See also entries למד, למדי, and העצם הדומה ללמד בכתיבת היוונים.
473 Ms מהתוספת emend. ed.: מהתוספות.
474 a ولما لم يكن للعضل Ms שהעצל emend. ed.: שאין לעצל.
475 a من العضل Ms מהעצבים emend. ed.: מהעצלים.
476 a (*K. al-Qānūn*, 1:51) طروخابطير: طروخانطير.
477 In addition to העצם הרחב, Nathan has עגז, a loan word from the Arabic (see entry).

אחד מהן בא מן <העצם>[478] הרחב (There are two muscles which abduct the thigh. One of these arises from the sacrum). Hebrew העצם הרחב does not feature in the current dictionaries. Zeraḥyah Ḥen translates the Arabic العظم العريض as העצם הרחב as well. This particular sentence is missing in Joseph Lorki, Ms Paris, BN, 1136, fol. 16a.

העצם השוה (*Sefer ha-Qanun*, Joseph Lorki) = Arabic الزورقي 'navicular or scaphoid bone'; cf. DKT 512–3, 818; FAL 173, no. 3701); cf. bk. 1 (fol. 13b): ועצמות כף הרגל כ״ו ... והעצם השוה ובו חלל הרגל הנקרא אכמץ (The foot has twenty-six bones ... the navicular (scaphoid) bone through which the hollow of the foot called ʾḪMṢ[479] is formed). For Hebrew העצם השוה, cf. SRP lxxxi, and 27 (176); for the other translator(s), see entry זורקי.

העצם שעל האמה (*Sefer ha-Qanun*, Zeraḥyah) = Arabic إعظام العانة 1. 'ossa innominata' (the hip bones); 2. 'ossa pubis' (pubic bones) (cf. DKT 506–7; 823; FAL 28, no. 529); cf. bk. 1, ch. 25 (fol. 22a): הפרק הכ״ה בניתוח העצם שעל האמה (Chapter twenty-five: On the anatomy of the hip bones). As featured in the *Sefer ha-Qanun*, Hebrew העצם שעל האמה is discussed in SRP 42 (326), and translated as 'the bone above the penis'. For the other translator(s), see entry עצמות גב הערוה.

העצם השפל (*Sefer ha-Qanun*, Zeraḥyah) = Arabic الزند الأسفل 'ulna' (cf. FAL 172, no. 3684); cf. bk. 1 (fol. 21a): ואמנם פרק היד הוא מחובר מפרק הזינד העליון והוא העצם הסמוך לעצם השפל שניהם מחוברים יחד (The elbow is formed by the articulation of the radius, which is the bone that is close to the ulna, [and] both are connected). Hebrew העצם השפל does not feature in the current dictionaries. For the other translator(s), cf. entry הזנאד התחתון.

עצם תרדי (*Sefer ha-Qanun*, Nathan) = Arabic عظم نردي 'cuboid bone' (cf. DKT 512–3, 823; FAL 29, no. 550); cf. bk. 1 (fol. 41b): ואחד מהם ע<צ>ם תרדי כמשושה[480] מונח על הצד החיצוני (One of these (i.e., of the tarsal bones) is the cuboid bone which resembles a hexagon [and] lies on the outer side [of the foot]). Hebrew תרדי is a corruption of נרדי, a transcription of Arabic نردي; cf. SRP 28 (180–2). Zeraḥyah Ḥen translates the Arabic عظم نردي as עצם דומה לעצמות הקוביא (see entry); Joseph Lorki transcribes the Arabic as ברדי (cf. SRP 28 (180)).

עצמות גב הערוה (*Sefer ha-Qanun*, Nathan) = Arabic إعظام العانة 1. 'ossa innominata' (the hip bones); 2. 'ossa pubis' (pubic bones) (cf. FAL 28, no. 529); DKT 506–7; 823); cf. bk. 1, ch. 25 (fol. 40a): הפרק עשרים וחמש בנתוח עצמות

478 a העצם> הרחב: العظم العريض a<.

479 ''ḪMṢ': I.e., Arabic أخمص (cf. DKT 512–3, 813; FAL 2, no. 24).

480 a כמשושה: كالمسدس a.

גב הערוה (Chapter twenty-five: On the anatomy of the hip bones). Hebrew עצמות גב הערוה features in MD 530 as עצם גב הערוה, s.v. 'os pubis'. For גב הערוה, cf. BM 668 (and ibid., n. 1), NM 2:33, and SRP 34–5 (235). Zeraḥyah Ḥen renders Arabic إعظام العانة as העצם שעל האמה (see entry).

עצמות קטנים (*Sefer ha-Qanun*, Zeraḥyah) = Arabic سلاميات 'phalanges' (cf. DKT 504–5, 819; FAL 144, no. 3118); cf. bk. 1 (fol. 22a): ונדבקו העצמות הקטנים הנקראים בער׳ סולימיית כלם בראשים מחודדים נכנס[481] בהם אותם הראשים וביניהם לחות ויזקוסו (All the phalanges that are called in Arabic *sulāmayāt* are articulated by sharp processes and by articular depressions which fit together and hold a viscous secretion). Hebrew עצם קטן, Plur. עצמות קטנים, does not feature in this sense in the current dictionaries. For the other translator(s), see entry פרק: פרקי האצבעות.

עוצר (עצר): See entries **כח** and **סם**.

עָקֵב (*Sefer ha-Qanun*, Nathan) = Arabic عَقِب 'calcaneus' (cf. DKT 512–3, 823; FAL 22, no. 398); cf. bk. 1 (fol. 41b): עצמות כף הרגל ששה[482]... ועקב בו משען קיום (The foot has six[483] bones ... the calcaneus which gives firm support [to the heel]...). In the sense of 'calcaneus', Hebrew עקב features as עצם העקב in MD 122; see also SRP 37 (267, 271).

עקב (*Sefer ha-Qanun*, Nathan) = Arabic عَقَب 'ligament, fibrous tissue' (cf. DKT 516–7, 823; FAL 22, no. 395; FL 3:190): 'nervi seu tendines, quibus chordae conficiuntur'; cf. bk. 1 (fol. 42b): ודקדק הבורא והצמיח מן העצמות דבר דומה בעצבים נקרא עקבים[484] וקשורים להתחברם עם העצבים ומסתבכים בו כדבר אחד (In his kindness the Creator made something grow on the bones resembling nerves—called [in Arabic] 'aqabim'—and ligaments. He has attached them to the nerves and interlaced them with the nerves). In the sense of 'ligament, fibrous tissue', Hebrew עקב is a non-attested loan word from the Arabic. Zeraḥyah Ḥen transcribes the Arabic عَقَب as עקבא, and Joseph Lorki as חזוק (see entry).

עקום: עקום הפה (*Sefer Ṣedat ha-Derakhim*) = Arabic لقوة 'paralysis of the facial nerve' (cf. WKAS 2.2:1134): 'paralysis of the facial nerve, facial paresis, paralysis of one side of the face, crooked mouth (*Spasmus cynicus, Risus sardonicus*)'; cf. bk. 1, ch. 23 (fol. 34a): והקשה ממנו מה שיחשך בו הדבור ויקרה עמו עקום הפה (And a severe [hemiplegia] is one in which one cannot speak and suffers from paralysis of the facial nerve). Hebrew עקום הפה does not feature in the current dictionaries. Hebrew synonyms featuring in medieval medical

---

481 a متداخلة :נכנס בהם אותם הראשים.

482 a ستّة وعشرون :ששה.

483 'six': The Arabic text has 'twenty-six'; cf. trans. Joseph Lorki, s.v. העצם השוה.

484 corr. Ms בעקבים Ms בנקבים emend. ed. :עקבים.

literature are עיקום (Moses Ibn Tibbon's translation of Maimonides, *Regimen of Health* 4.18, 27; עִוּוּת הפה (Zeraḥyah Ḥen's translation of Maimonides, *Medical Aphorisms* 20.69); עקימת הפה (*Sefer Hanhagat ha-Beri'ut*) (see next entry); עוות הפנים (cf. Isaac Todros, המאמר בלאקואה; cf. ed. Bos[485]); and נטית הפה (see entry).

עקימת הפה: עקימה (*Sefer Hanhagat ha-Beri'ut*)[486] = 'paralysis of the facial nerve'; cf. 8.5 (154): אז ינקה הגוף ממנה בסמים המנקים אותה נפרדים או מורכבים פן תוליד בו בטול כל הגוף או חציו ועקימת הפה (... then he should cleanse the body from it (i.e., the phlegm) with purgatives, simple or compound, so that they do not cause a total paralysis or a partial one (hemiplegia), and paralysis of the facial nerve). Hebrew עקימת הפה does not feature in the current dictionaries.

עקיצה (*Sefer ha-Shimmush*) = Arabic لذع 'burning, biting [pain]' (cf. WKAS 2.2:514b–517a); cf. fol. 137a, col. a: והם משקיטים העקיצה אשר תהיה באסטומכא (They (i.e., raisins) alleviate the burning (biting) [pain] in the stomach). In the sense of 'a burning (biting) [pain]' (in a part of the body), Hebrew עקיצה is a non-attested semantic borrowing from Arabic لذع, as Hebrew עקיצה only features in the current dictionaries in the sense of 'sting, cutting fruit by the stalk' (JD 1106), or 'biting or stinging (by an animal or insect)' (BM 4674). In his translation of Hippocrates' *Aphorisms* 5.41, Zeraḥyah Ḥen uses the term עקיצה to render Arabic مغص 'colic' (cf. NM 3:182), and the anonymous translator has the same term for Arabic قلق 'disturbance' (cf. ibid.).

(עקץ) עוקץ See entry **סם**.

עקר (*Sefer ha-Qanun*, Joseph Lorki) = Arabic مغرز 'the place of growth, insertion, base, root, origin'; cf. bk. 1 (fol. 14a): ואפשר שיקרב כנגד עקר האזן בקצת אנשים ויתדבק בו ומתחברים בו ויתנועע האזן (Sometimes they (i.e., fibers of the muscles of the cheek) come close to the root (origin) of the ear in some people and are attached and connected to it and move the ear). Hebrew עקר does not feature as an anatomical term in the current dictionaries, cf. BM 4685–8; KTP 3:166–7. In his translation of Hippocrates' *Aphorisms* 4.49, Moses Ibn Tibbon uses Plur. עקרים for Arabic مبادئ in the sense of the 'origins' (of the nerves) (cf. NM 3:183). For the other translator(s), see entry משקע.

עָרוּם (*Sefer ha-Shimmush*) = Arabic خبيث 'malignant'; cf. fol. 143a, col. a: בשר התיש המוכלח מגונה המזון מוליד דם שחורי ומביא מתמידו אל חליים שחוריים וכל שכן מי שהוא מעותד להם כגון השוטים[487] והנכפים ואל השחין הערום ודומיהם מן החליים הרעים (Meat of old he-goats is bad food; it produces melancholic blood and causes melancholic illnesses in the case of someone who consumes

485 Cf. Bos, 'Isaac Todros on Facial Paresis', 189.

486 Cf. entry עקום הפה.

487 השוטים: كالمالنخوليا a.

it frequently, especially someone who is susceptible to them, like people[488] suffering from melancholy and epilepsy, and [causes] malignant ulcers and similar bad afflictions). Hebrew עָרוּם features in the current dictionaries as 'deliberate, sensible, wise, prudent, crafty, shrewd' (BDB 791; JD 1115; BM 4718–9). It is not mentioned in a medical context.

עריפה: עריפת דם החוטם (*Sefer Ṣedat ha-Derakhim*)[489] = Arabic رعاف 'nosebleed'; cf. fol. 55b: עריפת דם החוטם פעמים יהיה לטוב ופעמים לרע והמתהוה ממנו למה שהוא טוב כמו עריפת הדם אשר יהיה בקדחת השורפת וחולי מורסת הראש על דרך הנקיון (Sometimes a nosebleed is good and sometimes it is bad. A good [nosebleed] is like one that occurs during a burning fever or the illness [called] phrenitis in the way of a crisis). Hebrew עריפת דם החוטם does not feature in the current dictionaries. The synonymous עריפת דם מהנחירים is mentioned by Ben Yehuda (BM 4724) in an attestation from Meir Aldabi, *Shevilei Emunah* (cf. next entry).

עריפת דם הנחירים (*Sefer Ṣedat ha-Derakhim*)[490] = Arabic رعاف 'nosebleed'; cf. bk. 2, ch. 15 (fol. 55a): השער החמשה עשר בעריפת דם הנחירים (Chapter fifteen: On nosebleeds). Hebrew עריפת דם הנחירים features in BM 4724 as עריפת דם מהנחירים in an attestation from Meir Aldabi, *Shevilei Emunah* (see previous entry).

ערעור (*Sefer ha-Shimmush*) = Arabic تغرغُر 'gargling'; cf. fol 136b, col. a: וערעור הגרון במים שנתבשלו בהם תאינים עוזר על התכת המורסות בקנה הריאה (If one gargles the throat with water in which figs have been boiled, it helps to dissolve the swellings in the windpipe). Hebrew ערעור features in BM 4739, a.o., in an attestation from Nathan ha-Me'ati's translation of Maimonides, *Medical Aphorisms* 2.11. Ben Yehuda defines the term as: שפשוף והדחה על ידי נוזל (rubbing and cleansing by means of a liquid), cf. NM 2:74.

ערער (*Sefer ha-Shimmush*) = Arabic حرشف 'artichoke (*Cynara cardunculus* L.)'; cf. fol. 135b, col. b: הערער ובו"ח העכביות יש ממנו שדי ויש ממנו פרדסי והפרדסי הוא הדרדר והשדי הוא הערער האמתי (Artichoke, Rabb. Hebr. 'KBYWT, has a wild and a garden variety. The garden variety is [called] DRDR, and the wild variety is the real artichoke). Hebrew ערער features in the Bible in Jer 17:6, and is interpreted as 'prob. a tree or bush; juniper?' (BDB 792, s.v. ערוער), or as 'a tree or shrub, trad. a tamarisk' (KB 887). The Targum on Jer 17:6 translated the term as Aram. עכוביתא (= Hebr. עכבית) 'a species of edible thistles, cardoon' (*Cynara Cardunculus* L. or *Cynara Syriaca* Boiss. or *Gundelia Tournefortii*); cf. SHS 1:380 (Ayin 6). Hebrew עכבית, Plur. עכביות, is identified

488 'people suffering from melancholy': Cf. entry שוטה.
489 Cf. entries זלוף הדם מן החוטם, and עריפת דם הנחירים.
490 Cf. entries זלוף הדם מן החוטם, and עריפת דם החוטם.

in Geonic literature as חרשף (i.e., Arabic حرشف 'artichoke'); cf. the Geonic commentary on *Tohorot* (EG 143): והעכביות פ׳ הרשף (= חרשף). Hebrew דרדר means 'thistle, artichoke' (KB 230; JD 32), it features in the Bible in Gen 3:18 and is explained in *Genesis Rabbah* 20:10[491] as 'KBYWT; see also IJ 167: وفي בראשית דר׳ הושעיה ודרדר אילו עכביות يريد العكوب وهو الخرشف. Cf. SHS 1 (ibid.).

ערק: עורקים שוכנים (*Sefer ha-Qanun*, Nathan) = Arabic عروق ساكنة 'veins' (cf. DKT 822; FAL 77, no. 1704); cf. bk. 1 (fol. 60a): ויעברו עם שריגי אלה העצבים[492] עורקים דופקים ושוכנים נכנסים במוצאיהם אל חוט השדרה (The branches of these nerves are companied by arteries and veins which go to the spinal cord and enter through the foramina [of the nerves]). In the sense of 'veins', Hebrew עורק שוכן, Plur. עורקים שוכנים, is a non-attested loan translation of Arabic عروق ساكنة. Zeraḥyah Ḥen translates Arabic عروق ساكنة as גידים בלתי דופקים, and Joseph Lorki as גידים נחים (cf. NM 1:81).

עשב: עשב הזכוכית (*Sefer Ṣedat ha-Derakhim*) = Arabic حشيشة الزجاج 'upright pellitory (*Parietaria officinalis* L.)' or 'spreading pellitory (*Parietaria ramiflora* L.)' (cf. DT 4:76); cf. bk. 1, ch. 7 (fol. 12a): או שישחק עמו קצת הסמים המנגבים[493] כמו שיקח עשב הזכוכית (Or pound it with a drying[494] drug, such as upright or spreading pellitory). Hebrew עשב הזכוכית is a non-attested calque of Arabic حشيشة الزجاج.

עשנות (*Sefer ha-Shimmush*) = Arabic دخانية 'smokiness'; cf. fol. 147a, col. b: ותשוב בכלל הדברים החריפים תשתנה באסטומ׳ אל העשנות וסוג המרה הכרכומית ותעצור המעים עצירה חזקה (And it (i.e., salted cheese) belongs to the sharp ingredients that change in the stomach into smokiness and a kind of yellow bile and have a strong constipating effect on the stomach). Hebrew עשנות does not feature in the current dictionaries. A synonym, derived from the same root, i.e., עשניות, features in BM 4756 in an attestation from the Torah commentary by Isaac Abarbanel.

(עתד) מעותד (*Sefer ha-Shimmush*) = Arabic مستعدّ 'predisposed, susceptible'; cf. fol. 143a, col. a: בשר התיש המוכלח מגונה המזון מוליד דם שחורי ומביא מתמידו אל חליים שחוריים וכל שכן מי שהוא מעותד להם כגון השוטים[495] והנכפים ואל השחין הערום ודומיהם מן החליים הרעים (Meat of old he-goats is bad food, it produces melancholic blood and causes melancholic illnesses in the case of someone who consumes it frequently, especially someone who is susceptible to them,

---

491 Cf. *Midrash Rabbah*, 11 vols., ed. by M. A. Mirkin (Tel Aviv 1968–74), 1:153.

492 a الأعصاب Ms העצלים emend. ed.: העצבים.

493 a המנגבים: الجالية.

494 'drying': 'cleansing' a.

495 a השוטים: كالمالنخوليا.

like people suffering from melancholy[496] and epilepsy, and [causes] malignant ulcers and similar bad afflictions). In a medical context, Hebrew מעותד features in BM 4784 in the sense of עלול ל- (prepared to, capable of).

פגימה (*Sefer ha-Qanun*, Nathan) = Arabic حزّ 'trochlea [of humerus]' (cf. DKT 496–7, n. 2); cf. bk. 1 (fol. 37b): וביניהם בלי ספק פגימה ובשתי קצוות אותה פגימה יש שתי נקרות מלמעלה לקדם ומתחת לאחור (Between them (i.e., the two apophyses at the lower end of the humerus) there is necessarily a trochlea and at the two ends of the trochlea are two cavities; one above at the front and one below at the back). Hebrew פגימה features in the current dictionaries in the sense of 'notch, concavity' (cf. JD 1133; BM 4812–3). Zeraḥyah Ḥen possibly reads the Arabic حزّ as حدّ and consequently renders it as גבול. Joseph Lorki, possibly reading Arabic حزّ as جزء, corrects Nathan's פגימה as חלק.

פי העורב :פה (*Sefer ha-Qanun*, Zeraḥyah) = Arabic منقار الغراب (lit., 'crow's beak'); i.e., 'coracoid process' (cf. FAL 94, no. 2075) (Greek κορακοειδής; cf. LSG 980)[497]; cf. bk. 1 (fol. 20b): ולה שתי תוספות אחת מהן למעלה ומאחור ויקרא היותר משמש ופי העורב ובה קשרי הכתף עם העצם הנקר' קטולא (It (i.e., scapula) has two processes, one above and [one] behind which is called 'who[498] serves better' and 'crow's beak'; through which the bone that is called QṬWL' (i.e., scapula) is connected to the clavicle). For Hebrew פי העורב, cf. BM 1758 in an attestation from the *Sefer ha-Qanun*: ולו שתי תוספות האחת מהן למעלה ומאחור ונקרא אגרס וחרטום ופי העורב ובהם קשרי הכתף עם השכם (= trans. Joseph Lorki, fol. 12a). The term is defined by Ben Yehuda as שם לחלק מעצם ההכתף (a name for a part of the scapula); see also SRP 21 (112). For the other translator(s), see entry חרטום העורב.

(פוג) מפיג See entry **סם**.

פורני (Aramaic) (*Sefer ha-Shimmush*) = Arabic فرن (from Greek φοῦρνος, via Aramaic פורני)[499] 'brick oven fuelled with wood, similar to glass-making furnaces' (NA 681–2)[500]; cf. fol. 125a, col. a: הלחם האפוי בתנור הוא יותר טוב מזה האפוי בפורני למהירות עכולו וצאתו מן האצטומכא (Bread baked in a *tannur* (i.e., domed clay oven)[501] is better than that baked in a *furni* (brick oven) because

496 'melancholy': Cf. entry שוטים.

497 In modern terminology, it is the 'anchor-shaped or 'sigmoid process'; cf. Galen, *On the Usefulness of the Parts of the Body* (trans. Tallmadge May, 2:615, n. 55); see also DKT 493, n. 12.

498 'who serves better' (היותר משמש): Zeraḥyah's translation results from reading Arabic الأخرم as الأخدم.

499 Cf. FA 27; SDA 892; HM 162–3, s.v. פורנה.

500 For a detailed description, cf. MT 61–3. See also KT 1:89.

501 '*tannur*' (תנור): Cf. KT 1:87; for the Arabic equivalent تنّور, cf. NA 697, RMA 53–5.

it is faster digested and excreted from the stomach).[502] Aramaic פורני features in SDA 892 and is explained by Sokoloff as 'oven', and by Jastrow (JD 1147) as 'a stationary large baking oven'. Aramaic פורני also features in the anonymous translations of Maimonides, *On Asthma* 3.1 (ed. Bos, 2:395) and Maimonides, *On the Elucidation of Some Symptoms* 27 (forthcoming ed. by G. Bos).

פחד (*Sefer ha-Qanun*, Nathan) = Arabic فخذ 'femur, thigh' (cf. DKT 824; FAL 57, no. 1230); cf. bk. 1 (fol. 67a): ומה שישאר מזה יבא אל הפחד ויתענף בו שריגים וענפים ואחד מהם מתחלק בעצלים אשר על מוקדם פחד הירך (The remainder of these [branches of the vena cava] go to the thigh in which they divide into branches, one of which spreads in the muscles situated in the front part of the thigh). In the sense of 'thigh', Hebrew פחד is attested in the Bible in Job 40:17 as גידי פחדו (the sinews of his thigh) (cf. BDB 808), and in the *Sefer ha-Qanun* (cf. BM 4874) also in the combination פחד הירך (see next entry), see also SRP 44 (340). Zeraḥyah Ḥen renders the Arabic فخذ as ירך.

פחד הירך (*Sefer ha-Qanun*, Nathan) = Arabic فخذ 'femur, thigh' (cf. DKT 824; FAL 57, no. 1230); cf. bk. 1 (fol. 67a): ומה שישאר מזה יבא אל הפחד ויתענף בו שריגים וענפים ואחד מהם מתחלק בעצלים אשר על מוקדם פחד הירך. In the sense of 'thigh', Hebrew פחד הירך features in BM 4874 in attestations from the *Sefer ha-Qanun*, cf. SRP 44 (340). Zeraḥyah Ḥen renders the Arabic فخذ as ירך.

פחד המים: פַּחַד (*Sefer ha-Shimmush*) = Arabic التفزّع من الماء 'hydrophobia'; cf. fol. 143b, col. b: בשר הכלב חמימותו מרובה מבשר זכר הבקר ומועטה מבשר האריה ומי שנשכו כלב שוטה מאכילין אותו מכבד כלב צלוי כי הוא מועיל מפחד המים (Meat of a dog is hotter than that of a male cow and less hot than that of a lion. If someone has been bitten by a mad dog one should feed him with the[503] roasted liver of a dog because it is good against hydrophobia). Hebrew פחד המים does not feature in the current dictionaries. Masie (MD 362) mentions the synonym כלבת or יראת מים. The term פחד המים also features in Moses Ibn Tibbon's *Sefer Ṣedat ha-Derakhim*, bk. 7, ch. 13.7 (cf. IJZ 146).

פלח (*Sefer Ṣedat ha-Derakhim*) = Arabic شقّ 'half [of the head]'; cf. bk. 1, ch. 10 (fols. 13b–14a): ואם היה הכאב מתילד מפני המרה האדומה ימצא החולה חום חזק בראשו ויובש בנחיריו ולשונו וימצאהו תעורה וצמא ויהיה רוב כאבו בפלח הימין מן הראש (If the pain [in the head] arises from yellow bile, the patient will suffer from a severe heat in his head, dryness in his nostrils and tongue, and he will be affected by sleeplessness and thirst. Most of the pain will be in the right half

---

502 Cf. NA 565, s.v. *khubz al-furn*: 'bread baked in commercial brick ovens. It is round, thick, and crusty bread that develops a dome wile baking … It is inferior to *khubz al-tannūr* because its pith remains doughy and under-baked.'

503 For a similar recipe, cf. Paul of Aegina, *Seven Books* 5.3 (trans. Adams, 2:165); IJZ 93.

of the head). In the sense of 'half [of the head]', Hebrew פלח features in BM 4944 in an attestation from the *Sefer ha-Qanun*: הפלות הוא כאב באחד מפלחי הראש (PLWḤ is a pain in one half (side) of the head).

פלח המח (*Sefer Ṣedat ha-Derakhim*) = Arabic شق الدماغ 'cerebral hemisphere'; cf. bk. 1, ch. 23 (fol. 33b): ואם הגיע החמר אל אחד מצדדי המוח ר״ל הפלח הימני או הפלח השמאלי יקרא הפלג ההוא חסר ויתיחס אל האבר אשר יסור הרגשו ותנועתו (And if the [putrid] matter reaches one of the sides of the brain, i.e., the right hemisphere or the left one, the hemiplegia is called 'incomplete' and relates to the organ that loses sensitivity and motion). Hebrew פלח המח features in BM 4944 in an attestation from Moses Narboni,[504] *Sefer Oraḥ Ḥayyim*.

הפלחי :פלחי (*Sefer Ṣedat ha-Derakhim*) = Arabic الشقيقة 'migraine'; cf. bk. 1, ch. 11 (fol. 19a): וכשנרצה לרפאות הפלחי נעיין ואם היה מפני מותר חם והורה על זה מה שזכרנו כבר מאותות כאב הראש שסבתו חום (If we want to cure migraine, we should examine: If it is caused by a hot superfluity which is indicated by [one of] the symptoms for headache caused by heat which I mentioned before ...). Hebrew פלחי, standing for כאב הראש הפלחי, does not feature in the current dictionaries.

שלשת הפלפלין :פלפל (*Sefer ha-Refu'ot ha-Libbiyot*) = Latin 'dyatrion pipereon'[505]; cf. fol. 252a: והרופאים הסכלים[506] עדיין חושבים שיש למטרודיטוס ולתריאק חום גובר ומפני זה בורחים לתת ממנה שעור חצי זהוב ואמנם לא יהיו נסוגים מלתת ד׳ זהובים מהדיאסימינום ומרקחת שלשת הפלפין (Ignorant[507] physicians still believe that both the Mithridates[508] and theriac are exceedingly hot and therefore refrain from administering [even] half an aureus, but they have no hesitation in prescribing four aurei of the dyaciminum[509] and dyatrion pipereon remedy). Hebrew שלשת הפלפלין does not feature in the current dictionaries. The anonymous author of *Sammim Libbiyim* translates the parallel Arabic الفلافلي as הפלפליי (see next entry).

---

504 On the author and the *Sefer Oraḥ Ḥayyim*, see Bos, 'R. Moshe Narboni, Philosopher and Physician', 219–51.

505 'dyatrion pipereon' (= Arabic الفلافلي; cf. next entry): A compound remedy; cf. BAN 36–8.

506 oppositores L (imperiti variant reading =) הסכלים.

507 'Ignorant' (= Latin variant: imperiti): 'opposing' L.

508 'Mithridates': An antidote ascribed to Mithridates VI. Eupator, king of Pontus (reg. 120–63 BC); see Ullmann, *Medizin im Islam*, 321; for its composition, see Ibn Ḥayyān, *Buch der Gifte* (trans. Siggel, 217); cf. entry זהוב.

509 'dyaciminum': Cf. entry הכמוני :כמון.

פלפלי: הפלפליי (*Sammim Libbiyim*) = Arabic الفلافلي 'the pepper [stomachic]'[510]; cf. fol. 133a: עוד החולקים מן הרופאים יחשבו שיש מן הטריאק והמטרידיטוס חום עובר הגבול ויעמדו מלהשתמש בשעור חצי משקל ממנו ולא יעמדו מלהשתמש בארבעה משקלים הכמוני ומן הפלפליי (The physicians that have a different opinion think that the theriac and the Mithridates[511] are exceedingly hot and therefore refrain from prescribing [even] half a *mithqāl*[512] of it, but they have no hesitation in prescribing four *mithqāls* of the cumin and pepper [stomachics]). Hebrew הפלפליי does not feature in the current dictionaries. The anonymous author of *Sefer ha-Refu'ot ha-Libbiyot* (fol. 252a) transcribes the parallel Latin 'dyatrion pipereon' as שלשת הפלפלין (cf. previous entry).

התפלץ (פלץ) (*Hanhagat ha-Beri'ut le-Abu 'Ali Ben Zuhr*) = 'to shiver, to suffer from rigor' (cf. Honofredi: 'rigeo'); cf. ch. 27: שער כ"ז בשווי הישיבות והטיולים. ראוי שלא יהיה אל אלו המקומות מחום מה שיזיע בו הגוף או [...] ולא גם כן מהקור מה שיתפלץ עמו הגוף (Ch. 27: On moderate sitting and walking. One should not live in those places that are so hot that the body has to sweat or [...], nor so cold that that the body starts to shiver). Hebrew התפלץ features in the current dictionaries in the sense of 'to shudder' (cf. BDB 814) and 'to shake (with fear); to tremble' (BM 4965). The noun פלצות, derived from the root פלץ, features in Moses' Ibn Tibbon's translation of Hippocrates' *Aphorisms* for Arabic اقشعرار 'shivering, rigor', or نافض 'rigor'; cf. NM 3:189.

פנים (*Sefer ha-Qanun*, Zeraḥyah)[513] = Arabic خدّ 'cheek'; cf. bk. 1 (fol. 24a): הפרק הששי בניתוח המושקלי של הפנים. הפנים לו שתי תנועות (Chapter six: The anatomy of the muscles of the cheeks. There are two [types of] movements in the cheeks). Hebrew פנים does not feature in this sense in the current dictionaries. For the other translator(s), cf. entry רקה.

פנימי: הפנימי (*Sefer ha-Qanun*, Joseph Lorki)[514] = Arabic الأجوف 'vena cava' (cf. DKT 830, s.v. الوريد الأجوف; cf. bk. 1 (fol. 19b): פרק ה' בנתוח הוריד הפנימי היורד כבר השלמנו מאמרינו בחלק העולה מ<ה>פנימי והוא היותר קטון שבשני חלקיו (Chapter five: On the anatomy of the inferior vena cava. We have finished the discussion of the ascending vena cava which is the smaller of the two).

510 'the pepper [stomachic]' (جوارشن الفلافلي): For this compound remedy, cf. Ibn Sīnā, *K. al-Qānūn*, 3:349.

511 'Mithridates': An antidote ascribed to Mithridates VI. Eupator, king of Pontus (reg. 120–63 BC); see Ullmann, *Medizin im Islam*, 321; for its composition, see Ibn Ḥayyān, *Buch der Gifte* (trans. Siggel, 217); cf. entry זהוב.

512 One *mithqāl* is 4.46 grams; cf. Hinz, *Islamische Maße und Gewichte*, 4–7.

513 Cf. entry יותר שניות: שניות.

514 In addition to הפנימי, Joseph Lorki has הוריד הפנימי (see entry) to indicate the 'vena cava', conform to Arabic الوريد الأجوف.

Hebrew הפנימי is not attested in the current dictionaries. For the other translator(s), see entry הנבוב.

פניס (*Sefer ha-Shimmush*) = Arabic فانيد; Persian *pānīd*, or *pānīḏ*: 'sugar-candy, a sweetmeat' (SC 233); 'purified, white sugar'; 'cane sugar', or 'a sweetmeat' (VL 1:324b; NA 596–7; esp. 597, 4); cf. fol. 141b, col. a: ודחית נזקם לאכלם על הצום ולאכול אחריהם בעל הלחה הלבנה מן הדבש ובעל החמימות מן הסוכר או מן הפניס (To prevent their harm (i.e., of coconuts) one should eat them on an empty stomach and someone with a phlegmatic temperament should then take honey, and someone with a hot temperament sugar or sugar-candy). The unattested Hebrew פניס is possibly a calque from Latin 'panis [zucri]' (sugar-loaf) (cf. LRM 329). The same Hebrew term features in *Hanhagat ha-Beri'ut le-Abu 'Ali Ben Zuhr*, ch. 9, where Honofredi's Latin translation has 'penidii' (cf. LRM 339: 'barley sugar'). It can also be found in the anonymous translation of Maimonides, *On Coitus* 8, while Zeraḥyah Ḥen and another anonymous translation have פ(א)ניד (= Arabic فانيد). Shem Tov Ben Isaac's contemporary Moses Ibn Tibbon renders the synonymous Arabic سكّر الفانيد as סוכר כנדי (cf. entry).

פקעיות (*Sefer ha-Shimmush*) = Arabic فقاع 'non-alcoholic beer' (cf. NA 551); cf. fol. 128a: השער השני במימות והשלג והמים הקפוים ומיני היין והשכר והפקעיות (Book two: On waters, snow, frozen waters, [different] kinds of wine, beverages and non-alcoholic beer). Hebrew פקעיות is possibly a non-attested calque of Arabic فقاع.

פֵּרוּך (*Sefer Hanhagat ha-Beri'ut*) = 'massage'; cf. 9.2 (165): ודע כי מיני הפירוך וחלקיהם רבים ממנו חזק וממנו רפה ואמצעי ביניהם (Know that there are many different sorts of massage, hard and soft and moderate). Hebrew פֵּרוּך (from פרך in the sense of 'to rub') does not feature in this sense in the current dictionaries. Ben Yehuda (BM 5146) only refers to פֵּרוּך as a Hebrew counterpart of Aramaic פרוכא 'barley groats'; cf. JD 1170.

פרח: פרח המלח (*Sefer Ṣedat ha-Derakhim*) = Arabic زهرة الملح 'salt efflorescence, salt scum'; cf. KM 684–6 (Greek ἄνθος ἁλός); cf bk. 1, ch. 24 (fol. 40a): וירחץ במים שנתבשלו בהם סמים חמים וימשח במה שזכרנו מן השמנים אחר שיצא ממים חמים שהושלך בהם פרח המלח (He should wash himself in water in which hot ingredients have been cooked and rub himself with oils that I mentioned once he has left the [bath with] hot water [mixed with] salt scum). Hebrew פרח המלח is a non-attested calque from Arabic زهرة الملح.

פרק: פרקי האצבעות (*Sefer ha-Qanun*, Nathan) = Arabic سلاميات 'phalanges' (cf. DKT 504–5, 819; FAL 144, no. 3118); cf. bk. 1 (fol. 40a): ונתחברו פרקי האצבעות כלם בזיזים[515] ונקרות נכנסים ביניהם לחות דבקה (All the phalanges are articulated

515 בזיזים: بحروف a.

by extremities (sharp processes) and by articular depressions which fit into each other and hold a viscous secretion). Hebrew פרקי האצבעות features in MD 565, s.v. 'phalanges'. Zeraḥyah Ḥen renders the Arabic سلاميات as העצמות הקטנים הנקראים בער׳ סולימיית (cf. entry), and Joseph Lorki as עצמות קטנות.

פרקי (*Sefer ha-Qanun*, Nathan) = Arabic مفصلي 'articular'; cf. bk. 1 (fol. 32b): והתוספות הפרקיות גם כן ענינם זה כי הוא מהודק קצתם בקצתם הדוק חזק בקשורים ומאסרים מכל הצדדים (The articular processes of the vertebrae have a similar disposition because they are solidly connected with each other through fasciae and ligaments from all sides). Hebrew פרקי features in BM 5241 in an attestation from the *Sefer ha-Qanun* and is explained by Ben Yehuda as לפרקים and משמש פרק. Zeraḥyah Ḥen renders the Arabic الزوائد المفصلية as תוספות הפרקים.

פשט (*Sefer ha-Qanun*, Zeraḥyah) = Arabic بسط 'to expand'; cf. bk. 1 (fol. 26a): אלו הם המושקלי הפושטים (These are the muscles that expand [the chest]). Hebrew פשט features in Rabbinic literature (cf. JD 1245; BM 5270) and modern literature (cf. EM 1492: פשט יד) in the sense of 'to stretch'; for the other translator(s), see entry (שטח) השטיח.

פשט הרוח (*Sammim Libbiyim*) = Arabic بسط الروح (to dilate the pneuma); cf. fols. 124b–125a, s.v. אבריסם הוא משי (silk): ולו סגולה לשמוח הלב ולחזקו ויעזור בזה דקדוקו ויפשט הרוח ויקשרהו[516] וינגבהו ויזככהו (And it has the specific property to gladden and strengthen the heart; it is supported in this by its refining property. It dilates the pneuma, makes[517] it translucid and clear). Hebrew פשט does not feature in this sense in the current dictionaries. Arabic بسط features as بسط النفس (to dilate, i.e., rejoice the soul) in Maimonides, *Medical Aphorisms* 8.32, where it is translated by Nathan ha-Me'ati as השטיח הנפש (cf. NM 2:87). The anonymous translator of *Sefer ha-Refu'ot ha-Libbiyot* translates Latin 'dilato spiritum' as המתיח הרוח (see entry).

הפשיט 1. (*Sammim Libbiyim*) = Arabic بسّط 'to rarefy' (cf. D 1:84); cf. fol. 126a: ויש לו עם זה דקות והוא בסבת הבושמיות אשר בו נאות לעצם הרוח [ו]למה שיש בו מן הקביצות עם הדקות מקשר אותו מנקה לעצמיותו מפשיט אותו (And it (i.e., the myrtle) has refining [power], and because of its aroma it is favorable to the substance of the pneuma. It strengthens, purefies and rarefies its substance (i.e., that of the pneuma) through its astringency and refining power). In the sense of 'to rarefy', Hebrew הפשיט is an unattested semantic borrowing

---

516 a وشدّه (= وشفّه): ויקשרהו וינגבהו.

517 'makes it translucid': Translated after the Arabic; cf. Ibn al-Bayṭār, *Traité des simples*, trans. by L. Leclerc, 3 vols. (Paris 1877–83), 1:15: 'Il dilate les esprits et, par sa propriété dessiccative, il les condense'; the Arabic text (ed. Beyrut 1992, 1:10) reads: فيبسط الروح ويشفه فينميه فينوره (It dilates the pneuma, makes it translucent, grow (expand), and clear).

from Arabic بسط. The anonymous translator of *Sefer ha-Refu'ot ha-Libbiyot* (fol. 249a) renders Latin 'simplicium' as פשוט; II. (*Sefer ha-Qanun*, Nathan) = Arabic بسط 'to extend, to stretch'; cf. bk. 1 (fol. 50a): וכשיתנועעו אלו השנים יפשיט<ו> הרסג פשוט עם מעט קבוב (When these two [muscles of the wrist] act together, they extend the carpus with some pronation). In the sense of 'to extend', Hebrew הפשיט is attested in Rabbinic literature (cf. BM 5272). Zeraḥyah Ḥen translates the Arabic بسط as שיטח, and Joseph Lorki as הרחיב.

פותח (פתח) See entry **סם**.

פתיחה (*Sammim Libbiyim*) = Arabic تفتيح 'deobstruent property' (of a remedy); cf. fol. 126b: בהמן: הוא באם חם בשנית יבש בראשונה וממנו לבן ואדום והאדום יותר חזק החום ובשניהם יחד קביצות עם דקדוק ופתיחה (Behen (*Centauria Behen* and *Statice limonium*); i.e., B'M, it is hot in the second [degree], dry in the first [degree]. It is of two kinds, white and red. The red kind is hotter. Both are astringent with refining and deobstruent properties). Hebrew פתיחה does not feature in this sense in the current dictionaries. The anonymous translator of *Sefer ha-Refu'ot ha-Libbiyot* (fol. 248a) renders Latin 'apertio' as פתיחה as well.

פתיחת האזן (*Sefer ha-Qanun*, Joseph Lorki) = Arabic صماخ '1. the inner cavity of the ear, the tympanic cavity, the middle ear'; 2. 'the external acoustic meatus' (cf. DKT 588–9, 821; FAL 139, no. 3005); cf. bk. 1 (fol. 17a): והחלק הראשון מכל זוג ממנו יכוון[518] אל הקרום <...> פתיחת האזן (The first part of each pair (i.e., of acoustic nerves) goes to the membrane [that covers] the inner cavity of the ear). Hebrew פתיחת האזן is not attested in the current dictionaries.

פתיחת העינים (*Sefer Issur ha-Qevurah le-Galienus*) = Arabic شخوص العينين 'staring eyes'; cf. par. 15: ואולם בסוף[519] זאת העלה יקרה לבעליה פתיחת העינים (From the onset[520] of this illness its victims will suffer from staring eyes ...). Hebrew פתיחת העינים does not feature in this sense in the current dictionaries.

פתיל: פתילים (*Sefer Ṣedat ha-Derakhim*) = Arabic خيوط 'tendrils'; cf. bk. 1, ch. 10 (Ms Oxford, Bodleian, Poc. 353, Uri Heb. 314, fol. 4b): וזכר גם כן שאם יכתשו עלי הגפנים ופתיליהם ויעשה מהם רטיה יועיל מכאב הראש הכרכומי (He (i.e., Dioscurides) also said that if leaves and tendrils of a vine are pounded, prepared as a linimen [and applied], it is good for headache caused by yellow bile). Hebrew פתיל, Plur. פתילים, does not feature in this sense in the current dictionaries; cf. NM 2:76. The term current in Rabbinic literature is קנוקנת, Plur. קנוקנות; cf. FM 187.

518 Ms יתרון emend. ed.: יכוון.

519 a[1] عند وقت أخذ: عند وقت آخر) = בסוף).

520 'From the onset': Translated after the Arabic عند وقت أخذ.

פתילה (*Sefer ha-Shimmush*) = Arabic شيافة 'suppository'[521]; cf. fol. 144a, col. a: ואם יתחדש בבטן הברה ואומץ המעים ראוי לעשות לו פתילה מורידה הצואה או פדלקון בבורית וחלב פקועות ופניס וכיוצא בהם (But if he suffers from intestinal rumblings and constipation one should in order to excrete the feces apply a suppository or a clyster with borax and colocynth pulp and sugar-candy and the like). In the sense of 'suppository', Hebrew פתילה features in BM 5325 in attestations subsequent to Shem Tov Ben Isaac, namely from the *Sefer ha-Qanun* and other sources.

צאת: אחרי צאת המאכל מן האצטומכא (*Sefer Ṣedat ha-Derakhim*) = Arabic على الريق 'on an empty stomach'; cf. bk. 1, ch. 23 (fol. 36a): הלקיחה ממנו ד' שקלים במים חמים אחרי צאת המאכל מן האצטומכא (One should take a dosis of four *shekels*[522] on an empty stomach). Hebrew אחרי צאת המאכל מן האצטומכא does not feature in the current dictionaries. The same Arabic term is rendered by Nathan ha-Me'ati as בריקות נפש in his translation of Maimonides, *Medical Aphorisms* 22.36, and by Zeraḥyah Ḥen as קודם אכילה (cf. NM 2:86).

צבה: הצבא (*Sefer Ṣedat ha-Derakhim*) = Arabic النافخة '[the illness called] gassy, windy, flatulent'; Greek φυσώδης; cf. bk. 1, ch. 18 (fol. 27b): כמו אשר יקרה זה בחולי אשר יקרא הצבא אלנפכא בערבי (Similarly to what happens in the illness called HṢB', in Arabic 'L-NPK'). Hebrew הצבא does not feature in the current dictionaries. Arabic العلّة النافخة (the gassy illness) features in Maimonides, *Medical Aphorisms* 9.44, and is rendered by Nathan ha-Me'ati as העלה הנופחת, and by Zeraḥyah Ḥen as המחלה הנופחת.

צד: צדי האמה (*Sefer Issur ha-Qevurah le-Galienus*) = Arabic حالب 'ureter' (cf. FAL 68, no. 1508 and 168, no. 3617; DKT 816; UWS 1:815)[523]; cf. par. 31: והמקום השלישי העורק בין צדי האמה והאמה כשיהודקו הדוק חזק ירגיש האדם כמו התלהבות האש ואם תראה זה הנה הוא חי (Third, there is an artery between ureter and urethra which, when firmly palpated, feels to the (investigating) person as if a fire were burning inside it—if this is what you find, then [the patient] is alive). Hebrew צדי האמה, possibly meaning 'ureter', does not feature in the current dictionaries.

צהוב: על גבו ציהוב (*Sefer ha-Shimmush*) I. = Arabic مزغب الجسم 'covered with yellow fuzz'; cf. fol. 138b, col. a: ויש ממנו מין לבן רב החמימות ועל גבו ציהוב והוא בלתי מתפלח (... and there is a white variety of it (i.e., of peaches) that is very hot and that is covered with yellow (golden) fuzz and that cannot be split).

---

521 For Arabic شياف in the sense of 'eye-salve (collyrium)', cf. entry עגול.

522 '*shekels* (Arabic *miṯqāls*)': One *mithqāl* is 4.46 grams; cf. Hinz, *Islamische Maße und Gewichte*, 4–7.

523 See also entry חולב: החולבים.

Hebrew ציהוב features in Shem Tov Ben Isaac's glossary to the *Sefer ha-Shimmush* (SHS 1:437 (Ṣade 16)): ציהוב כמו שער דק ב״ה זגב (ṢYHWB is like fine hair; ZGB in Arabic (i.e., زغب)); II. = Arabic زِئبِر (cf. D 1:616: 'surface velue d'une étoffe' (hairy surface of a fabric) (= زئبر); cf. L 1211: 'The nap or villous substance of a garment or piece of cloth'); cf. fol. 150, col. b: כל לבוש מתלהט[524] חלק חומו בכלל לגופות יותר מועט משאר הלבוש וראוי ללבוש אותו בקיץ ומה שיש לו כובד או ציהוב והיתה אריגתו מתחלחלת או שיהיה עב בלתי מתלהט הוא מחמם הגוף יותר וראוי ללבשו בסתו (Every garment [from smooth and flatwoven fabric] is generally less hot on bodies than garments [from other fabrics]. One should wear such a garment during the summer, but garments that are heavy or hairy or finely woven or coarse and not smooth have a stronger heating effect on the body and should be worn during the winter).

צחצוחי חלב :צחצוח (*Sefer ha-Shimmush*) = Arabic لِبأ 'colostrum, beestings, first milk' (WKAS 2.1:96a–97a); cf. fol. 147b, col. a: צחצוחי חלב יותר עבים מהגבנה ויותר מתאחרים להתעכל ויותר רחוקים לרדת (Colustrum is thicker than cheese, slower to digest and further away to go down (slower to pass through the stomach)). Hebrew צחצוחי חלב features in Rabbinic literature and is rendered by Jastrow as 'particles of diluted milk (in the holes of cheese)' (JD 1273); cf. LW 4:182: 'Milchtropfen, die im Käse zurückbleiben' (drops of milk that remain in the cheese).

צירים בבטן :ציר (*Sefer ha-Shimmush*)[525] = Arabic مغص, Plur. أمغاص 'colics'; cf. fol. 143b, col. b: בשר הזאב[526] יותר חם מבשר הכלב אלא שהוא עב וקשה להתעכל מאד ומוליד צירים בבטן (The meat of a wolf[527] is hotter than that of a dog, but it is thick and very hard to digest and produces colics). Hebrew צירים בבטן does not feature in the current dictionaries. Hebrew ציר, Plur. צירים, features in the current dictionaries as 'pain' in general and 'labour-pains' in particular (cf. BM 5474–5); it is used by Moses Ibn Tibbon to render Arabic مغص in his translation of Hippocrates' *Aphorisms* 4.11, 5.41 (cf. NM 3:191–2, 220).

צירים וחבלים (*Sefer ha-Shimmush*)[528] = Arabic مغس 'colic'; cf. fol. 142a, col. a: ותקונם ודחית נזקם למי שיולידו לו צירים וחבלים באצטומכא למצוץ עליהם מן הרמונים הקוססים (To improve [their quality] and undo their harm (i.e., of [small] pine seeds) in the case of someone in whom their consumption causes a colic in the stomach, he should suck pomegranate [juice] that is

524 a מתלהט: صقيل.

525 Another translation by Shem Tov of Arabic مغص, variant reading of مغس, is צירים וחבלים (cf. next entry).

526 a הזאב: سعب.

527 'wolf': 'beast of prey' a.

528 Another translation by Shem Tov of Arabic مغس, variant reading of مغص, is צירים בבטן (cf. previous entry).

somewhat sweet and somewhat sour). Hebrew צירים וחבלים does not feature in this sense in the current dictionaries. However, both terms are used separately to render Arabic مغصّ, a variant reading of مغس, in medieval medical literature. Hebrew צירים features in Moses Ibn Tibbon's translation of Hippocrates' *Aphorisms* 4.11, 5.41, and חבלים in Nathan ha-Me'ati's translation of this aphorism (cf. NM 3:78, 191–2, 220).

צילבחא: צלבחא (Aramaic) (*Sefer ha-Shimmush*) = Arabic سلباح (from Aramaic צלבחא, cf. FA 122) 'eel' (cf. D 1:671); cf. fol 150a, col. a: הצילבחא היא מין הדגים אלא שהיא מתילד במקומות מעופשים וביצה (Eel: It is a kind of fish although it originates from putrid marshy places). Aramaic צלבחא features as צלובחא or צלופחא in Rabbinic literature in the sense of 'eel' (cf. SDA 963; LFA 10).

צלובחא: See entry **צלבחא**.

צלי: צלי אש (*Sefer Ṣedat ha-Derakhim*) = Arabic القليّة المشوية (cf. NA 614, s.v. *qaliyya*: 'a dish of fried meat which has been diced or sliced and fried with onion, a small amount of vinegar or *murrī*[529] (liquid fermented sauce) and some spices and herbs'[530]); cf. bk. 1, ch. 19 (29b): ויהיה מזונו צלי קדר וצלי אש וכרוב מבושל בבשר צאן או כרוב שלוק מתוקן במוריס ושמן טוב (He[531] should feed himself with a dish[532] of sliced and braced red meat [...], or a dish of fried meat [...] or cabbage boiled with meat of small cattle or cabbage boiled [and] prepared with *murrī* and oil from unripe olives). Hebrew צלי אש only features in the current dictionaries in the general sense of 'roasted' (of flesh) (BDB 852); 'roasted by fire' (JD 1283).

צלי הפורני (*Sefer ha-Shimmush*) = Arabic شوي الفرن (lit., '[a dish of meat] roasted in the oven'), also called راهبي (lit., 'monastic'); i.e., 'a dish consisting of meat, onions, honey, rosewater, coriander, a lot of saffron, and a few cooked almonds' (cf. D 1:562); cf. fol. 145b: צלי הפורני רב המזון קשה להתעכל ולרדת מן האסטומ' נוטה להוליד המרה השחורה (A dish of meat [...] roasted in the oven is very nutritious, hard to digest and to pass through the stomach, and tends to produce black bile). Hebrew-Romance צלי הפורני does not feature as a technical term for a compound dish in the current dictionaries.

צלי קדר (*Sefer Ṣedat ha-Derakhim*) = Arabic طباهجة; cf. NA 617–8: 'a dish of sliced and braised red meat of quadrupeds, marinated in sauce, and slowly

529 '*murrī*' (liquid fermented sauce)': This term is normally translated as 'garum', i.e., a fish sauce common in the classical Mediterranean world during Greco-Roman times. But there were actually two varieties of *murrī* in the Arabic/Islamic tradition, one made from fish, and the other from cereals. Cf. SHS 1:435 (Ṣade 12).

530 For some recipes, see ISW 210–5 (ch. 84); NA 343–9.

531 I.e., someone who is drunk and has a cold temperament.

532 'dish of sliced and braced red meat': Cf. entry צלי קדר.

simmered in a small amount of liquid with oil, spices, and herbs, and sometimes vegetables'[533]; cf. bk. 1, ch. 19 (fol. 29b): ויהיה מזונו צלי קדר וצלי אש וכרוב מבושל בבשר צאן או כרוב שלוק מתוקן במוריס ושמן טוב (He[534] should feed himself with a dish of sliced and braced red meat […], or a dish[535] of fried meat […] or cabbage boiled with meat of small cattle or cabbage boiled [and] prepared with *murrī*[536] and oil from unripe olives). Hebrew צלי קדר is only attested for Rabbinic literature in the general sense of 'roasted through the heat of the pot' (cf. JD 1318; BM 5491).

צלילה (*Sefer Ṣedat ha-Derakhim*) = Arabic دويّ 'ringing in the ears (tinnitus)' (Greek ἦχος; cf. UWS 1:452); cf. bk. 2, ch. 8 (fol. 49a): ואם היתה הצלילה מפני חולי שהחליש האבר הנה יועילהו חומץ חם עם סחיטת אישנץ (If the ringing in the ears (tinnitus) is caused by an illness that weakened the organ, hot vinegar with absinthe extract is good for it). Hebrew צלילה features as צלילת האזנים in BM 5493 in an attestation from Moses Narboni,[537] *Sefer Oraḥ Ḥayyim*. See also MD 722, s.v. 'tinnitus': צלילה/צלצול/צלילת האזנים.

צלעות אמצע החזה: צלע (*Sefer ha-Qanun*, Joseph Lorki) = Arabic أضلاع الزور 'false ribs' (cf. DKT 821, FAL 53, no. 1143); cf. bk. 1 (fol. 12a): ואמנם הה׳ הקצרים[538] הנשארים הם עצמות האחור וצלעות אמצע החזה נבראו ראשיהם דבקים נבדלים[539] כדי להיות בטוחים מהשבירה בשעת ההכאה (As for the remaining five short [ribs], i.e., the posterior bones or false ribs, their extremities have been made attached to[540] cartilages to protect them from being fractured when they suffer from blows). Hebrew צלעות אמצע החזה is not attested in the current dictionaries. For the other translator(s), see entry צלעות הכוזבות; see also entry אמצע החזה.

צלעות כוזבות (*Sefer ha-Qanun*, Nathan) = Arabic أضلاع الزور 'false ribs' (cf. DKT 821, FAL 53, no. 1143); cf. bk. 1 (fol. 36b): ואמנם החמשה המקוצרות הנשארות הנה הם עצמות האחור וצלעות הכוזבות נבראו ראשיהם מחוברים בשחוסים לבטוח מן ההשבר בעת הנגיפה. In the sense of 'false ribs', Hebrew צלעות כוזבות features in MD 633, s.v. 'costae spuriae'. Ben Yehuda (BM 5503) mentions the term without any further explanation. Zeraḥyah Ḥen renders the Arabic

---

533 For some recipes, cf. ISW 219–23 (ch. 86); NA 355–9.

534 I.e., someone who is drunk and has a cold temperament.

535 'dish of fried meat […]': Cf. entry צלי אש.

536 '*murrī*': See entry צלי אש.

537 On the author and the *Sefer Oraḥ Ḥayyim*, see Bos, 'R. Moshe Narboni, Philosopher and Physician', 219–51.

538 Ms הקשרים emend. ed.: הקצרים.

539 a נבדלים: بغضاريف.

540 'to cartilages': Translated according to a.

أضلاع الزور as (?)העצם הנק' הַוְוֹרָק[541], and Joseph Lorki as צלעות אמצע החזה (see entry).

צמוק: צמוקי ההר (*Sefer Ṣedat ha-Derakhim*) = Arabic زبيب الجبل (lit., 'mountain raisins'), a calque of Greek σταφὶς ἀγρία (DT 4:141 (657) 'stavesacre' (*Delphinium staphisagria* L.; *Ranunculaceae*); cf. bk. 1, ch. 1 (fol. 6b): או יטוח אותו בבשר קולוקונטידא אחר שיודק בחומץ ושמן או יטוח בצמוקי ההר כמו כן (He may also smear pulp of colocynth on it (i.e., the spot affected by alopecia) once it has been pounded in vinegar and [olive] oil; or mountain-raisins [applied] in the same way). Hebrew צמוקי ההר is a non-attested calque of Arabic زبيب الجبل. The term features as a loan translation of the Arabic حبّ الرأس in the *Sefer ha-Shimmush* (cf. SHS 1:429–430 (Ṣade 2)), composed by Moses Ibn Tibbon's contemporary Shem Tov Ben Isaac, and in the latter's *Sefer Almansur* (cf. NM 2:17). It can also be found in Judah Ben Solomon Natan, *Kelal Qaṣar mi ha-Sammim ha-Nifradim* (= Hebrew translation of Abū Ṣalt's *K. al-Adwiya al-mufrada* (cf. JNK 169).

הצמוקים השמשיים (*Hanhagat ha-Beri'ut le-Abu 'Ali Ben Zuhr*)[542] 'raisins' (Latin Honofredi: 'uvae passae'); cf. ch. 10: אולם שמירת האצטומ' יהיה בעשית הקיא פעם אחת בחדש שהוא ינקה אותה ממותרי המאכל ומהליחות הרעות, ובאכילת הצמוקין השמשיים בגרעיניו על הצום שהוא יחזק אותה ויתקן המזגים הרעים אשר בה ([The health of] the stomach can be preserved by applying emesis once a month as it cleanses the stomach from the food residues and bad humours, and by the consumption of raisins with their seeds on an empty stomach. This strengthens [the stomach] and corrects its bad temperaments). Hebrew הצמוקים השמשיים does not feature in the current dictionaries. The second element of the term השמשיים possibly results from reading Arabic كشمش (raisins, esp. small seedless raisins; cf. FL 4:40) as كشمس (like the sun).

הצטמק (צמק) (*Sefer ha-Shimmush*) = Arabic طبخ 'to boil down, to thicken'; cf. fol. 127a, col. b: העדשים המבושלים בבשר החי ראוי לבשלם על זה התאר והוא לקחת מן הבשר השמן ולבשלו במה שיכסהו מן המים שתי פעמים ולהסיר חלאתו ולבשל מן העדשים הלבנים הקלופים בעשרה כמותם ממים מתוקים בקדרה אחרת ולתבל הבשר בכוסבר הלח ובצלים ועץ של שבת ושרשי כרשין וכשיצטמקו העדשים לשפוך מימיהם ולרחצם במים אחרים חמים (Lentils and raw meat should be boiled as follows: Take fat meat, cook it twice in water that covers it [completely], then remove the foam, cook white peeled lentils in another pot in an amount of

---

541 The term הַוְוֹרָק is possibly a corruption of הזורק, which in turn is a corruption of הזוֹר, which is Arabic الزور; cf. fol. 31b, where Zeraḥyah translates the Arabic أضلاع الزور as צלעות המקום הנקרא אלזור.

542 Cf. entry (צרד) הצריד.

sweet water that is ten times as much and season them with fresh coriander, onions, aneth stems, and leek root. When the lentils are boiled down, pour the [remaining water out], and wash them with new hot water). In the sense of 'to boil down', Hebrew הצטמק is attested in Rabbinic literature in BM 5533.

צנור הכיור: צנור (*Sefer Ṣedat ha-Derakhim*) = Arabic أنبوب 'spout' (cf. D 1:632–3); cf. bk. 1, ch. 10 (fol. 16b): וירחץ הראש במים שנתבשלו בהם קמומילא ואניט[543] וקורונא ריאל ותהיה יציאת המים מצנור הכיור כדי שיפליג תוך הראש יותר (And wash the head with water in which camomile, aneth,[544] and melilot have been cooked, and let the water pass through a spout (narrow pipe) so that it penetrates the head as much as possible).[545] Hebrew צנור הכיור does not feature in the current dictionaries.

צנורות הגידים (*Sefer ha-Qanun*, Joseph Lorki) = Arabic جداول العروق 'mesentery' (DKT 815): cf. bk. 1 (fol 18b): וא״כ יחלק מן הגיד הדופק הגדול הזה שני גידים דופקים יפרדו בצנורות הגידים אשר סביב המעי הישר (From this large artery [other] arteries detach themselves which spread along the mesentery which surrounds the rectum). Hebrew צנורות הגידים does not feature in the current dictionaries. For the other translator(s), see entry תעלות העורקים.

ציניי ותריסי: צִנִּי (*Sefer ha-Qanun*, Nathan) = Arabic درقي 'shield-shaped; thyroid [cartilage]' (cf. DKT 534–5, 824 (s.v. الغضرف الدرقي)[546]; FAL 64, no. 1424); cf. bk. 1 (fol. 46b): והוא מחובר משחוסים שלשה אחד מהם שחוס אשר ישיגהו החוש קדם הגרון ותחת הזקן ונקרא הדרקי הציניי והתריסי בהיות מקוער מפנים מגובן החוץ ודומה הצנה והתריס[547] (It (i.e., the larynx) consists of three cartilages. The first is the one that can be touched (seen) at the foreside of the throat, beneath the chin and is called [in Arabic] DRQY [i.e., Hebrew] ṢNYY and TRYSY. It is concave on the inner side and convex at the outer, resembling a shield). Hebrew צִנִּי, adjective coined from צִנָּה ('large shield'; cf. BM 5541) and תריסי, adjective coined from תריס, do not feature in the current dictionaries. Zeraḥyah Ḥen translates the Arabic درقي as (!)הזקני, and Joseph Lorki as צנה.

---

543 add. a ואניט: ومرزنجوش.

544 'aneth': 'and marjoram' add. a.

545 For this recommendation, cf. Abu Marwān Ibn Zuhr, *Kitāb al-taisīr fīl-mudawāt wal-tadbīr*, ed. by M. al-Khouri (Damascus 1983), 29: فإن كان الوجع من سبب حار فإن زيت الورد المبرد في البإر يربء منه إذا صبّ على الرأس من أنبوب ضيق; *Le traité médical* Kitab al-taysir *par Ibn Zuhr de Séville*, trans. by F. Bouamrane (Paris 2010), 100: 'Si la douleur est due à un principe chaud, l'huile de rose, refroidie dans le puits, et versée sur la tête à l'aide d'un tube étroit, la supprime'.

546 Arabic درقي is coined from درقة 'a shield composed of leather without wood' (cf. FL 2:24). The Arabic term stands for the Greek θυρεός; cf. LSG 805: 'an oblong shield'.

547 Ms והתרסים emend. ed.: והתריס.

צער (*Sefer Ṣedat ha-Derakhim*) = Arabic أرق 'sleeplessness'; cf. bk.1, ch.18 (fol. 26a): מורסת הראש במאמר מוחלט היא מורסא חמה תקרה בקצת קרומות המוח ישיגהו תמיד צער ושגעון וערבוב השכל (In an absolute sense phrenitis is an inflammation in one of the meninges of the brain whereby [the patient] is always affected by sleeplessness, raving, and mental confusion (delirium)). Hebrew צער, a variant reading of סער (cf. entry), does not feature in this sense in the current dictionaries. In his translation of Hippocrates' *Aphorisms* 7.12, Ibn Tibbon uses the same Hebrew term for Arabic اضطراب 'disturbance' (cf. NM 3:196).

צער באסטומכא (*Sefer ha-Shimmush*) = Arabic قلق في المعدة 'an upset stomach'; cf. fol. 144a, col. a: ואם לא יתעכל וירגיש בכבדות וצער באסטומכא וגעש נפסד ותעורה וצרות הנשימה ורוגז ראוי לעורר הקיא (If the [meat from the head of an animal] is not digested and one feels a heavy and upset stomach and suffers from putrid eructations, sleeplessness, orthopnea and distress, one should vomit). Hebrew צער באסטומכא does not feature in this sense in the current dictionaries.

צופד (צפד) (*Shemot ha-Mashqim*) = Latin 'glutinativus' (gluey, agglutinant); cf. 19 (59): דיאה דרגאגאן דרגאגאן שרף קר בשנייה לח בראשונה צופד ומדבק (Dyadragagantum, tragacanth, a gum, cold in the second, moist in the first [degree], agglutinant, and viscous). Hebrew צפד features in the current dictionaries in the sense of 1) 'to be pressed; to cleave'; 2) 'to press, to contract' (JD 1295) and 'to adhere, to dry, to contract, to harden' (BM 5577).

צפורן סוסית :צפרן (*Shemot ha-Mashqim*) = Latin 'ungula caballina' (coltsfoot; *Tussilago farfara* L.) (cf. SLN 4:217); cf. 26 (73): נינופארנום נינופאר פרח צפורן[548] סוסית קרה ולחה בשלישית (NYNWP'RNWM, [i.e.,] water lily, the flowers of coltsfoot; cold and moist in the third [degree]). In the sense of 'coltsfoot', Hebrew צפורן סוסית is a non-attested calque of the Latin 'ungula caballina'.

הצריד (צרד) (*Hanhagat ha-Beri'ut le-Abu 'Ali Ben Zuhr*) = 'to make [the voice] hoarse' (cf. Honofredi: 'rautifico'); cf. ch. 9: ואמרו הרופאים: אכילת אזביב[549] השמשיים בבלתי גרעין על הצום יחזק קנה שלו ובהרחקת תבשילים מלוחים מאד שהם ישאירו לכלוך בקנה ויצרידו הקול (The Sages said: the consumption of seedless raisins on an empty stomach strengthens the trachea; [the same is achieved] through the avoidance of very salty dishes which leave the trachea unclean

548 faulty reading ed. McVaugh-Ferre צפורן: צפירן.

549 'raisins' (אזביב השמשיים): This is a mixed term, i.e., Arabic الزبيب (raisin) and Hebrew השמשיים (sunny), a faulty translation, possibly resulting from reading Arabic كشمش (raisins, esp., small seedless raisins) as كشمس (like the sun); in addition to אזביב השמשיים, Jacob Ibn Tibbon has הצמוקים השמשיים (see entry).

and make the voice hoarse). In the sense of 'to make [the voice] hoarse', Hebrew הצריד is only attested as a modern term in EM 1549.

צרות הנשימה :צרות (*Sefer ha-Shimmush*) = Arabic ضيق النفس 'orthopnea'; cf. fol. 132a, col. b: והחוג והרעישה וכבדות כל הגוף וצרות הנשימה הממית בעליו באורך הזמן (And dizziness, trembling, heaviness of the whole body, and orthopnea which will be fatal when it lasts for a long time). Hebrew צרות הנשימה features in BM 3826 (s.v. נשימה) in an attestation subsequent to Shem Tov Ben Isaac, namely from Nathan ha-Me'ati's translation of Maimonides, *Medical Aphorisms* 3.76. Ben Yehuda's translation of the Hebrew term as 'asthma' is not precise as this condition is rendered by Maimonides with the standard Arabic ربو. Zeraḥyah Ḥen renders ضيق النفس in aphorism 3.76 as צרות הניפוש (cf. NM 1:182).

צֳרִי (*Sefer ha-Refu'ot ha-Libbiyot*)[550] = Latin 'tiriaca' (theriac, antidote); cf. fols. 248b–249a: דרוניקש: חם ויבש בתחלת המדרגה השנית ובו סגולה חזקה מאד בחזוק הלב ולשמחו ולה[551] אינו מנגד שום הפעולות ועוזרת בצריותו ומה שיש בו מעפיצות דק ומפני זה הוא צרי כל הארסים (Leopard's bane (*Doronicum pardalianches*): It is hot and dry in the beginning of the second degree; it has a very strong specific property of strengthening and exhilarating the heart. Its[552] excessive heat does not oppose it (does not have a negative effect on it). It is supported by its theriacal[553] property and fine astringency. For this reason it is a theriac (antidote) for all poisons). Hebrew צרי does not feature in this sense in the current dictionaries. The anonymous author of *Sammim Libbiyim* (fol. 127a) renders the parallel Arabic ترياق (theriac) as טריאק.

צֳרִיּוּת (*Sefer ha-Refu'ot ha-Libbiyot*) = Latin 'tiriacalitas' (having theriacal (antidotal) property); cf. fol. 246b: והסמים המחזקים לצריותם נכנסים בכל רפואת הלב לפי שהם נאותים בסגולה לטבע האנושי (All the tonic remedies that have the property of an antidote are part (fall under the category) of cardiacs because they are suited to human nature by their specific property). Hebrew צֳרִיּוּת does not feature in the current dictionaries. The anonymous author of *Sammim Libbiyim* renders the Arabic ترياقيّة as טריאקיות (see entry).

(קבב) קיבב 1. (*Sefer Ṣedat ha-Derakhim*) = Arabic انكبّ 'to bend one's head'; cf. bk. 2, ch. 14 (fol. 54b): ואם היה מפני חום נצוה החולה לעשות דברים קרים דקים כמו קבוב על אד המים שנתבשל בהם קאממילא ורדים והדס או יקבב על עשן אבן מחוממת אחר שיזה עליו חומץ יין (If the [rheum] is caused by heat we let the patient

550 In addition to צרי, the anonymous author has סם צרי (see entry).

551 cui non repugnat excessus caliditatis L :ולה אינו מנגד שום הפעולות.

552 'Its excessive heat does not oppose it': Translated after L.

553 'theriacal property': See next entry.

bend his head over cooling, refining ingredients, for instance over the vapor (steam) of water in which camomile, roses and myrtle have been boiled or over the vapor of a stone that has been heated once wine vinegar has been sprinkled on it). In a medical context, Hebrew קיבב features in BM 5668 in attestations from the *Sefer ha-Qanun* only (see also NM 2:119, 158 (Qof 12));

II. (*Sefer ha-Qanun*, Nathan) = Arabic أكبّ 'to produce pronation (cf. DKT 825, s.v. كبّ); cf. bk. 1 (fol. 50a): ואמנם המקבב הוא זוג המונח[554] מחוץ (The pronators [of the forearm] are a pair [of muscles] placed on the outer side [of the forearm]). Joseph Lorki translates Arabic أكبّ as משפיעים (see entry).

קִבּוּב (*Sefer ha-Qanun*, Nathan) = Arabic كبّ 'pronation'; cf. bk. 1 (fol. 50a): וכשיתנועעו אלו השנים יפשיט<ו> הרסג פשוט עם מעט קבוב (When these two [muscles of the wrist] act together, they extend the carpus with some pronation). Hebrew קבוב does not feature in this sense in the current dictionaries. Joseph Lorki translates Arabic كبّ as שיפוע (see entry).

קִבּוּץ (*Sefer ha-Qanun*, Zeraḥyah) = Arabic انقباض 'flexion'; cf. bk. 1 (fol. 27b): והושם האצבע[555] מקצר בקבוץ על מושקלי אחד (For flexion the thumb[556] only needs one muscle). Hebrew קבוץ does not feature in this sense in the current dictionaries. In his translation of Maimonides, *Medical Aphorisms*, Zeraḥyah uses the same Hebrew term for Arabic قَبْض in the sense of 'astringency, contraction'. For the other translator(s), see entry התקבצות.

קביצות (*Sefer ha-Qanun*, Nathan) = Arabic قبض 'flexion'; cf. bk. 1 (fol. 51b): ואמנם התחתון ממנו הנה קביצותם עם ירידה והשפלה ואמנם העליון הנה קביצותו עם מעט הגבהה והרמה (The lower [muscles produce] flexion [of the fingers] while lowering them, and the higher [muscles produce] flexion [of the fingers] while raising them somewhat). Hebrew קביצות does not feature in this sense in the current dictionaries. In his translation of Maimonides, *Medical Aphorisms* 9.71, Nathan uses the same Hebrew term for Arabic قبض in the sense of 'astringency' (cf. NM 2:78). Zeraḥyah Ḥen translates the Arabic قبض as קבלה (see entry), and Joseph Lorki as קבוץ.

קבלה (*Sefer ha-Qanun*, Zeraḥyah) = Arabic قبض 'flexion'; cf. bk. 1 (fol. 27b): והנמוך מהם קבלתו עם הכנעה וחוסר והעליון קבלתו עם מעט הרמה ונשיאות. Hebrew קבלה does not feature in this sense in the current dictionaries. For the other translator(s), see entry קביצות.

קבסא: גרם קבסא (*Sefer ha-Shimmush*) = Arabic أتخم 'to cause indigestion'; cf. fol 139a, col. a: ובעל מזג חם אין ראוי לתקנם על הרוב אם לא יגרמו לו קבסא (And

554 a موضوع Ms המוח emend. ed. :המונח.

555 a الإبهام :האצבע.

556 'thumb': Translated after the Arabic.

someone with a hot temperament does not need to [take anything else to correct their effect] (i.e., that of cherries), unless their consumption causes indigestion). Aramaic קבסא features in SDA 1009 in the sense of 'vomit'. The Hebrew counterpart קבסה is translated by Jastrow (JD 5707) as: 'Brechdurchfall, cholerine'. Subsequent to Shem Tov Ben Isaac, קבסא features in the sense of 'indigestion' in Nathan ha-Me'ati's translation of Maimonides, *Medical Aphorisms* 2.24 (cf. NM 2:78–9). Shem Tov's contemporary Moses Ibn Tibbon has Hebrew קבסא for Arab. غثيان 'nausea' (cf. NM 1:66).

קבץ (*Sefer ha-Qanun*, Nathan) = Arabic قبض 'to draw together, to flex'; cf. bk. 1 (fol. 55a): ואמנם העצלים המניעים האצבעות בקובצים[557] (Among the muscles that move the toes, those that flex them ...). In the sense of 'to draw together, to flex' Hebrew קבץ is a non-attested semantic borrowing from Arabic قبض.

קיבץ (*Sefer ha-Qanun*, Nathan) = Arabic قبض 'to draw together, to flex'; cf. bk. 1 (fol. 49b): העצלים המניעים הקנה יש מהם שיקבצוהו ומהם שימתחוהו (Some of the muscles which move the forearm flex it and others stretch it). Ben Yehuda (BM 5717) quotes the parallel translation by Joseph Lorki and interprets it as meaning 'to contract' (כוץ וצמצם).

קובץ: See entry **סם**.

קָבוּץ (*Sefer Ṣedat ha-Derakhim*) = Arabic منقبض 'contracted, shrivelled'; cf. bk. 2, ch. 17 (fol. 57a): ואם ראינו הלשון אדומה מאד הנה הוא אות חום ואם לבנה מאד הנה הוא אות הקור ואם תהיה רכה עם לחות הרבה בה הוא אות לחות ואם היתה נגובה מאד קבוצה הוא אות יובש (If we see that the tongue is very red it is an indication of heat and if it is very white it is an indication of cold and if it is soft with much moisture it is an indication of moisture and if it is very dry [and] shrivelled it is an indication of dryness). In the sense of 'shrivelled', Hebrew קבוץ is a non-attested semantic borrowing from the Arabic منقبض.

קדם: See entry **קודם**.

קדר: See entry **צלי**.

קדרה (*Sefer ha-Qanun*, Nathan) = Arabic قحف 'skull' (cf. FAL 123, no. 2711); cf. bk. 1 (fol. 28b): הפרק השני בנתוח קדרת המוח (Chapter two: On the anatomy of the skull of the brain). Hebrew קדרה features in BM 5774 in the sense of 'brainpan' in attestations from Rabbinic literature (cf. JD 1318) and halakhic literature, i.e., Israel Isserlein, *Terumat ha-Deshen*. For an extensive discussion of the term as featuring in the *Sefer ha-Qanun*, cf. SRP 29; RTT 145. Zeraḥyah Ḥen and Joseph Lorki translate Arabic قحف as גלגלת.

557 a בקובצים: فالقوابض.

קוֹדֵם: הקודם מן הראש (*Sefer Ṣedat ha-Derakhim*) = Arabic مقدّم الرأس 'the front of the head'; cf. bk. 1, ch. 10 (fol. 16b): ואם היה כאב הראש מחום השמש ושריפתו ראוי שיוצק על הקודם מן הראש שמן ורדים מעורב במים קרים או בחומץ יין (And if the headache arises from the burning heat of the sun, pour on the front of the head olive oil mixed with cold water or wine vinegar). Hebrew הקודם מן הראש does not feature in the current dictionaries.

קִוּוּץ (*Sefer Ṣedat ha-Derakhim*) = Arabic كزاز ; 'spasme, tétanos' (D 2:462); cf. UW 626, s.v. σπάσμα, σπάσμος: 'Krampf, Konvulsion, Zuckung' (spasm, convulsion); UW 671, s.v. τέτανος: 'Starrkrampf' (tetanus);[558] cf. bk. 1, ch. 23 (fol. 35a): תאר גרגרי קבאשיה לפי מה שתקנתיהו ונסיתיהו והוא מועיל מן הפלג ועקום הפה ומן הקווץ והוא אלכזאז ומכל חולי שסבתו קור ומהנקרס והקולון והרוחות העבות (Recipe of pepperweed pills that I revised and tried and that is good for hemiplegia, paralysis of the facial nerve, spasms, i.e. [Arabic] *al-kuzāz*, every illness that is caused by cold, podagra, colic, and thick winds). Hebrew קִוּוּץ features in BM 5824 in an attestation from the commentary by the otherwise unknown Jacob bar Joseph Ibn Zabara on Hippocrates' *Aphorisms*. For the composition of this commentary, Ibn Zabara extensively used Moses Ibn Tibbon's Hebrew translation of Maimonides' commentary on the *Aphorisms* (cf. NM 3:11). Ben Yehuda (ibid.) explains the term as synonymous with קויצה (cf. BM 5827), in an attestation from the *Sefer ha-Qanun*: בקויצה הנקראת תשנג ובלטי׳ אשפאשמו היא עלה עצביית יתנועעו העצלים בה אל התחלתם ויקשו יהתפשט (On QWYṢH called TŠNG (i.e., Arabic *tašannuǧ*; cf. NM 1:37, 66) and in Latin 'ŠP'ŠMW; it is an illness of the nerves in which the muscles move towards their beginning (i.e., contract) and hardly stretch). In his translation of Maimonides, *Medical Aphorisms* 22.16 Nathan translates Arabic كزاز as רפיון האברים (cf. NM 2:87).

קוּסֵס: See קסס.

קוּסְסוּת (*Sefer ha-Shimmush*) = Arabic مزازة 'having a taste between sweet and sour' (cf. L 2710); cf. fol. 138a, col. b: והחשוב שבמין האגס מה שיהיה ממנו בעל בשר דק הקלפה ושיש בטעמו מעט קוססות וקביצות (The best kind of plum[559] is that which has flesh with a thin skin and that is a little bit sweet and sour and astringent). Hebrew קוּסְסוּת, coined from קסס (see entry), does not feature in the current dictionaries.

קוֹץ (*Sefer ha-Qanun*, Nathan) = Arabic شوك 'spine (i.e., spinous process)'; cf. bk. 1 (fol. 32a): ובעד השנית שהשדרה מחסה ומגן לאיברים הנכבדים המונחים לפניה ולכן ברא לה קוצים וסנסנים ([The second use] of the spinal cord is that it covers

558 Cf. also FL 32: 'Morbus ex frigore, aliis Tremor ex frigore'; WKAS 1:166: 'starke Erkältung, Schüttelfrost/bad cold, shivers, ague'.

559 'plum' (אגס): For Hebrew אגס in the sense of 'plum', cf. SHS 1:128 (Alef 53).

and protects the noble organs that lie in front of it. For this reason He created spines and spinous processes for it). Hebrew קוץ does not feature as an anatomical term in the current dictionaries.[560] Zeraḥyah Ḥen renders the Arabic شوك وسناسن as קוצים.

קוץ ערבי (Anonymous glossary; Ms Oxford, Bodleian, Mich. Add. 22) (lit., 'Arabian thorn'); i.e., 'thistle'; cf. fol. 5b: איברא קוץ הרועה קוץ ערבי ([Arab] *ʾibrat* [*ar-rāʿī*]; [Hebrew] QWṢ HRWʿH or QWṢ ʿRBY). Hebrew קוץ ערבי is a non-attested calque of the Arabic *šawka ʿarabiyya*.[561]

קוץ הרועה (Ms Oxford, Bodleian, Mich. Add. 22) (lit., 'needle of the shepherd'); i.e., 'thistle'; cf. fol. 5b: איברא קוץ הרועה קוץ ערבי ([Arab] *ʾibrat* [*ar-rāʿī*]; [Hebrew] QWṢ HRWʿH or QWṢ ʿRBY). Hebrew קוץ הרועה is a non-attested calque of the Arabic *ʾibrat ar-rāʿī*.[562]

קטן (*Sefer ha-Qanun*, Nathan)[563] = Arabic قطن 'loins'; cf. bk. 1 (fol. 35b): והקטן עם העגז הוא כמושב[564] כן לשדרה כלה והוא משענת ונושא לעצם[565] הערוה עאנה ומקום צמיחת עצבי הרגל (The loins and the sacrum are like the basis for the whole spine. They support and bear the pubic bone, [Arabic] *ʿānah*, and are the place from which the nerves for the legs emerge). In the sense of 'loins', Hebrew קטן is a loan word from Arabic قطن (cf. SRP 43 (332)). Zeraḥyah Ḥen renders the Arabic as קוטן,[566] and Joseph Lorki as מתנים.

קטני: See entry **עיצב**.

קיא: See entry **שלשול**.

קיום 1. (*Sefer ha-Refuʾot ha-Libbiyot*) = Latin 'soliditas' (compactness, firmness, solidity); cf. fol. 246a: הסם העוצר והמדביק נכנס ברפואות הלב שהם יתנו לעצם הרוח קיום ודבוק נאות (Astringent and viscous (agglutinant) remedies

---

560 Hebrew קוצים וסנסנים stands for Arabic شوك وسناسن, which in turn stands for Greek ἄκανθαι (spinous processes). Thus it seems that קוצים וסנסנים are in fact synonymous terms; cf. entries כנף and סנסן as well.

561 Cf. MIG 988. Arabic *šawka ʿarabiyya* is a calque of Greek ἄκανθα Ἀραβική, which actually refers to the smaller milk thistle (*Notobasis syriaca* L. (cf. PDA 3:13 (185)). The Arabic sources often equated *šawka ʿarabiyya* with the Persian loan word *bāḏāward*, which refers to the 'soldier thistle'.

562 Arabic *ʾibrat al-rāʿī* is regarded as a synonym of *šukāʿā*, a generic name for 'thistle'; especially Scotch thistle, *Onopordum acanthium* L., and plume thistle, *Cirsium ferox* L.; Dietrich (DT 3:13 (358–9), n. 11) suggested that *ibrat al-rāʿī* might in fact be the name of the 'storksbill' (herb-robert, *Geranium robertianum* L.); cf. DT 3:13 (357–9); 4:15 (528–9); MIG 12, 949.

563 In addition to קטן, we find the spelling קטון (cf. fol. 60a).

564 a כמושב כן: كالقاعدة.

565 add. Ms לעצם: נם.

566 In his translation of Maimonides' *Medical Aphorisms* 12.23, 16.5, 17.14, 19.13, Zeraḥyah renders Arabic قطن as העצם הנקרא קוטן/העצם העומד למטה מכל השדרה הנקרא קוטון/עצה/עצם העגבות (cf. NM 1:177).

are used as cardiacs as they give the substance of the pneuma appropriate (sound) compactness and continuity). Hebrew קיום features in BM 5903–5 in the sense of 'conservation, confirmation, existence, affirmation', and in KTP 3:279–80 as 'Bejahung; Bekräftigung; Existenz; Dauer'. The anonymous translator of *Sammim Libbiyim* renders the parallel Arabic متانة as התקשרות (see entry); II. (*Sefer Ṣedat ha-Derakhim*) = Arabic ثبات 'firmness, solidity'; cf. bk. 1, ch. 14 (fols. 20b–21a): השער הארבעה עשר בחולי השכחה: טוב השמירה וקלות הזכרנות הדברים ההוים בנפש יורה כי עצם החלק האחרון מן המוח אשר יקראוהו הרופאים הזכרון הוא עצם יש לו קיום ושווי ואם יהיה עצמו נגר שלא יהיה לו קיום יהיה בעליו שכחן גדול עם רוחק ההבנה והסח הדעת ואיחור השכל (Chapter fourteen: On the illness of forgetfulness: A good and easy memory of the things that are in the soul indicates that the substance of the posterior part of the brain which the physicians call 'memory' is firm (solid) and balanced. But if its substance is fluid and not firm (solid), someone [with such a brain] will be very forgetful, dull-witted, absentminded and slow to understand).

קִיטוֹר I. (*Sefer ha-Refu'ot ha-Libbiyot*) = Latin 'vapor' (vapour); cf. fol. 250a: לאפיש ארמיני: יש לו סגולה לחזק הלב ולשמחו מפריד ביותר הקיטור השחוריי והע־שני מהרוח וגם מנקה הגוף מליחה שחוריית (Armenian stone: It has the specific property to strengthen and exhilarate the heart and moreover to ward off the melancholic smoky vapour from the pneuma and to purify the body from the melancholic humour). Hebrew קיטור features as a biblical term in the sense of 'thick smoke' (cf. BDB 882), as a Rabbinic term in the sense of 'smoke' (cf. JD 1357–8), and as a modern term in the sense of 'steam' (cf. EM 1597). The anonymous author of *Sammim Libbiyim* (fol. 128a) renders Arabic دخان as אד. See also NM 3:268 (section 'Corrections and additions to NM 2)'; II. (*Sefer ha-Shimmush*) = Arabic بخار 'vapour'; cf. fol. 127a, col. a: והמזון המתילד מהם על הכלל עב קשה להתעכל מתאחר לרדת מולידים דם שחורי וכל שכן כשיאכלו בקליפיהם ולפיכך הם ממלאים מוח מתמידם מקטורים עבים שחוריים מכאיבים[567] (The food prepared from them (i.e., lentils) is in general thick, difficult to digest and slow to descend from the stomach. They produce melancholic blood especially when they are eaten with their skins, and therefore fill the brain of those who eat it frequently with thick melancholic vapours that[568] cause headache).

קִיפָאל: הקיפאל (*Sefer ha-Qanun*, Nathan) = Arabic القيفال 'cephalic vein' (cf. DKT 825; FAL 123, no. 2710); cf. bk. 1 (fol. 66a): והרביעי והוא הגדול שבהם והוא אותו אשר יראה ויעלה וישתלח ענף מאסף עמו שריג מן הקיפאל ויתהוה ממנו האכחל ושאריתו הוא הבאסליק (The fourth [branch of the axillary vein], the largest of

567 a מכאיבים: ويصدّع.

568 'that cause headache': Translated after the Arabic.

all, is the one that goes up along the outer part and sends out branches that join a branch of the cephalic vein and from these branches the median vein is formed. The remaining part is the basilic vein). Hebrew הקיפאל is a non-attested loan word from Arabic القيفال. Zeraḥyah Ḥen transcribes the Arabic القيفال as הקיפל.

קיפל: See entry **קיפאל**.

מוקץ (קיץ) (*Sefer Ṣedat ha-Derakhim*) = Arabic منتبه 'being awake, esp., a kind of illness that arouses and keeps awake'; cf. D 2:638: 'espèce de maladie, qui excite, qui tient réveillé', following Dugat, *Études*, 221 (341)[569]; cf. Latin 'quas expergefacio'; cf. bk. 1, ch. 15 (fols. 22a–b): השער הט״ו בחולי הנקרא המוקץ כשיתחדש במאוחר מן המוח ליחה לבנה עם מרה אדומה וימזגו יחד יקרה מזה שיהיה החולה מושלך על ערפו כמת ועיניו[570] פתוחות עד אצל שלא יגיע ממנו אל הנפש נזק ולא צער ויהיה שקט החולה ומנוחתו מפני קור הליחה הלבנה ולחותה ויהיה תעורתו[571] והקצתו מפני יובש המרה האדומה וחדודה ולכן אמר גאלינוס כי הכונה ברפואת החולי הזה הנקרא המוקץ נקוי המוח משתי אלו הליחות המתהפכות בעצמיהם ר״ל ליחה לבנה ומרה אדומה (Chapter fifteen: On the illness called 'being awake': When the posterior part of the brain is affected by phlegm and yellow bile and they mix together, it causes the patient to lie on his back as if he is dead while his eyes are open and[572] staring, but his soul does not suffer any harm or distress. The calmness and tranquillity of the patient originate from the coldness and moisture of the phlegm; his staring[573] and wakefullness is induced by the dryness and sharpness of the yellow bile. For this reason Galen said that to heal this illness called 'being awake' one should aim to cleanse the brain from these two humours that are opposite in their substance, i.e.,

---

569 G. Dugat, 'Études sur le *Traité de Médecine* d'Abou Djafar Ahmad, intitulé: *Zad al-Moçafir*, La Provision du Voyageur', *Journal Asiatique* 1 (1853), repr. in Beiträge zur Geschichte der arabisch-Islamischen Medizin. Aufsätze, vol. 1 (1819–69), ed. by F. Sezgin, in collab. with M. Amawi, D. Bischoff, E. Neubauer, (Frankfurt 1987), 169–233 (290–353), esp. 220–33 (340–53); Ibn Sīnā, *K. al-Qānūn*, 2:53, calls this illness: السبات السهري 'sleepless torpor, stupor' (cf. Avicenna, *The Canon of Medicine*, vol. 3: *Special Pathologies*, trans. by P. Adeli Sardo (Chicago 2014), 3:105: 'lethargic sleeplessness'), and remarks that some physicians call it شخوص (staring), but are mistaken, since شخوص (staring) is a kind of stiffness (الشخوص هو نوع من الجمود).

570 ועיניו פתוחות: مفتوح العينين شاخصًا a.

571 תעורתו: شخوصه a.

572 'and staring': Trans. according to a.

573 'staring': Trans. according to a.

phlegm and yellow bile).[574] Hebrew מוקץ does not feature as the name of an illness in the current dictionaries.

קלוח (*Sefer Ṣedat ha-Derakhim*) = Arabic حقنة 'clyster'; cf. bk. 1, ch. 15 (fols. 22b–23a): ואם תהיה המרה האדומה יותר גוברת ירבה מן השמנים הקרים וימעיט מן החמים ואם הליחה הלבנה יותר גוברת ירבה מן השמנים החמים וימעיט מן הקרים ויקח זה למשל ולדמיון בכל מה שירפאו בו החולי הזה מקלוח הנקרא קלישטירי או פתילות אם נעצר הטבע או רפואה משלשלת או משקה או מזון (If the yellow bile dominates, one should [rub the head] more with cold oils and less with hot oils, but if phlegm dominates [one should rub the head] more with hot oils and less with cold oils, and one should apply all things with which this kind of illness[575] is treated, such as a clyster called (in Romance) QLYŠṬYRY or a suppository in case the patient suffers from constipation, or a purging medicine, drink or food). In the sense of clyster, Hebrew קלוח features in BM 5940 in attestations from Meir Aldabi, *Shevilei Emunah*. In addition to קלוח, Moses Ibn Tibbon renders the Arabic with a variant term from the same root, i.e., מקלח (see entry).

קלח: See entry **מקלח**.

קלפה (*Sefer ha-Qanun*, Nathan)[576] = Arabic الدرز القشري 'squamous (aquamosal) suture' (cf. DKT 459, n. 8); cf. bk. 1 (fol. 29a): ואמנם שני השלבים הכוזבים המה לוקחים באורך הראש על נכחיות החציי משני צדדים ואינם שוקעים בעצם תכלית השקיעה ואלו השנים נקראים שתי קלפות (The two false sutures run longitudinally at both sides of the head parallel to the sagittal [suture] and do not enter the bone completely and are [therefore] called 'squamous (squamosal) [sutures]'). Hebrew קלפה does not feature in this sense in the current dictionaries. Joseph Lorki translates الدرز القشري as קלפין. In his translation of Maimonides, *Medical Aphorisms* 13.37, Nathan uses the same Hebrew term to render Arabic قشر in the sense of 'epithelial debris, scale' (cf. NM 2:82), Moses Ibn Tibbon uses the same Hebrew term for Arabic قشر in the sense of 'scab' (cf. NM 2:67), and Shem Tov Ben Isaac for Arabic خشكريشة 'eschar' (NM 2:112).

קְלָפִי: See entry **שלב**.

קְלָפִי (*Sefer ha-Qanun*, Zeraḥyah) = Arabic غضروفي 'cartiliginous'; cf. bk. 1 (fol. 20a): עצם העצה מֻחובר מחוליות שלשה קלפיי אין לו תוספת (The coccyx is made of

---

574 Ibn al-Jazzār knew the (lost) commentary on humours, where Galen will have talked about bile as the cause of sleeplessness (as he does elsewhere). However, where talking about cures, he seems to have used exactly the words quoted at *De sanitate tuenda* 3.12 (ed. Kühn, 6:226); in such diseases one should aim to rebalance the fluids in the constitution by using contraries. I thank Vivian Nutton for this elucidation.

575 I.e., the illness called منتبه; cf. entry מוקץ above.

576 Nathan also renders the Arabic الدرز القشري as השלב הקלפי (see entry).

three cartiliginous vertebrae that do not have processes). Hebrew קלפי only features in the current dictionaries in the sense of 'parchment-like' (cf. BM 5971). For its occurrence in Zeraḥyah's translation of the *K. al-Qanun* in the sense of 'cartiliginous', cf. SRP 40. For the other translator(s), cf. entry שחוסי.

קנה (*Sefer ha-Qanun*, Nathan) = Arabic ساعد 'forearm'; cf. bk. 1 (fol 37b): והנקרה החיצונית היא הגדולה ממנה ומה שנלוה לנקרה הפנימי בלתי חלק ובלתי עגול החפירה אבל כגדר הישר עד שיתנועע בו תוספת הקנה אל הצד החיצוני יגיע אליו ויעמד אצלו (The external cavity (of the humeral trochlea) is the largest, that which is adjoining the internal cavity is neither smooth nor hollow in a spherical way but is like a straight wall so that the apophysis of the forearm, when it moves [in this cavity] to the outside, stops when it reaches it). As an anatomical term, Hebrew קנה features in the Bible in the sense of 'shoulder-joint' (BDB 889), in Rabbinic literature in the sense of 'forearm' or 'windpipe' (JD 1338–9); according to LOW LXXVII it is used for: 'forearm, or any bone which resembles a reed. Therefore: קנה הזרוע; *ulna*, bone of forearm (Avicenna); קנה גדולה: shin bone (Avicenna); קנה קטנה: *fibula* (Avicenna)'. Ben Yehuda (BM 6019) defines the קנה של זרוע as העצם העליונה שלזרוע. See also SRP 24 (138) and entry שני הקנים. Zeraḥyah Ḥen renders the Arabic ساعد as זרוע; Joseph Lorki corrects Nathan's קנה as קנה הזרוע.

הקנה הגדול (*Sefer ha-Qanun*, Nathan)[577] = Arabic القصبة الكبرى 'tibia' (cf. DKT 508–9, 825: FAL 123, no. 2700); cf. bk. 1 (fol. 41a): השוק היא כמו הקנה מחוברת משני עצמים אחד מהם יותר גדול ויותר ארוך והוא פנימי ונקרא הקנה הגדול והשני יותר קטון ויותר קצר ... ונקרא הקנה הקטון (Like the forearm, the leg is composed of two bones, one is bigger and longer and is situated at the inside and is called 'tibia', the second [bone] is smaller and shorter ... it is called 'fibula'). Hebrew הקנה הגדול features in MD 720, s.v. 'tibia', with a reference to the *Sefer ha-Qanun*; see also LOW LXXVII: 'קנה גדולה: shin bone (Avicenna)', and SRP 36–7 (252, 256, 262).

קנה החוטם (*Sefer Ṣedat ha-Derakhim*, Ms Oxford, Bodleian, Poc. 353, Uri Heb. 314) = Arabic قصبة الأنف (lit., 'tube(s) of the nose'; i.e., 'passage(s) of the nose' (nostrils))[578]; cf. Latin 'canales narium' (nasal passages); cf. bk. 1, ch. 21 (fol. 9a): ופעמים יבא פתאום מבלתי חולי וזה כי קנה חוטם האדם קצר ויגיעו בעבור זה מהר דברים מזיקים מחוץ למוח כמו אבק ועשן וקור חזק וזריחת השמש ומה שדומה להם (Sometimes [sneezing] occurs all of a sudden without an illness because the nostrils of a human being are short, and for this reason harmful things quickly reach the brain from the outside such as dust, smoke, severe

577 Another term used by Nathan to refer to the 'tibia' is הקנה הפנימי (see entry).

578 Cf. FL 3:450, s.v. قصبة: 'cartilago sive imbrex nasi; os nasi'; L 2530, s.v. قصبة الأنف: 'the nasal bone'.

cold, smoke, sunbeams and the like). Hebrew קנה החוטם does not feature in the current dictionaries.

הקנה החיצוני (*Sefer ha-Qanun*, Nathan)[579] = Arabic القصبة الوحشية 'fibula' (cf. DKT 574–5, 825; FAL 123, no. 2703); cf. bk. 1 (fol. 54b): ועצל מסתבך ממנו שני מיתרים אחד מהם מקבץ כף הרגל והשני מפשיט הבהן וזה שהעצל הזה צמיחתו מראש הקנה הפנימי מקום שפוגע החיצוני וימשך ביניהם ומשתרג לשני מיתרים (Another muscle [of the foot] is divided into two tendons, one of which flexes the foot and the other stretches the big toe, because this muscle originating from the head of the tibia at the place where it is connected to the fibula, descends between these two [bones] and is divided into two tendons). Hebrew הקנה החיצוני is not attested in the current dictionaries. Zeraḥyah Ḥen translates the Arabic القصبة الوحشية mistakenly as הקנה הפנימי (i.e., the tibia, see entry), and Joseph Lorki as הקנה הימני (see entry).

קנה הטוב (*Hanhagat ha-Beri'ut le-Abu 'Ali Ben Zuhr*) = Arabic قصب الطيب or قصب الذريرة (Greek κάλαμος ἀρωματικός) 'lemon grass (*Cymbopogon martini*)'; cf. MIG 846; cf. ch. 5: והתמדת הרחת המוסרחים והעכורים יעכירו הרוח הנפשי וינצחו אותו ולזה יתחיב להריח הריח הטוב ולהתמידו ולהתעשן בעשן הבשמים כעשן הליגנאלובין והענבר וקנה הטוב (Continuous inhalation of putrid, foul [air] overcomes the psychical pneuma and makes it impure. For this reason one should frequently inhale [air] that smells good, and fumigate [the house?] with fragrant spices, like aloeswood, ambergris, and lemon grass). Hebrew קנה הטוב does not feature in the current dictionaries. Nathan ha-Me'ati renders the Arabic قصب الذريرة as קנה בושם in his translation of Maimonides, *Medical Aphorisms* 21.42 (cf. IJ 638, 29–30: קנה בשם قصب الطيب وهو قصب الذريرة الداخل في الطيوب), and Zeraḥyah Ḥen as קלמו ארומטיקו. See also MIG 846.

הקנה הימני (*Sefer ha-Qanun*, Joseph Lorki) = Arabic القصبة الوحشية 'fibula' (cf. DKT 574–5, 825; FAL 123, no. 2703); cf. bk. 1 (fol. 16b): ועצל אחד ישתרגו ממנו שני יתרים האחד מהם יקבץ הרגל והשני יפשט הבהן וזה <ש>העצל הזה תולדתו מראש הקנה השמאלי באיזה מקום שפוגע הימני ויולד[580] ממנו וישתרג לשני יתרים (Another muscle [of the foot] is divided into two tendons, one of which flexes the foot and the other stretches the big toe, because this muscle originating from the head of the tibia at the place where it is connected to the fibula, descends[581] between these two [bones] and is divided into two tendons). Hebrew הקנה הימני is not attested in the current dictionaries. For the other translator(s), see entry הקנה החיצוני.

579 Another term used by Nathan to refer to the 'fibula' is הקנה הקטן (see entry).
580 a ויולד ממנו: وتحدر بينهما.
581 'descends between': Translated after the Arabic وتحدر بينهما.

קנה הסוכר (*Sefer ha-Shimmush*) = Arabic قصب السكّر 'sugar cane'; cf. fol. 139b, col. b: קני הסוכר בטבעם ומזגם קרובים מטבע המוזי (Sugar canes are in their nature and temperament close to the nature of bananas). Hebrew קנה הסוכר features as a modern term in EM 1616.

הקנה הפנימי (*Sefer ha-Qanun*, Nathan)[582]= Arabic القصبة الانسية 'tibia' (cf. DKT 574–5, 825; FAL 123, no. 2698); cf. bk. 1 (fol. 54b): אמנם המגביהים יש מהם עצל גדול מונח קדם הקנה הפנימי (Of the [muscles] that raise [the foot] there is a large muscle that lies at the front side of the tibia). Hebrew הקנה הפנימי is not attested in the current dictionaries. Joseph Lorki translates Arabic القصبة الانسية as הקנה השמאלי (see entry).

הקנה הקטן (*Sefer ha-Qanun*, Nathan)[583] = Arabic القصبة الصغرى 'fibula' (cf. DKT 508–9, 825: FAL 123, no. 2702); cf. bk. 1 (fol. 41a): השוק היא כמו הקנה מחוברת משני עצמים אחד מהם יותר גדול ויותר ארוך והוא פנימי ונקרא הקנה הגדול והשני יותר קטון ויותר קצר ... ונקרא הקנה הקטון (Like the forearm, the leg is composed of two bones, one is bigger and longer and is situated at the inside and is called 'tibia', the second [bone] is smaller and shorter ... it is called 'fibula'). Hebrew הקנה הקטן features in MD 291, s.v. 'fibula', with a reference to the *Sefer ha-Qanun*; see also SRP 36 (258, 262).

הקנה השמאלי (*Sefer ha-Qanun*, Joseph Lorki) = Arabic القصبة الانسية 'tibia' (cf. DKT 574–5, 825; FAL 123, no. 2698); cf. bk. 1 (fol. 16b): ואמנם המרימים מהם עצל גדול מונח לפני הקנה השמאלי (Of the [muscles] that raise [the foot] there is a large muscle that lies at the front side of the tibia). Hebrew הקנה השמאלי is not attested in the current dictionaries. For the other translator(s), see entry הקנה הפנימי.

שני הקנים (*Sefer ha-Qanun*, Nathan) = Arabic القصبتان 'the two bones [of the leg, i.e., tibia and fibula]' (cf. FL 3:450 'Duo ossa cruris, quorum exterior appellatur القصبة الكبرى, interior القصبة الصغرى'); cf. bk. 1 (fol. 42a): והקרסול מונח בין שתי הקצות הבולטים משני הקנים מקיפים עליו מצדדיו ר״ל מעליונו ותחתיתו (The astragalus is located between the two projecting ends of the two bones [of the leg] (i.e., tibia and fibula) which surround it from [different] sides, i.e., from above and below). As an anatomical term, Hebrew קנה features in the Bible in the sense of 'shoulder-joint' (BDB 889), in Rabbinic literature in the sense of 'forearm' or 'windpipe' (JD 1338–9); according to LOW LXXVII it is used for: 'forearm, or any bone which resembles a reed. Therefore: קנה הזרוע; ulna, bone of forearm (Avicenna); קנה גדולה: shin bone (Avicenna); קנה קטנה: fibula (Avicenna)'. Ben Yehuda (BM 6019) defines the קנה של זרוע

582 Another term used by Nathan to refer to the 'tibia' is הקנה הגדול (see entry).

583 Another term used by Nathan to refer to the 'fibula' is הקנה החיצוני (see entry).

as העצם העליונה שלזרוע. See also SRP 24 (138) and entry קנה. Zeraḥyah Ḥen translates the Arabic القصبتان as שתי הקנים.

קוסס: קסס (*Sefer ha-Shimmush*) = Arabic مُزّ 'having a taste between sweet and sour' (cf. L 2710; RR 176, n. 1: '*muzz*, which, according to the classical dictionaries, means 'half way between sour and sweet' when applied to drinks and to the pomegranate'); cf. fol. 137b, col. b: והמבושל ישתנה בפעולתו כפי טעמו כי יש ממנו עפוץ ויש ממנו חמוץ ויש ממנו קוסס ויש ממנו מתוק ויש ממנו תפל (Boiled [quinces] vary in their effects according to their taste, for they can be astringent and bitter, or sour, or sweet and sour, or sweet, or tasteless). Hebrew קסס features in the Bible in Ez 17:9 (cf. KB 1116; LF 1:101), in Rabbinic literature (JD 1396), and in modern literature (EM 1621) in the context of wine in the sense of 'to bite, to have a pungent taste, to be sourish', or 'to turn sour, to become somewhat spoiled' (BM 6046); Löw (FL 1:101) relates the term to קשקשת 'Fischschuppe' and explains it as 'kahmig werden' (to become mouldy).

קערורית האצטומכא: קערורית (*Hanhagat ha-Beri'ut le-Abu 'Ali Ben Zuhr*) 'the concave part (bottom) of the stomach' (Honofredi: 'fundus stomaci'); cf. ch. 8: והרחקת אכילת העצמים הדקים כמו עצם העוף והפרדיץ והצפרים והתרנגולים ואכילת הדגים הקוציים, זולת עצמי השיות והתישים הסריסים כאשר יותך מהם לעיסותם ממה שירכך הקנה והאוילה וירכך הושט וישלשל המעברות ויעזור לירידת המאכל בקערורית האצטומכא (One should avoid the consumption of fine bones such as those of birds, partridges, small birds (sparrows?), chickens and of spiny fish except for the bones of (young) sheep, and castrated billy-goats; when these are chewed so that they become soft it is something that mollifies the trachea, uvula and esophagus, cleanses the passages and helps the food to descend to the concave part (bottom) of the stomach). Hebrew קערורית features in BM 6051 in the sense of 'concavity' as an astronomical, geographical term in some attestations from medieval literature. As a medical term it features as קערורית הכבד (the concave side of the liver) in Nathan ha-Me'ati's translation of Maimonides, *Medical Aphorisms* (cf. NM 1:18–9).

קצה העין מצד האזן: קצה (*Sefer ha-Qanun*, Joseph Lorki) = Arabic لحاظ 'external angle of the eye'; cf. DKT 586–7, 826; FAL 82, no. 1806); cf. bk. 1 (fol. 17a): והחלק הב׳ עובר בנקב הנברא אצל קצה העין מצד האזן (The second part (i.e., of the third branch of the trochlear pair of nerves) penetrates the hole that has been created close to the external[584] angle of the eye). Hebrew קצה העין מצד האזן is not attested in the current dictionaries. For the other translator(s), see entry סקירה.

584 'the external angle': Read: 'the internal angle'; cf. DKT 586–7.

הקצוות אשר הדמע יורד מהן (*Sefer ha-Qanun*, Zeraḥyah) = Arabic مأقان 'the inner and outer angle (canthi) of the eye' (cf. DKT 827; FAL 88, nos. 1945–7); cf. bk. 1 (fol. 23b): אמנם זה המושקולי ד׳ מהם בצדדיו הד׳ למעלה ולמטה ושתי הק־צוות אשר הדמע יורד מהן הנקרא בערבי מאקין (These [six] muscles [that move the eyeball], four of them are situated at the four sides, above, below, and in the two angles from which tears stream down (i.e., canthi) that are called in Arabic M'QYN). Hebrew הקצוות אשר הדמע יורד מהן does not feature in the current dictionaries. For the other translator(s), see entry קצה: קצוות העין.

קצוות העין (*Sefer ha-Qanun*, Nathan) = Arabic مأقان 'the inner and outer angle (canthi) of the eye' (cf. DKT 827; FAL 88, nos. 1945–7); cf. bk. 1 (fol. 43a): הפרק הרביעי בנתוח עצלי כלל העין ואמנם העצלים המניעים לכלל[585] העין הם עצלים ששה ארבעה מהם בצד הם הארבעה למעלה ולמטה בשתי קצוות העין הנקרא מאקים (Chapter four: The anatomy of the muscles of the eyeball. There are six muscles that move the eyeball. Four of them are situated at the four sides, above, below, and in the two angles (canthi) of the eye that are called M'QYM). Hebrew קצה העין, Plur. קצוות העין, does not feature in the current dictionaries. Zeraḥyah Ḥen translates the Arabic مأقان as הקצוות אשר הדמע יורד מהן (see entry), and Joseph Lorki as זנבות העין, a term also featuring in Sing. זנב העין in Shem Tov Ben Isaac's *Sefer ha-Shimmush* (cf. NM 1:90). In his translation of Maimonides, *Medical Aphorisms* 15.21 and 23.72, Nathan ha-Me'ati renders the Arabic مأق العين as קצוות העין הנקרא מאק and מאק שבעין, and Zeraḥyah as קצה העין הנקרא בערבי מאק and קצוות העיניים. In his translation of Maimonides, *Medical Aphorisms* 15.73, Nathan ha-Me'ati renders the Arabic المأق الأكبر 'the inner angle of the eye' as קצה העין הגדול, and Zeraḥyah as קצה העין לצד האף (cf. NM 2:83).

קצוי: קצויות (*Sefer ha-Qanun*, Nathan)[586] = Arabic ناجذ, Plur. نواجذ 'wisdom teeth'; cf. bk. 1 (fol. 31b): והקצויות יצמחו ברוב באמצע זמן הגדול והוא אחר ההמרצה אל ההעמדה וזה כי ההעמדה קרובה מל׳ שנה ולכן נקראים שני אלחלם כלו׳ החלימה (In most cases wisdom teeth appear during the time of growth, after one reaches maturity. For [one reaches] maturity at about thirty years and therefore [these teeth] are called 'wisdom teeth'). Hebrew קצוי does not feature in this sense in the current dictionaries. Zeraḥyah Ḥen renders the Arabic نواجذ as שינים, and Joseph Lorki as קצויות הנקראות נואג׳ד.

קרב: קרב בעל השתים עשרה אצבעות (*Sefer Hanhagat ha-Beri'ut*) = 'duodenum'; cf. 8.1 (144): ונקרא הקרב הזה הדבק בשוער בעל שתים עשרה אצבעות כי שעורו מכל אדם שתים עשרה אצבעות מאצבעות ידיו (And this intestine that adheres to the pylorus is called 'duodenum' because with all people it measures twelve fingers

585 a للمقلة Ms לכלל: לעצלי.

586 See also entry שן: שני אלחלם כלו׳ החלימה.

from the fingers of his hands). Hebrew קרב בעל השתים עשרה אצבעות does not feature in the current dictionaries. Another term common in medieval Hebrew literature is המעי השנים עשר, which Ben Yehuda (BM 3166) quotes from Meir Aldabi, *Shevilei Emunah*.

קָרוּי: בלתי קרוי (*Sefer Issur ha-Qevurah le-Galienus*) = Arabic لا سقف له 'roofless'; cf. par. 45: ויכניסו החולה ויסגרו בעדו בבית בלתי קרוי (and they shall put the patient into a roofless house and lock him up). Hebrew קָרוּי (Pass. Part. Qal) is not attested in this sense in the current dictionaries. The regular form for 'roofed' is מְקוֹרֶה (Part. Pu'al); cf. BM 6158.

קרום: קרום הלב (*Sefer Issur ha-Qevurah le-Galienus*) = Arabic حجاب القلب 'pericardium'[587]; cf. par. 187: והמין האחר מפני השינה וזה שהאדם רב המילוי ממאכלים או מהדברים הלחים ויכבד זה על טבעו וישן על צדו האחד ויטו המאכלים והכימוסים אל <הלב>[588] וילחצו קרומו (The other kind of [someone being apparently dead] occurs because of sleep, namely when [his stomach] is more than full with moist foodstuff or [other] moist things that are a burden for his nature. He sleeps on one side and the foodstuff and chyles turn to the heart and press upon the pericardium). Hebrew קרום הלב does not feature in the current dictionaries. A similar term, i.e., קרום שעל הלב features in Zeraḥyah Ḥen's translation of Maimonides, *Medical Aphorisms* 4.27–8; 25.72, whereas Nathan ha-Me'ati has כיס הלב (cf. entry). In Rabbinic literature, 'pericardium' is rendered as Aramaic טרפשא דלבא (cf. LOW LIV).

הקרום הקשה (*Sefer ha-Qanun*, Nathan) = Arabic الغشاء الصلب 'the hard membrane, i.e., dura mater' (cf. DKT 824, s.v. الغشاء الصفيق); cf. bk. 1 (fol. 65b): ומתפרד ממנו שריגים בשני קרומי המוח לזונם ושיקשר הקרום הקשה במה שסביבותיו ולמעלה הימנו (Some of its branches (i.e., of the jugular vein) spread out in the two meninges to feed them and to fasten the dura mater to the parts around and above it). In the sense of 'dura mater', Hebrew הקרום הקשה features in MD 237, s.v. 'dura mater'. <י>

קרומ<י> המוח (*Sefer ha-Shimmush*) = Arabic حجب الدماغ 'meninges' (cf. UW 420, s.v. μῆνιγξ); cf. fol. 127a, col. b: ומחדשים חלומות רעים וממלאים האסטומ' והמעים רוחות מנפחות ומולידים סתומים ומתיחה ועצירת הבטן ומזיקים אל הריאה והטרפשה ואל קרומ<י> המוח ויתר העצבים והקרומות (They (i.e., lentils) cause bad dreams, fill the stomach and intestines with flatulent winds, produce blockages, tension (tetanus) and constipation and are harmful for the lungs, diaphragm, meninges, and all the other nerves and membranes). Hebrew קרום המוח, Plur. קרומי המוח, features in BM 6170 without any further explication.

---

587 For the Arabic synonym غلاف القلب, cf. entry כיס הלב.
588 a القلب: <הלב>.

קרסל: קרסול (*Sefer ha-Qanun*, Nathan) = Arabic كعب 'astragalus, talus, ankle-bone' (cf. DKT 512–3, 826; FAL 79, no. 1753); cf. bk. 1 (fol. 41b): עצמות כף הרגל ששה[589] קרסול שבו ישלם הפרק עם השוק (The foot has six[590] bones: the astragalus which together with [the bones of] the leg forms the articulation [of the foot]). Hebrew קרסל features in the current dictionaries and secondary literature in the sense of 'ankle' (BDB 902; BM 6202); 'bent, joint, ankle'; 'articulation of the ankle' (LOW LXXVIII); in the sense of 'astragalus', it features in MD 75, s.v. 'astragalus', a.o., as עצם הקרסל; see also SRP 26–7 (166, 168–9). Zeraḥyah Ḥen (fol. 23a) renders the Arabic كعب as עקב.

קשוא: קשואים מרים (*Sefer Ṣedat ha-Derakhim*) = Arabic قثّاء الحمار 'squirting cucumber' (*Ecballium Elaterium* L.) (cf. MIG 826); cf. bk. 2, ch. 18 (fol. 61a): תואר רפואה חברתיה ונסיתיה ומצאתיה מועילה לכאב השנים והטוחנות מקור ורוח עבה ערובו יקח פליטרי ואישוף ופולי ושרש קשואים מרים (Composition of a remedy that I made and tried and found to be good for pain affecting the teeth and molars caused by cold and thick wind: Take pellitory, hyssop, mint, and root of squirting cucumber). Hebrew קשוא מר, Plur. קשואים מרים (lit., bitter cucumbers), does not feature in the current dictionaries or botanical literature. The current name for 'squirting cucumber' is קשוא החמור or ירוקת החמור (cf. BM 6228, s.v. קשא; LF 1:549–50). Note however, that the Arabic synonym of قثّاء الحمار is علقم, which—according to Meyerhof (M 292)—designates bitter kinds of *Cucurbitaceae*. He adds that bitterness is not a property of the squirting cucumber except for the variety that grows in Spain.

קשי: קושי (*Sefer ha-Shimmush*) = Arabic إنعاظ 'erection'; cf. fol. 131b, col. b: שכר החטה: יש ששותים אותו מתוק חדש ויש ששותים אותו ישן והמתוק רב המזון קשה להתעכל רב הרוחות והנפח ומוסיף בתאות המשגל והקושי תוספת גדולה (Wheat wine: Some drink it when it is young and sweet, others when it is old. When it is sweet it is very nutritious and hard to digest; it produces many winds and much flatulence, greatly increases the libido and erection). The term קשי features in the sense of 'hardness of the member' (קשיו של אבר) in BM 6248 in an attestation from tb*Sanhedrin* 55a. In medieval medical literature, it features in the sense of 'erection' in Zeraḥyah Ḥen's translation of Maimonides, *Medical Aphorisms* 22.61 (cf. NM 1:186; 2:84), and in Moses Ibn Tibbon' translation of Hippocrates' *Aphorisms* 5.49 (cf. NM 3:211). In the latter translation, Ibn Tibbon also uses the term קשי to render Arabic توتّر 'tension' (cf. NM 3:211).

קושי השתן (*Sefer Issur ha-Qevurah le-Galienus*) = 'difficult urination (dysuria)' (Honofredi: 'difficultas urinandi'); cf. par. 26: ואין ראוי שיעצר דבר מן השתן

589 a ששה: ستّة وعشرون.

590 'six': The Arabic text has 'twenty-six'.

כי עצירת השתן מביא קושי השתן וחולי במקוה ורפיונה (One should not withhold urinating in any way for doing so leads to difficult urination and a sick and weak bladder). Hebrew קושי השתן does not feature in the current dictionaries. The anonymous translator of Hippocrates' *Aphorisms* 6.36 uses the same Hebrew term to render the Arabic parallel term عسر البول (cf. NM 3:211), and in his translation of *Aphorisms* 3.5, he renders the same Arabic term as קושי ההשתנה (cf. ibid.). Nathan ha-Me'ati renders عسر البول as קשי יציאת השתן in his translation of Hippocrates' *Aphorisms* 6.36 (cf. ibid.).

קשקשי: הקשקשי (*Sefer ha-Shimmush*) = Arabic ما له فلوس 'that which has scales, that which is scaly'; cf. fol. 149b, col. b: והקשקשי הוא בכלל יותר חשוב ממה שאין לו קשקשת (Scaly [fish] is generally better than fish that does not have scales). Hebrew קשקשי features in EM 1657 as a modern term.

(קשר) מקשר (*Sammim Libbiyim*)[591] = Arabic ممتّن (fortifying); cf. fol. 125a: ויהיה סם מקשר לרוח (And it (i.e., emblic myrobalan) is a remedy that fortifies the pneuma). Hebrew קישר, Part. מקשר, does not feature in this sense in the current dictionaries. The anonymous translator of *Sefer ha-Refu'ot ha-Libbiyot* (fol. 247b) renders the parallel Latin 'solidativus' as מחזק.[592]

קֶשֶׁר (*Sefer Ṣedat ha-Derakhim*) = Arabic عقدة (Greek: συστροφή; cf. LSG 1736 and IJZ 121, n. 262) 'tumor'; cf. bk. 2, ch. 13 (fol. 53b): או יקח מן הרפואה הזאת כי היא תמהר בריאות הנואסיר[593] והקשרים המתהוים בחוטם (Or take this medicine because it quickly heals the polyps and tumors that develop in the nose). Hebrew קֶשֶׁר does not feature in this sense in the current dictionaries.

(ראה) נִרְאֶה (*Sefer Ṣedat ha-Derakhim*) = Arabic ظاهر 'clear, evident'; cf. bk. 2, ch. 17 (fol. 57b): ואם קרה העדר התנועה והפסק הדבור מן הלשון מבלתי שאר אברי הגוף ולא נראה בלשון חולי נראה ידענו כי זה מפני כאב העצב אשר יעבור בו כח התנועה מן המוח אל הלשון (If loss of movement and speech of the tongue occur without the other organs [being affected] and we do not see that the tongue is clearly ill, we know that this [happens] because of the pain the nerves through which the power of movement [of the tongue] streams from the brain to the tongue). In the sense of 'clear, evident' (נגלה/גלוי), Hebrew נִרְאֶה features in BM 6293 in an attestation from the *Sefer ha-Kuzari* (trans. Judah Ibn Tibbon).

ראות (*Sefer Ṣedat ha-Derakhim*) = Arabic ناظر 'pupil'; cf. bk. 2, ch. 4 (fol. 45a): תאר אבק יחזק הראות ויסיר הדמע (Recipe of a powder that strengthens the

591 Cf. entry התקשרות.

592 In addition to מחזק, the anonymous author of *Sefer ha-Refu'ot ha-Libbiyot* has מחבש (see entry (חבש) חיבש).

593 a הנואסיר: البواسير.

pupil and cures epiphora). Hebrew ראות does not feature in this sense in the current dictionaries. Arabic ناظر is also translated as ראות by Moses Ibn Tibbon's contemporary Shem Tov Ben Isaac (cf. NM 1:113–4). In his translation of Maimonides, *Medical Aphorisms* 15.30, Nathan ha-Me'ati renders Arabic ناظر as רואה, and Zeraḥyah Ḥen as שומר (cf. NM 2:85 and NM 1:190).

ראש (*Sefer ha-Qanun*, Nathan) = Arabic رأس 'root [of a tooth]' (cf. DKT 818); cf. bk. 1 (fol. 31b): ואמנם המלתעות הנעוצות בלחי בתחתון הפחות שיהיה לכל אחד מהם שני ראשים ולפעמים יותר (The molars that are inserted in the lower jaw, each of them has at least two roots, and sometimes more). In the sense of 'root', Hebrew ראש is a non-attested semantic borrowing from Arabic رأس. Zeraḥyah Ḥen renders Arabic رأس as עיקר.

ראש הכתף (*Sefer ha-Qanun*, Nathan) = Arabic رأس الكتف 'acromion process, superior process of scapula' (cf. DKT 492–3, 818; FAL 126, no. 2762) (= Greek ἀκρώμιον; cf. LSG 58); cf. bk. 1 (fol. 37a): ונוטה אל הצד החיצוני ומחוברת בראש הכתף ונקשרת בה הכתף ובהם יחדו נקשר הזרוע (Then it (i.e., clavicle) goes to the outside and articulates with the acromion process so that the scapula is connected to it, and the humerus to both of them). Hebrew ראש הכתף does not feature in the current dictionaries. Masie (MD 10, s.v. 'acromion'), referring to the *Sefer ha-Qanun*, mentions מרום השכמה as Hebrew equivalent.

ראש הלב (*Sefer ha-Qanun*, Nathan) = Arabic رأس القلب 'the apex of the heart' (cf. FAL 126, no. 2767); cf. bk. 1 (fol. 62a): ואמנם החלק היורד מן אוריטי הנה הוא הולך תחלה אל יושר עד שיסמך אל החוליא החמשית כי היא הנחתה נכח הנחת ראש[594] הלב (The descending part of the aortus goes down, first of all, in a straight direction (vertically) until it leans on the fifth [dorsal] vertebra because it is located opposite the apex of the heart). Hebrew ראש הלב is not attested in the current dictionaries.

רבה (*Sefer ha-Shimmush*) = Arabic كثيراء 'gum tragacanth' (cf. WKAS 1:547); cf. fol. 123b, col. a: ומתועלות הקמח הדק על דרך הסם כי כשלשין אותו מבלי מלח היטב כראוי ורוחצין אותו במים עד שיצא חלבו וכחו ואחר כן מבשלין החלב ההוא היטב בשזיפין ורבה עד שובם בגדר המזון (As a remedy, fine meal is good when it is well and properly kneaded without salt and washed with water until the milky part comes out with its strength. Then this milky part should be well cooked with prunes and gum tragacanth until they turn into a kind of foodstuff). In the sense of 'gum tragacanth', Hebrew רבה is a non-attested loan translation from Arabic كثيراء, by deriving the latter term from كثير (Heb. רב).

רביכות: רביכה (*Sefer ha-Shimmush*) = Arabic ثرائد, Sing. ثريد or ثريدة 'a dish consisting of broken pieces of bread sopped in broth with meat and/or vegetables,'

594 Ms הראש emend. ed.: ראש.

cf. FL 1:214; L 334–5; NA 618 (for some recipes, cf. ISW 162 (ch. 61), 204–9 (ch. 83); NA 287–8, 337–42); cf. fol. 123b, col. 2–124a, col. 1: הרביכות: הרביכה זנה מועט וממהרת להתעכל ולרדת מן האסטומ׳ יותר מן הלחם הטבול במרק ולפי כך ראוי להנזר מן הרביכות בעלי היגיעה והטיול והרוצה להנעים גופו (RBYKWT: RBYKH has less nutrition, is quicker digested and descends quicker than bread dipped in soup; therefore, those who strain themselves and do physical exercise and want to fatten their body should refrain from it). Hebrew רביכה features in Rabbinic literature in the sense of 'a pulp of flour mixed with hot water and oil' (JD 1442; BM 6380–1). Ben Yehuda mentions Plur. רביכין, referring to Levi Ben Gershom. Arabic ثرائد also features in Maimonides, *On Hemorrhoids* 2.3 (ed. and trans. Bos, 23) and is translated by Zeraḥyah Ḥen (ibid., 53, ll. 24–5) as הלחם השרוי עם המרק וחתיכות בשר זה נקרא תראיד (bread sopped in broth and pieces of meat; this is [the dish] called TR'YD); and in Maimonides, *On Poisons* 64 (ed. and trans. Bos, 41) it is translated by Moses Ibn Tibbon as שופש פתים 'bread [broth], i.e., Occitan ŠWPŠ'[595] (ibid., 98, ll. 4–5). And in *On Poisons* 76, 89, we find Arabic Sing. ثردة, which is translated by Ibn Tibbon (ibid., 105, l. 8; 113, l. 3) as פתים '[pieces of] bread'.

רֹגֶז (*Sefer ha-Shimmush*) = Arabic كرب 'distress'; cf. fol. 136a, col. a: אם יקרה מאכילתן צרות הנשימה ורגז ועלוף ראוי למהר ולשתות מן המוריס ומן הבורית[596] ואחר ממי הדבש (If someone suffers as a result of the consumption [of mushrooms] from orthopnea, distress, and fainting, he should hurry to take *murrī* (liquid fermented sauce)[597], borax, and then honey-water (hydromel)). Hebrew רגז features in the current dictionaries in the sense 'agitation, excitement, raging' (cf. BDB 919), 'excitement, commotion, anger, trouble' (JD 1456), and 'fright, anger' (BM 6407–8). The same Arabic term is translated as צער by Moses Ibn Tibbon (cf. IJZ 9.2, 7 (138–40)).

הרגיל (רגל) (*Sefer Ṣedat ha-Derakhim*)[598] = Arabic استعمل 'to apply'; cf. bk. 2, ch. 4 (fol. 44b): והעושה הגרגרים ימשח ידו בשמן ורדים וירגיל בהם (He who prepares the pills should anoint his hands with rose oil and apply [one of] these). Hebrew הרגיל does not feature in this sense in the current dictionaries. Moses Ibn Tibbon's contemporary Shem Tov Ben Isaac uses the same Hebrew term to render Arabic استعمل (cf. NM 1:114–5), and Hillel of Verona employs it for Latin 'utor' (to use, to apply) (cf. NM 1:39). Subsequently,

595 For Old Occ. 'sopa' (Plur. 'sopas'), cf. FEW 17:284b: 'dünne Brotscheibe, auf die Brühe gegossen wird'; conform the German Etymon '*sŭppa', 'eingetunkte Brotschnitte' (FEW l.c.). I thank Julia Zwink for this reference.

596 a (cf. SHS 1:133) הבורית: البورق.

597 '*murrī* (liquid fermented sauce)': Cf. entry צלי אש.

598 Ms Munich, Bayerische Staatsbibliothek 295, fol. 83a, has a variant reading עשה; a term that is also employed by Moses Ibn Tibbon for Arabic استعمل; cf. NM 1:65.

Bonfos Bonafil Astruc uses the same term for Latin 'utor' in his translation of the treatise *On the Treatment of Small Children* that was attributed to al-Rāzī (cf. NM 2:181).

רגל: רגל יונים (Anonymous; Ms Vatican 361) (lit., 'pigeon's foot') = 'alkanet (*Alkanna tinctoria* L.; *Anchusa tinctoria* L.)'[599]; cf. fol. 181a: רגל יונים ע' רג'ל חמאמה לע' פיקולומין ([Hebr.] RGL YWNYM; Arabic RĞL ḤM'MH; vern. PYQWLWMYN). Hebrew רגל יונים, which does not feature in the current dictionaries, is attested as רגלי היונים in the *Sefer ha-Roqeḥim* by Saladino di Ascoli (ed. by S. Muntner, 113, no. 199b).[600]

רדם: See entries **מרדים** and **סם**.

רוח: הרוח החיה (*Sefer Hanhagat ha-Beri'ut*) = 'the vital pneuma'; cf. 2.1 (117): גם הכח המוליד לא יהיה תמיד תמים פעלו זולתו כי הוא צריך אל הרוח החיה ואל החום הטבעי (Also the activity of the procreative faculty is not always perfect on its own because it needs the vital pneuma and the natural heat). Hebrew הרוח החיה does not feature in the current dictionaries. A more common synonymous term is הרוח החיוני (cf. BM 6493, KTP 4:26, EP 110).

רוחי: See entry **אבר**.

רוחני: See entries **אבר** and **עלה**.

(רחב) נִרְחָב (*Sefer ha-Qanun*, Joseph Lorki) = Arabic بِاطح 'supinated'; cf. bk. 1 (fol. 15b): ואם יעזור אותו עצל הבוהן אשר נזכור אותו אחר זה ישלים הפכת <בהן> הכף נרחב (If [this muscle] is assisted by the muscle attached to the thumb which I will mention later on the hand will be completely supinated). Hebrew נרחב does not feature in this sense in the current dictionaries. For the other translator(s), see entryשטוח על ערפו.

הרחיב (*Sefer ha-Qanun*, Joseph Lorki) = Arabic بِطح 'to supinate'; cf. bk. 1 (fol. 15b): ואמנם המרחיב הזרוע זוג האחד ממנו מונח מחוץ בין שני העמודים הנקראים זנדין (The supinator [muscles] of the forearm are a pair. One of these lies on the outer side between the two muscles of the forearm that are called ZNDYN [in Arabic]). Hebrew השטיח על ערפו does not feature in the current dictionaries. For the other translator(s), see entry (שטח) שטיח על ערפו.

הרחיב את הנפש (*Sefer Ṣedat ha-Derakhim*) = Arabic بِسط النفس 'to dilate the soul', i.e., 'to rejoice the soul'; cf. bk.1, ch. 20 (fol. 30b): ואמר רופוש אין היין לבדו כשישתה בשווי מרחיב הנפש ומסיר ממנה הדאגה (Rufus said: Not only a moderate consumption of wine dilates the soul (i.e., rejoices the soul) and removes sorrow). Hebrew הרחיב את הנפש does not feature in the current

---

599 For the identification, cf. M 376, s.v. شنجار (alkanet): 'It is 'donkey lettuce' (*ḫass al-ḥimār*) and the 'pigeon's foot' (*riğl al-ḥamām*), a well-known plant'; see also MIG 908.

600 Cf. Saladino di Ascoli, *Compendium Aromatariorum. The Book of the Pharmacists. Based on a Hebrew Ms. of the early XV. Century*, ed. by S. Muntner (Tel Aviv 1953).

dictionaries. The same Hebrew term (for بسط النفس) features in two anonymous translations of Maimonides, *On Coitus* 3.4, whereas Zeraḥyah Ḥen has שימח. The Hebrew term (for بسط النفس) also features in the two anonymous translations of Maimonides, *On the Elucidation of Some Symptoms and the Response to Them* 2.4. A variant reading بسط الروح features in Ibn Sīnā, *K. al-adwiya al-qalbiya* 13 (14), and is translated by the anonymous author of *Sammim Libbiyim* (fol. 125a) as פשט את הרוח.

רֹחַב (*Sefer ha-Qanun*, Joseph Lorki) = Arabic بَطْخٌ 'supination'; cf. bk. 1 (fol. 15b): ואלו הקובצים והמותחים הם עצמם פועלים השפוע והרחב (The same muscles that flex and extend [the wrist] produce [its] pronation and supination). Hebrew רחב does not feature in this sense in the current dictionaries. For the other translator(s), see entry שטיחה: שטיחה על העורף.

רחבי: See entry **שלב**.

רוחץ (רחץ): See entry **סם**.

ריח: ריח הפה (*Sefer Ṣedat ha-Derakhim*) = Arabic بخر 'bad breath' (cf. FL 1:90: 'foetor oris'); cf. introduction (fol. 2b): השער הכ״ג בריח הפה (Chapter twenty-three: On bad breath). Hebrew ריח הפה is only attested for Rabbinic literature (cf. BM 6572; LW 4:446).

ריחניות (*Sefer ha-Refu'ot ha-Libbiyot*) = Latin 'aromaticitas' (aroma; fragrance); cf. 249a: ועם זה יש בו דקות והנה נאות ברוח לריחניותו ועפיצותו (Besides, it (i.e., the myrtle) has refining [power] and it is favorable to the pneuma because of its aroma and astringency). Hebrew ריחניות features in EM 1712 in the sense of 'fragrance' as a novel term. For the anonymous author of *Sammim Libbiyim*, see entry בְּשָׂמִיּוּת.

רסג (*Sefer ha-Qanun*, Nathan) = Arabic رسغ 'carpus, tarsus' (cf. DKT 500–1, 818; FAL 126, no. 2778); cf. bk. 1 (fol. 38b): הרסג מחובר מעצמים רבים שלא יכללהו פגע (The carpus is formed from many bones so that an injury does not extend to the whole carpus). Hebrew רסג, a loan word from Arabic رسغ, features in MD 135, s.v. 'carpus', referring to the *Sefer ha-Qanun*. See also SRP lxxxi, 25 (152). Zeraḥyah Ḥen renders Arabic رسغ as ריסג.

רֹעַ: רוע בשול (*Hanhagat ha-Beri'ut le-Abu 'Ali Ben Zuhr*) = 'indigestion' (Honofredi: 'indigestio'); cf. ch. 24: וראוי שירחיק רוע בשול וימעט המאכל ביום ההוא ויקל המזון כאשר ימשך (One should avoid indigestion and eat a small amount of light food on the day [it happens] and lasts for a long time). Hebrew רוע בשול is not attested in the current dictionaries. Cf. next entry.

רוע האצטומכא (*Sefer Ṣedat ha-Derakhim*) = Arabic تُخَم (Greek ἀπεψία; cf. UW 117) 'indigestion'; cf. introduction (fols. 3a–3b): השער הט' ברוע בשול האצטומכא הוא אלתכם (Chapter nine: On indigestion, [Arabic] ʾLTKM). Hebrew רוע בשול האצטומכא is not attested in the current dictionaries.

Zeraḥyah Ḥen translates Arabic تخم(ة), featuring in Maimonides, *Medical Aphorisms*, as אמפונימינטו והוא המילוי הנקרא תכמה or אמפונימינטו בערבי תכמה or המילוי הנקרא תכמה בערבי, while Nathan ha-Me'ati translates it as קבסא (cf. NM 2:78–9).

רעד (*Sefer Ṣedat ha-Derakhim*) = Arabic اختلاج 'twitching of muscles and their tendons' (cf. SN 102: 'Sehnenhüpfen. Subsultus tendinum')[601]; cf. bk. 1; ch. 24 (fol. 39b): ואולם הרעד הנקרא בערבי איכתילאג׳ הוא התפשטות יוצא מן הטבע ויתחדש בכל האיברים אשר מדרכם שיתפשטו (Twitching of muscles and their tendons called *iḫtilāǧ* in Arabic is an unnatural stretching that occurs in all the limbs that can stretch). Hebrew רעד features in the current dictionaries in the general sense of 'quivering, trembling'; cf. BDB 944; BM 6641. Ibn Tibbon's contemporary, Shem Tov Ben Isaac, translates Arabic اختلاج as רפפות (cf. SHS 1:485–6 (Resh 12)). Subsequent to Moses Ibn Tibbon and Shem Tov Ben Isaac, Hebrew רפפות (for Arabic اختلاج) recurs in Zeraḥyah Ḥen's translation of Maimonides, *Medical Aphorisms* 3.55, while Nathan ha-Me'ati uses the term רפרוף (cf. NM 2:87). About this term, Nathan remarks in the glossary to the *Sefer ha-Qanun* (cf. NM 2:120, 161 (Resh 11)): שמשתי בתנועת השפה או העין הבלתי רצונית או משאר האיברים רפרוף וכן שמשו בו רז״ל באמרם רפרף בגפו (I used RPRWP for the unvoluntary movement of the lip or eye or other limbs, and so did the Rabbis, of blessed memory, employ it when they said [with regard to a bird, that] 'flapped (RPRP) its tail'). Regarding the term רפפות, he remarks (cf. ibid.): הם כלים שמנשבים בהם לנשב הרוח ובלעז ונטאלש וכן שמשו בו רז״ל באמרם הרפפות במשנת אהלות (These are devices used to ventilate, to blow (to fan) the air, and in the vernacular (Romance) WNṬ'LŠ. Thus it (the term) was used by our Rabbis, of blessed memory, when they referred to RPPWT in *Mishnah Ohalot* [13:1]).

רעישה (*Sefer ha-Shimmush*) = Arabic ارتعاش 'tremor' (cf. UWS 2:490: 'Zittern, Beben'); cf. fol. 134b, col. b: ומתועלותיו גם כן על דרך הסם שהוא מועיל מן הרעישה וחולשת הראות (As a remedy it (i.e., cabbage) is also good for tremors and weakness of vision). As a medical term, Hebrew רעישה features as רעישת האברים in BM 6654 in an attestation from Meir Aldabi, *Shevilei Emunah*; cf. NM 3:220.

מרפה (רפה) See entry **סם**.

רצפה (*Sefer ha-Qanun*, Zeraḥyah) = Arabic رضفة 'patella' (cf. DKT 570–5, 818; FAL 126, no. 2777); cf. bk. 1 (fol. 28b): ולו שני קצוות האחד מהם בשריי ויתדבק ברצפה קודם היותו יתר והאחר קרומי יתחבר בקצה הפנימי מקצויי[602] הירך ([This

601 The same Arabic term is translated as 'convulsion' in Avicenna, *Canon of Medicine* (trans. Adeli Sardo, 3:206).

602 Ms מקצה emend. ed.: מקצויי.

muscle] (i.e., of the knee joint) has two ends, one is fleshy and inserted on the patella before becoming a tendon, and the other which is membranous is inserted on the inner end of the thigh bone). Hebrew רצפה is a non-attested loan word from Arabic رصفة. For the other translator(s), cf. entry עגול הארכובה.

(רצץ) רֻצַּץ (*Sefer Ṣedat ha-Derakhim*) = Arabic رُضَّ 'to be crushed'; cf. bk. 1, ch. 23 (fol. 37a): ירוצץ כל זה ויושם בשמן וירתיחהו על האש עד שיקח השמן כח הסמים (All this (these ingredients) should be crushed and put in olive oil and boiled on the fire until the oil assumes the power of the ingredients). Hebrew רֻצַּץ only features as a Puʿal of the verb רצץ in EM 1743, but not as a pharmaceutical term.

רקה (*Sefer ha-Qanun*, Nathan) = Arabic خدّ 'cheek'; cf. bk. 1 (fol. 44a: הפרק הששי בנתוח עצלי הרקה. הרקה יש לה שתי תנועות (Chapter six: The anatomy of the muscles of the cheeks. There are two [types of] movements in the cheeks). Hebrew רקה only features in the current dictionaries in the sense of 'temple'; cf. BDB 956; BM 6728–9, EM 1744; cf. LOW LXXX: 'parietal bones, temples of the head'. Zeraḥyah Ḥen translates the Arabic خدّ as פנים, and Joseph Lorki as לחיים.

רקוח: רקוחים (*Sammim Libbiyim*) = Arabic جوارشن, Plur. جوارشنات 'stomachics'; cf. fol. 133a: ואולם אשר בו רוע מזג חם ובמזגים[603] החמים והארצות החמות הנה לא[604] יקל אליהם בהם ולא בשאר המרקחות והריקוחים החמים אלא בעת ההכרח הנגלה (But if a person has a bad hot temperament and in the hot seasons[605] and hot places, he[606] is not allowed [to use] any hot electuary and hot stomachic, unless it is clearly necessary at that time). Hebrew רקוח features in the Bible (BDB 955) and *Piyyut* literature (EM 1744) in the sense of 'perfumery, unguent'. In modern literature, it is attested in the sense of 'fruit preserve, concoction' (EM 1744). This passage is missing in *Sefer ha-Refuʾot ha-Libbiyim*, Mss Munich 373 and Vienna Hebr. 59.

(רתע) הרתיע (*Sefer ha-Shimmush*)[607] = Arabic قمع 'to restrain, suppress, subdue'; cf. fol. 137b, col. b: ומסגלתו שהוא מדקדק החלטים ומגיר השתן בדקות ומרתיע המרה הכרכומית (One of its specific properties (i.e., of the pomegranate) is that it refines the humours, makes the urine flow by its thinning effect and restrains the yellow bile …). Hebrew הרתיע is attested in a medical context in BM 6771 in attestations from the *Sefer ha-Qanun*, a.o., as הרתיע את הפצע,

---

603 a وفي الفصول :ובמזגים.

604 a فلا رخصة له :לא יקל אליהם.

605 'seasons': Trans. after a.

606 'he is not allowed': Trans. after a.

607 See also entry סם מרתיע.

and is rendered by Ben Yehuda as גרם לנסיגת הפצע והקטנתו (to reduce the size of the wound and to make it smaller). In the *Sefer Almansur*, Shem Tov Ben Isaac uses הרתיע לאחור to translate the synonymous Arabic ردع 'to suppress'; cf. NM 1:116.

שְׁבָכָה (*Sefer ha-Qanun*, Nathan) = Arabic شبكة 'rete mirabile' (cf. DKT 610–1, 820; FAL 136, no. 2956); cf. bk. 1 (fol. 62a): ולכן נפרשה השבכה תחת המוח להחזיר הדם השרייני והרוח בו ויתדמה במזג המוחיי אחרי הבשול (For this reason, the rete mirabile spreads beneath the brain to circulate the arterial blood and pneuma in it and [so that] it resembles the temperament of the brain, once it has been cooked). Hebrew שבכה features in BM 7515, a.o., in the sense of 'circulus arteriosus Willisii' in an attestation from Meir Aldabi, *Shevilei Emunah*. Joseph Lorki has סבכה.

השבכה השליית (*Sefer ha-Qanun*, Nathan) = Arabic الشبكة المشيمية 'choroid plexus' (cf. DKT 632–3; FAL 136, no. 2956); cf. bk. 1 (fol. 65b): ואחר נמתח מן החדר האמצעי אל שני החדרים המוקדמים ופוגע בעורקים הדופקים העולים שם ומתארג <הידוע> כשכבה השליית הקרום (Then [these branches] (i.e., of the vena cava) spread from the middle ventricle [of the brain] into the two anterior ventricles and join with the arteries that ascend to this place and form a network known as the choroid plexus). Hebrew השבכה השליית does not feature in the current dictionaries.

נשבר (שבר) (*Sefer Ṣedat ha-Derakhim*) = Arabic انكسر (lit., 'to be broken'), but also 'to cease, to abate' (cf. WKAS 1:181a–b), cf. bk. 1, ch. 18 (fol. 26b): ואולם אשר יתערבב שכלם בסבת כאב המוח לבד הנה ערבובם יתוסף ויגדל מעט מעט ויתמיד בהם אחר מנוחת הכאב והשבר הקדחת ולא יפסק כלל כי החולי במוח עצמו (But those who suffer from mental confusion (i.e. in the case of phrenitis) especially because of the pain in their brain, their confusion will slowly increase and become greater and persistent once the pain has subsided and the fever has abated. It will not at all come to an end because the illness is in the brain itself). In the sense of 'to cease, to abate', Hebrew נשבר is an unattested semantic borrowing from Arabic انكسر.

שובר: See entry **סם**.

מְשַׁבֵּר: See entry **סם**.

שגל (*Sefer Issur ha-Qevurah le-Galienus*) = Arabic جامع 'to have sexual intercourse'; cf. par. 109: והמין האחר הוא מפני אכילת המטעמים אשר לא נאכלו מזמן ארוך כמי שחסר לו לחם ימים רבים ואחר אכלו או מפני המשגל שעמד זמן ארוך ואחר שגל (As regards the other type (of psychological coma), it may be due to the consumption of food which a person has not had for a long time, like someone who has been deprived of bread for a long time and then [suddenly] eats it. Or it may be due to sexual intercourse, if someone has not had it for a long time and then [suddenly] has it). Biblical Hebrew שגל (cf. BDB 993) is attested for medieval literature in an attestation from Meir Aldabi, *Shevilei Emunah* (cf. BM 6896).

שגעון (*Sefer Ṣedat ha-Derakhim*) = Arabic هذيان 'raving'[608]; cf. bk. 1, ch.18 (fol. 26a): מורסת הראש במאמר מוחלט היא מורסא חמה תקרה בקצת קרומות המוח ישיגהו תמיד צער ושגעון וערבוב השכל (In an absolute sense phrenitis is an inflammation in one of the meninges of the brain whereby the patient is always affected by sleeplessness, raving, and mental confusion (delirium)). Hebrew שגעון features in BM 6898 in the sense of 'rage, raving'. In his translation of Hippocrates' *Aphorisms* 7.9, Ibn Tibbon transcribes the same Arabic term as הדיאן (cf. NM 3:60). In his translation of al-Rāzī's medical encyclopaedia *K. al-Manṣūrī*, Shem Tov Ben Isaac uses Hebrew שגעון for Arabic مالنخوليا 'melancholy' (cf. BMZ 7, 16–7, l. 10).

השגעון השחור (*Sefer Ṣedat ha-Derakhim*) = Arabic الوسواس السوداوي 'melancholic delusion'[609]; cf. bk. 1, ch. 18 (fol. 26b): וכבר זכר גאלינוס שכל הערבובים נמשכים אחר הליחות החדות העוקצות ואין דבר מהם שתהיה הסבה בו ליחה קרה זולת הערבוב אשר יקרא השגעון השחור[610] והוא בערבי אלוסואס אלסודאוי (Galen mentioned that all [mental] confusions (deliria) result from acute, biting humours and that none of them is caused by a cold humour, except for the [mental] confusion (delirium) that is called 'melancholic delusion', i.e., Arabic *al-waswās al-sawdāwī*). Hebrew השגעון השחור does not feature in the current dictionaries. In his translation of Hippocrates' *Aphorisms* 3.22, Moses Ibn Tibbon translates the same Arabic term as הוסואס השחורי (cf. NM 3:219; see also NM 1:193; 2:31–32).

שָׂדִי (*Sefer ha-Shimmush*) = Arabic بَرّي 'wild'; cf. fol. 126b, col. b: השדיים מכל מיני האפונין פעולותיהם יותר חזקים מן הפרדסיים (Of all the [different] kinds of chickpeas, wild [chickpeas] have a stronger effect than cultivated ones). Hebrew שָׂדִי does not feature in the current dictionaries. Both, Nathan ha-Me'ati and Zeraḥyah Ḥen, translate Arabic بَرّي as מדברי in their translations of Maimonides, *Medical Aphorisms* 9.71.

משתדף (שדף) (*Sefer ha-Shimmush*) = Arabic ضامر 'meager'; cf. fol. 125b, col. a: ויש ממנו מין שלישי דק משתדף עב מעט הלובן לא נתבשל בשבלים כל צרכו וזה המין מגונה מאד לא יאות לעשות ממנו שרף ולא לחם כלל (There is a third kind of it (i.e.,

608 Cf. M. W. Dols, *Majnūn: The Madman in Medieval Islamic Society*, ed. by D. E. Immisch (Oxford 1992), 57; S. Stroumsa, *Maimonides in His World. Portrait of a Mediterrean Thinker* (Princeton 2009), 138–152.

609 Cf. Dols, *Majnūn*, 50.

610 Ms Oxford, Bodleian, Poc. 353, Uri Heb. 314, fol. 7b השחור: השחורי.

wheat) which is thin, meager, rough, and a little bit white that is not sufficiently ripened in its ears. This kind is very bad, it is not good for making broth nor any bread at all). Hebrew השתדף, Part. משתדף, only features in the current dictionaries in the sense of 'to be blighted' (BDB 995), 'to be blasted' (JD 1525), 'to be blackened' (BM 6918).

שוטה: שוטים (*Sefer ha-Shimmush*) = Arabic <ذو> المالنخوليا '[those suffering from] melancholy'; cf. fol. 143a, col. a: בשר התיש המוכלח מגונה המזון מוליד דם שחורי ומביא מתמידו אל חליים שחוריים וכל שכן מי שהוא מעותד להם כגון השוטים[611] והנכפים ואל השחין הערום ודומיהם מן החליים הרעים (Meat of old he-goats is bad food, it produces melancholic blood and causes melancholic illnesses in the case of someone who consumes it frequently, especially someone who is susceptible to them, like people suffering from melancholy and epilepsy, and [causes] malignant ulcers and similar bad afflictions). Hebrew שוטה features in the current dictionaries only in the sense of 'madman, fool, wild (of plants)' (cf. JD 1531–2; BM 6961–3; EM 1789–90). For the noun שטות, used by Shem Tov Ben Isaac in the sense of 'melancholy', cf. NM 1:117; for שטות in the sense of 'mental confusion, delirium', cf. NM 3:226.

שוער: שער (*Sefer ha-Qanun*, Nathan) = Arabic بوّاب; (lit., 'gate-keeper'), i.e., 'pylorus' (cf. DKT 815; FAL 32, no. 618); cf. bk. 1 (fol. 63b): והחלק השני מתפרק בשיפולי האסטומ׳ ואצל השער אשר הוא פי האסטומכא (The second branch (i.e., of the branches of the portal vein) is distributed to the lower parts of the stomach and to the pylorus, i.e., the [lower] orifice of the stomach). In the sense of 'pylorus', Hebrew שוער features in MD 614, s.v. 'pylorus'; see also SRP 4. The same term features in Joseph Ibn Zabara, *Batei ha-Nefesh* (ed. by I. Davidson, 160, l. 52)[612]: ומעה שם עלי פתחה לשוער (An entrail hath he placed at its mouth (i.e., of the stomach) as a doorkeeper).[613]

שוקד: See entry **שקד**.

שור: שור הבר (*Sefer ha-Shimmush*) = Arabic البقر الوحشية 'wild cow (ox)'; cf. fol. 143b, col. a: וכן צריך לעשות בכל בשר עב כבשר שור הבר (The same should be done (i.e., to quickly purge the black bile) in the case of [someone who eats] any fat meat, such as that of the wild cow (ox) …). Hebrew שור הבר features in Rabbinic literature, for instance in m*Kil'ayim* 8.6 (cf. JD 1541: 'wild ox, aurochs'; BM 6993; LZ 127–8 (no. 158)).

---

611 השוטים: كالمالنخوليا a.

612 Cf. Joseph Ben Meir Zabara, *Sepher Shaashuim*, ed. by I. Davidson (New York 1914).

613 Idem, *The Book of Delight*, trans. by M. Hadas, with an introduction by M. Sherwood (New York 1932), 173, l. 52.

שחוס: למטה משחוס החזה (*Sefer Ṣedat ha-Derakhim*) = Arabic ما دون الشراسيف 'hypochondrium' (cf. UW 715)[614]; cf. bk. 2, ch. 15: ואם לא יפסק הדם במה שזכרנו וירבה ההגרה נקשור הידים והרגלים מלמעלה למטה ונשים למטה משחוס החזה מצד הנחיר אשר נגר ממנו הדם כלי המציצה (If the bleeding [from the nose] does not stop by the [treatment] that we mentioned but becomes worse we bind the arms and legs from top to bottom and we put a cupping glass on the hypochondrium). Hebrew למטה משחוס החזה does not feature in the current dictionaries. ما دون الشراسيف is translated as תחת החלצים in Shem Tov Ben Isaac's *Sefer ha-Shimmush* (cf. NM 1:93), and as מתחת החלצים in Zeraḥyah Ḥen's translation of Maimonides, *Medical Aphorisms* 6.52 (cf. NM 1:149).

שחוסי (*Sefer ha-Qanun*, Nathan) = Arabic غضروفي 'cartiliginous'; cf. bk. 1 (fol. 35b): העצה מחובר מחוליות שחוסיים[615] אין תוספות אליהם (The coccyx is made of [three] cartiliginous vertebrae that do not have processes). Hebrew שחוסי is an adjective coined from שחוס, which is a variant reading of סחוס, which features in printed editions of the Mishnah and Talmud next to חסחוס (cf. JD 486–7). Hebrew שחוסי features as a modern term in EM 1230 (cf. MD 136). For its occurrence in the *Sefer ha-Qanun*, cf. SRP 39–40 (294). Zeraḥyah Ḥen renders the Arabic غضروفي as קלפי (see entry), and Joseph Lorki as בדלי (see entry).

שחורי (*Sefer ha-Shimmush*) = Arabic سوداوي 'black bilious, melancholic'; cf. fol. 131b, col. b: שכר התמרים עב מוליד דם שחורי (Date wine is thick [and] produces black bilious (melancholic) blood). Hebrew שחורי features in EM 1801 with a reference to Judah ha-Levi's *Sefer ha-Kuzari* (Hebrew translation by Judah Ibn Tibbon), and is translated by Even Shoshan as 'someone suffering from melancholy, depression', following Ibn Tibbon's Hebrew translation: ... אדם גברה עליו מרה שחורה (Someone ... overcome by melancholy). However, the Arabic text (ed. by D. Baneth (Jerusalem 1977), 210) reads: מן ... וערצה וסואס סודאני (*סודאוי) (Someone ... suffering from melancholic delusion; i.e., delusion caused by a surplus of black bile) (cf. trans. Touati (Leuven 1994), 215: 'est atteint de démence').

שחיי: השחיי (*Sefer ha-Qanun*, Zeraḥyah) = Arabic الابطي 'the axillary vein' (cf. DKT 813; FAL 72 (no. 1612)); cf. bk. 1 (fol. 34b): והשני ישתלח אל מקום כפל הקוברי בנראה של הזרוע ויתערבו בו שעיפים מן השחיי (The second [branch of the branches of the cephalic vein] proceeds to the elbow pit (cubital fossa) at the outer part of the forearm and joins with branches of the axillary vein). Hebrew השחיי is not attested in the current dictionaries. For the other translator(s), see entry אַצִּילִי: האצילי.

614 For Arabic شراسيف in the sense of 'costal cartilages', see entry חלץ: חלצים.
615 Ms שחוציים emend. ed.: שחוסיים.

שחין (*Sefer Ṣedat ha-Derakhim*) = Arabic بثر 'pustule' (Greek ἐξανθήμα; cf. UW 248: 'Hautausschlag'[616]; LSG 585: 'efflorescence, eruption, pustule'); cf. bk. 2, ch. 1 (fol. 42b): תאר עגולים שלישיים לבנים מועילים מן הנגעים והקצידא והשחין וכבר נסיתים (Further examples of recipes of white collyria that are good for ulcers, ophthalmia, and pustules that I have tried). Hebrew שחין features in the current dictionaries in the sense of an 'external affliction of the skin, a boil, eruption, leprosy, inflammation, abscess, ulcer' (cf. BDB 1006; JD 1547; LOW LXXXII; BM 7020). Shem Tov Ben Isaac, Moses Ibn Tibbon's contemporary, renders the Arabic بثور also as שחין in the *Sefer ha-Shimmush* (cf. NM 1:117–8). In his translation of Hippocrates' *Aphorisms* 6.9, Moses Ibn Tibbon renders Arabic بثور as גרב, and the anonymous translator as כתמים (cf. NM 3:47). Nathan ha-Me'ati renders the term, as featuring in the Hippocratic *Aphorism*, as צמחים (cf. ibid.).

שחין דק (*Sefer ha-Shimmush*) I. = Arabic قلاع (Greek ἄφθα; Plur. ἄφθαι; cf. UW 151) 'aphthae'; cf. fol. 141a, col. a: ומזיקים אל הדרדני ומחדדים שחין דק בפה ומולידים האפר בעינים (... and they (i.e., dates) are harmful for the gums and cause aphthae in the mouth and ophthalmia). Hebrew שחין דק does not feature in the current dictionaries. In his translation of Hippocrates' *Aphorisms* 3.24, Moses Ibn Tibbon renders Arabic قلاع as השחין אשר בפה, and Zeraḥyah Ḥen as חולי הפה הנקרא קלאע (cf. NM 3:225). Nathan ha-Me'ati renders the Arabic as featuring in the Hippocratic *Aphorism* as נגעי הפה (cf. NM 3:151); II. = Arabic بثر, Plur. بثور 'pustules' (see previous entry); cf. fol. 147b, col. a: קום החלב משלשל המרה הכרכומית ומועיל מן הבהק והגרב[617] והשחין הדק (Whey purges the yellow bile and is good for *bahaq* (alphos), scabies,[618] and pustules ...).

משחין (שחן): See entry **סם**.

שטוח על ערפו: שָׁטוּח (*Sefer ha-Qanun*, Nathan) = Arabic باطح 'supinated'; cf. bk. 1 (fol. 50b): ואם יעזרהו עצל הבוהן אשר נזכיר אחר זה ישלם הפוך הכף שטוח על ערפו (If [this muscle] is assisted by the muscle attached to the thumb which I will mention later on the hand will be completely supinated). Hebrew שטוח על ערפו does not feature in the current dictionaries. Zeraḥyah Ḥen does not translate the Arabic باطح. Joseph Lorki translates the Arabic as נרחב (see entry).

616 The term بثر seems to have been used for a wide variety of skin diseases; see also UW 806 (index); UWS 2:760 (index).

617 והגרב: والجرب a.

618 For the term גרב, cf. NM 3:47 and entry חרס above.

שטח (*Sefer Ṣedat ha-Derakhim*) = Arabic طلى 'to plaster, smear, rub'; cf. bk. 1, ch. 1 (fol. 6b): או יקח רודא מדברית או גרעיניה וישחק בחומץ יין[619] ויטוח בו או[620] יטוח בליברוס לבן או שחור או בשל ניטרי אחר שישחק בחומץ יין וישטחהו עליו שעה אחר שעה ואחר כך יקנחהו במטלית (Or take wild rue or its seeds, pound it with wine[621] vinegar and plaster it on the spot (affected by alopecia) or[622] plaster it with white or black hellebore or natron, after pounding it with wine vinegar, every hour and then clean it with a cloth). Hebrew שטח does not feature in this sense in the current dictionaries; cf. BM 7051: 'to spread, stretch'.

השטיח (*Sefer ha-Qanun*, Nathan) = Arabic بسط 'to expand'; cf. bk. 1 (fol. 48a): אלו הם העצלים המשטיחות (These are the muscles that expand [the chest]). Hebrew השטיח does not feature in a medical context in the current dictionaries; see also NM 1:117; 2:87. Zeraḥyah Ḥen translates the Arabic بسط as פשט (see entry), and Joseph Lorki as מתח.

השטיח על ערפו (*Sefer ha-Qanun*, Nathan) = Arabic بطح 'to supinate'; cf. bk. 1 (fol. 49b): ואמנם המשטיח לקנה על ערפו הוא זוג אחד נפרד ומונח מחוץ בין שני הזנאדים (The supinator [muscles] of the forearm are a pair. One of these lies on the outer side between the two muscles of the forearm). Hebrew השטיח על ערפו does not feature in the current dictionaries. Zeraḥyah Ḥen translates the Arabic بطح as היפך על פניו (see entry), and Joseph Lorki as הרחיב (see entry).

שטיחה: שטיחה על העורף (*Sefer ha-Qanun*, Nathan) = Arabic بَطْحٌ 'supination'; cf. bk. 1 (fol. 50b): ואלו המקבצים והמפשיטים הם בעצמם פועלים הקבוב והשטיחה[623] על העורף (The same muscles that flex and extend [the wrist] produce [its pronation and supination]). Hebrew שטיחה על העורף does not feature in the current dictionaries. Zeraḥyah Ḥen translates the Arabic بَطْحٌ as חיתוך (see entry), and Joseph Lorki as רחב (see entry).

שיבוטא: שבוטא (Aramaic) (*Sefer ha-Shimmush*) = Arabic شَبّوط (from Aramaic שיבוטא; cf. FA 122; LFA 11) 'fish of uncertain identity', cf. L 1496: 'A species of cyprinus, or carp; or. accord. to Golius, a fish resembling the alosa, or shad, but three times larger ...; a species of fish slender in the tail, wide in the middle part, soft to the feel, small in the head, resembling a بربط or Persian lute'; D 1:721: 'καλλιώνυμος, Uranoscopus scaber, dans l'Euphrate et dans le Tigre; carpe; turbot'; JAD 121: 'A species of Cyprinus or carp'; cf. fol. 149b,

619 om. a :יין.
620 om. a :או יטוח בליברוס לבן או שחור.
621 'wine': om. a.
622 'or plaster it with white or black hellebore': om. a.
623 Ms והשחיטה emend. ed. :והשטיחה.

col. b: החשוב יותר ממיני הדג הוא המין הנודע בשבוטא הנקרא[624] אצל המצריים אל בלטי (The best kind of fish is that known as ŠBWṬʾ and [the species] known[625] under the inhabitants of Egypt as ʾLBLṬY …) (cf. L 249, s.v. بلطيّ 'The labrus Niloticus; a kind of fish that is found in the nile, said to eat of the leaves of Paradise: it is the best of fish'. Aramaic שיבוטא features in Rabbinic literature in the sense of 'a scaled fish' (SDA 1131); see also the extensive account of all interpretations of the term in LFA 10–2.

שם בנחיריו: שים (*Sefer Ṣedat ha-Derakhim*)[626] = Arabic سعط 'to apply an errhine'; cf. bk. 1, ch. 10 (fol. 15b): ויושם בנחיריו מיץ מברילה עם חלב אשה ילדה בת ושמן ורדים או שמן ויאולד (And apply an errhine of black nightshade juice with the milk of a woman that has given birth to a girl and rose oil or violet oil). Hebrew שם בנחיריו does not feature in the current dictionaries.

שכם (*Sefer ha-Qanun*, Joseph Lorki) = Arabic ترقوة 'collar bone (clavicle)'; cf. DKT 815; FAL 150, no. 3226; cf. bk. 1 (fol. 12a): פרק י״ו בנתוח השכם. השכם עצם מונח על כל אחד משני צדי עליון החזה (Chapter sixteen. On the anatomy of the collar bone. The collar bone is a bone that lies on each side of the higher part of the sternum). Hebrew שכם features in the current dictionaries in the sense of 'shoulder' or in general 'back' (cf. BDB 1014; BM 7102–3) For its occurrence in the *Sefer ha-Qanun* in the sense of 'collar bone', see SRP 20 (107). For the other translator(s), see entry תרקוה.

שכרון (*Hanhagat ha-Beriʾut le-Abu ʿAli Ben Zuhr*) = 'intoxication' (Honofredi: 'ebrietas'); cf. ch. 24: וראוי לו שלא ידחה האכילה כאשר תבא התאוה אם לא שתהיה התאוה כוזבת כאשר התעורר בשכרון לבעלי הקבסא (One should not postpone eating when one has an appetite; unless the appetite is false as happens in the case of someone who is drunk and suffers from eructation). Hebrew שכרון features in the current dictionaries in the sense of 'intoxication' in the Bible and modern literature only, cf. BDB 1016; BM 7112; EM 1828).

השלב הארוכיי: שלב (*Sefer ha-Qanun*, Nathan) = Arabic الدرز الطولي 'the longitudinal suture'; cf. bk. 1 (fol. 29a): ויהיה השלב הרחבי באמצע הרוחב מן האוזן אל האזן כמו שהשלב הארוכיי באמצע האורך (The transverse suture is in the middle of the width, from ear to ear, just as the longitudinal suture is in the middle of the length). Hebrew השלב הארוכיי does not feature in the current dictionaries. Zeraḥyah Ḥen renders the Arabic الدرز الطولي as החוליא ההולכת באורך (see entry). Joseph Lorki has השליבה(?) אשר לארך.

---

624 a הנקרא אצל המצריים אל בלטי: والمعروف عند أهل المصر بالبلطي.

625 'known under': Translated after a.

626 In addition to שם בנחיריו, Moses Ibn Tibbon has משח נחיריו for Arabic سعط; see entry.

השלב הקְלָפִיי (*Sefer ha-Qanun*, Nathan)[627] = Arabic الدرز القشري 'the squamosal suture'; cf. bk. 1 (fol. 29b: ושני הגדרים אשר ימין ושמאל הם העצמות אשר יש בהם האזנים הנקראים אלחגריין כלומ' האבנים לקשים כאבן ונאחז כל אחד מהם מלמעלה השלב הקלפיי (The walls on the right and left side [of the skull] are the petroid bones which are called like that because they are hard as a stone. Each of them is bounded above by the squamosal suture ...). Hebrew השלב הקלפיי does not feature in the current dictionaries. The term קלפי features in BM 5971 in an attestation from Simon Ben Zemah Duran, *Magen Avot*. For its occurrence in the *Sefer ha-Qanun*, see RTT 147. Zeraḥyah Ḥen translates the Arabic as החוליה הקלפית (see entry).

השלב הרחבי (*Sefer ha-Qanun*, Nathan) = Arabic. الدرز العردي 'the transverse suture'; cf. bk. 1 (fol. 29a): ויהיה השלב הרחבי באמצע הרוחב מן האוזן אל האזן כמו שהשלב הארוכיי באמצע האורך (The transverse suture is in the middle of the width, from ear to ear, just as the longitudinal suture is in the middle of the length). In the sense of the 'transverse suture', Hebrew השלב הרחבי features in MD 695 as a subentry to 'suture'. The term רחבי features in EM 1703 as a modern term. Zeraḥyah Ḥen renders the Arabic الدرز العردي as החוליה ההולכת ברוחב (see entry), and Joseph Lorki as השלוב אשר לרוחב.

שלבים (*Sefer ha-Qanun*, Nathan) = Arabic. شأن, Plur. شؤون 'cranial sutures' (cf. DKT 456–7); cf. bk. 1 (fol. 28b): ולכמו התבנית הזה יש שלבים ג' אמתיים ושני שלבים כוזבים (A skull with such a shape has three 'true' sutures and two 'false' sutures). For Hebrew שלב in the sense of 'suture' and its occurrence in the *Sefer ha-Qanun*, cf. SRP 38 (274) and RTT 146. Zeraḥyah Ḥen renders the Arabic شأن, Plur. شؤون, as חליה, Plur. חליות (see entry).

(שלח) שָׁלוּחַ מן (*Sefer Ṣedat ha-Derakhim*) = Arabic منبعث من 'coming from'; cf. bk. 2, ch. 17: ואם היה החולי מן המוח והורה על זה המופת אשר הקדמנו או מפני העצב השלוח מן המוח אשר יעבור בו כח התנועה אל הלשון נצוה החולה שישתה הגיראש הגדולות אשר דרכם לנקות המוח (If the illness (i.e., of the tongue) originates from the brain—and this is indicated by the symptoms mentioned before—or from the nerves that come from the brain through which the power of motion streams to the tongue we tell the patient to ingest [one] of the great hieras which have the property to cleanse the brain). In the sense of 'coming from', Hebrew שלוח מן is a non-attested semantic borrowing from the Arabic منبعث من.

שליה (*Sefer ha-Qanun*, Nathan) = Arabic مشيمة '1. chorion; 2. chorioid plexus; 3. after-birth (placenta + umbilical cord + foetal membranes)'; cf. DKT 616–7, 828; FAL 88 (no. 1965); cf. bk. 1 (63a): והנוטה אל האצילי ושני הנרדמים מקום

627 In addition to השלב הקלפיי, Nathan renders the Arabic as קלפה (see entry).

שיתפרדו בשבכה ובשליה (And the [artery] that goes to the [left] axilla (i.e., the left axillary artery), and the two carotid [arteries] at the spot where they spread into rete mirabile and the chorion …). Hebrew שליה only features in the current dictionaries in the sense of 'afterbirth, placenta'; cf. JD 1582; LOW LXXXIII; BM 7157–8.

שליי: See entry **השבכה השליית**.

משליך (שלך): See entry **כח**.

שלשול (*Sefer Ṣedat ha-Derakhim*) = Arabic إسهال 'purgation'; cf. bk. 2, ch. 1 (fol. 41b): וירגיל להכנס במרחץ אחר נקוי הגוף אם בהקזה או בשלשול (He should make it his habit to go to the bathhouse once he has cleansed his body either through bleeding or through purgation). Hebrew שלשול only features in the current dictionaries in the sense of 'diarrhoea' (cf. BM 7196; EM 1844; LOW LXXXIII, and JD 1589: 'slimy abdominal secretion'). Subsequent to Ibn Tibbon, the same Hebrew term (for Arabic إسهال) features in Nathan ha-Me'ati's Hebrew translation of Maimonides, *Medical Aphorisms* 3.110 (cf. NM 2:88).

שלשול וקיא (*Sefer ha-Shimmush*) = Arabic هيضة 'cholera' (Greek χολέρα; cf. UWS 2:691); cf. fol. 136a, col. a: ויש פחד מן הפטריות שאינם ממיתים שלא יקרה מהן חניקה וגנוח ועלוף וקרירות הידים והרגלים ועל הרוב ירדוף אותן שלשול וקיא חזקים (And if someone takes mushrooms that cause non-fatal [poisonings], he has to fear that he will suffer from quinsy, asthma, fainting, cold hands and feet, and in most cases he will be attacked by severe cholera). Hebrew שלשול וקיא does not feature in the current dictionaries. A parallel שלשול היוצא הקיא features in an anonymous translation of Hippocrates' *Aphorisms* 3.30 (cf. NM 3:229). Other Hebrew synonyms, featuring in translations of the *Aphorisms*, are: הרקת הירוקה מלמעלה ומלמטה (Joseph Delmedigo); כאב הקיבה (Anonymous); שפיכה (Moses Ibn Tibbon) (cf. NM 3:73, 116, 235). In his translation of Maimonides, *Medical Aphorisms* 3.60, 7.42 and 23.83, Nathan ha-Me'ati renders Arabic هيضة as ליאנטריא הנק' היצא or חולי היצא הנקרא ליאנטריא, and Zeraḥyah Ḥen as האנשטיאון בער' היצה and אינגישטיאון הנקרא בערבי היצה.

משלשל (שלשל): See entry **סם**.

שמיר (*Sefer ha-Shimmush*) = Arabic فالوذ 'steel'; cf. fol. 146b, col. a: והצלוי בחלוקי אבנים או בחתיכות השמיר עד שתכלה מימיותו יעזור על עצירת הבטן (And [milk of sheep] that is roasted on smooth stones or pieces of steel until the watery part dissolves is good for constipation). Hebrew שמיר only features in the current dictionaries in the sense of 'thorn flint, diamond, adamant' (BDB 1038; JD 1596; BM 7248–9).

שמירה: See entry **מעבר**.

שממון (*Hanhagat ha-Beri'ut le-Abu 'Ali Ben Zuhr*) = Arabic كرب/ كآبة[628] (Honofredi: 'tristitia'[629]) 'grief, affliction, distress, sadness'; cf. ch. 12: ואולם הטחול הוא כלי השחוק כמו שאמ׳ פיתגורש לפי שהוא ינקה הדם השחור וכאשר לא ינוקה ממנו יזון הלב בדם שחור עכור ויחודש ממנו השממון (The spleen is the organ of laughter as Pythagoras said since it cleanses the black blood [from it]; but if it is not cleansed from [the spleen] it feeds the heart with black, turbid blood which causes sadness ...). Hebrew שממון features in the current dictionaries in the sense of 'appalment, horror' (cf. BDB 1031); 'grief, depression, boredom' (EM 1853), and 'state of depression, desolateness' (BM 7254).

שמן טוב: שמן (*Sefer Ṣedat ha-Derakhim*) = Arabic الزيت الأنفاق 'oil from unripe olives (Greek: το ὀμφάκινον [ἔλαιον]; cf. UW 459; D 1:41–2); cf. fol. 29b: ויהיה מזונו צלי קדר וצלי אש וכרוב מבושל בבשר צאן או כרוב שלוק מתוקן במוריס ושמן טוב (He[630] should feed himself with a dish of sliced and braced red meat [...], or a dish[631] of fried meat [...] or cabbage boiled with meat of small cattle or cabbage boiled [and] prepared with *murrī*[632] (liquid fermented sauce) and oil from unripe olives). Hebrew שמן טוב does not feature in this sense in the current dictionaries; in the Bible, we find שמן הטוב in 2 Kings 20:13, which is rendered as 'the fragrant oil' (trans. JPS) or 'the precious ointment' (King James Bible).

שומשמני: שמשמני (*Sefer ha-Qanun*, Nathan) = Arabic سمسماني 'sesamoid'; cf. bk. 1 (fol. 40a): ונמלא הריוח בפרקיהם לתוספת ההדוק בעצמות קטנים נקראים שומשמניים (The interstices between the [phalangeal] joints are filled with small bones that are called 'sesamoid' to make them more stable). Hebrew שמשמני features as a modern term in EM 1858; see also MD 653, s.v. 'sesamoid'. Joseph Lorki translates Arabic سمسماني as סמסניא.

שני החלומות: שן (*Sefer ha-Qanun*, Zeraḥyah) = Arabic أسنان الحلم 'wisdom teeth' (cf. DKT 468–9, 819); cf. bk. 1 (fol. 18a): וארבעה שנים וברוב הם צומחות באמצע זמן הגדול והוא אחר היותו רואה קרי עד שיגיע אל העמידה כי העמידה קרובה משלשים

628 Cf. KZ 38.

629 In addition to 'tristitia', Honofredi has 'desperatio' (despair) and 'stupor' (stupor) as parallel terms to Hebrew שממון, cf. ch. 13: 'cor habet duos nocivos hostes, scilicet desperationem et tristitiam' (Jacob Ibn Tibbon: ללב שני מזיקין השממון והיגון), and ibid.: 'Et dicunt sapientes quod audire instrumenta expellit fletum ab anima et a corde tristitiam et stuporem' (Jacob Ibn Tibbon: ואמרו חכמים: שמע הנגונים יגרש מן הנפש האבל ויסיר היגון והשממון מן הלב).

630 I.e., someone who is drunk and has a cold temperament.

631 'dish of fried meat [...]': Cf. entry צלי אש.

632 '*murrī* (liquid fermented sauce)': See entry צלי אש.

שנה ועל כן נקראות שני החלומות (And four teeth [wisdom teeth]; these appear mostly during the time of growth, namely from the time that one has a noctornal pollution until one reaches maturity. For [one reaches] maturity at about thirty years and therefore [these teeth] are called 'wisdom teeth'). Hebrew שני החלומות (lit., 'dream teeth') results from reading أسنان الحِلْم (wisdom teeth) as أسنان الحُلُم (dream teeth). For the other translator(s), see entry שני החלם כלומר החלימה.

שני החלימה (*Sefer ha-Qanun*, Joseph Lorki) = Arabic أسنان الحِلْم 'wisdom teeth' (cf. DKT 468–9, 819); cf. bk. 1 (fol. 11a): והקצויות הנקראות נואגיד צומחות ברוב באמצע זמן הגדול והוא אחר הגיע אל העמידה כי העמידה קרוב משלשים שנה לכן נקראים שני החלימה ובער׳ אסנאן אלחלם (In most cases [wisdom teeth] appear during the time of growth, i.e., after one reaches maturity. For [one reaches] maturity at about thirty years and therefore [these teeth] are called 'wisdom teeth', in Arabic *asnān al-ḥilm*). Hebrew שני החלימה is attested in BM 1575, s.v. חלימה, in a quotation of Lorki's translation. Ben Yehuda explains the term as 'strong, healthy teeth', as he derives חלימה from 2) חלם), meaning 'to be sane, strong' (cf. BM 1584). For the other translator(s), see entry שני החלם כלומר החלימה.

שני החלם כלומר החלימה (*Sefer ha-Qanun*, Nathan)[633] = Arabic أسنان الحِلْم 'wisdom teeth' (cf. DKT 468–9, 819); cf. bk. 1 (fol. 31b): והקצויות יצמחו ברוב באמצע זמן הגדול והוא אחר ההמרצה אל ההעמדה וזה כי ההעמדה קרובה מל׳ שנה ולכן נקראים שני אלחלם כלו׳ החלימה (In most cases wisdom teeth appear during the time of growth, i.e., after one reaches maturity. For [one reaches] maturity at about thirty years and therefore [these teeth] are called 'wisdom teeth' (*shinnei al-ḥilm*, i.e., *ha-ḥalimah*)). The term שני אלחלם כלו׳ החלימה is not attested in the current dictionaries. For Hebrew חלימה, cf. entry שני החלימה. Zeraḥyah Hen translates Arabic أسنان الحِلْم as שני החלומות (see entry), and Joseph Lorki as שני החלימה (see entry).

שינונים :שנון: See entry **סינונים :סנון**.

יותר שניות :שניות (*Sefer ha-Qanun*, Zeraḥyah) = Arabic أكثر تكررا 'more frequent'; cf. bk. 1 (fol. 24b): כי תנועות איברי הפנים[634] והשפתים יותר מנין ויותר שניות והתמדה (… because the movements of the [different] parts of the cheeks[635] and lips are more numerous and more frequent and last longer). Hebrew שניות features in the current dictionaries in the sense of 'duplicity' and 'dualism' (cf. BM 7325). For the other translator(s), cf. entry נכפל (כפל).

633 See also entry קצוי :קצויות.

634 a הפנים: الخدّ.

635 'cheeks': Trans. after Arabic خدّ. Cf. entry פנים.

שעיף (*Sefer ha-Qanun*, Zeraḥyah) = Arabic شعبة 'branch (of a nerve)'; cf. FAL 138 (no. 2990); cf. bk. 1 (fol. 31b): והשני זוגות השפלים ישלחו שעיף גדול אל צד השוקים ויתערב עמם שעיף מן הזוג השלישי ושעיף ראשון מעצבי העצם הנק׳ הזקן (The two lower pairs [of lumbar nerves] send large branches to the side of the legs and they (i.e., these pairs) mix with a branch of the third pair [of lumbar nerves] and a branch of the first nerve of the sacrum). In the sense of 'branch (of a nerve)', Hebrew שעיף is a non-attested variant of סעיף, which features in the same sense in MD 113. Nathan ha-Me'ati translates the Arabic شعبة as שריג (cf. BM 7618).

שעירות (*Sefer Ṣedat ha-Derakhim*) = Arabic خشونة 'roughness'; cf. bk. 1; ch. 18 (fol. 26a): ויקרה לחולה עם עלות החולי וקרוב חזקתו מקרים מפחידים כמו צמא חזק ונגוב פה ושעירות לשון ושחרותה וסער ודפיקת לב (And when the illlness becomes severe and burning hot, the patient suffers from frightening afflictions such as severe thirst, dryness of the mouth, roughness and blackness of the tongue, distress and cardialgia). Hebrew שעירות only features in the current dictionaries in the sense of 'hairiness' (cf. BM 7594–5). The same Hebrew term features in Hillel of Verona's *Sefer Keritut* as a translation of Latin 'asperitas' (roughness); cf. NM 1:40, and in the *Hanhagat ha-Beri'ut le-Abu 'Ali Ben Zuhr*, ch. 9, where the Latin parallel is 'asperitas'.

שעמום (*Sefer Issur ha-Qevurah le-Galienus*)[636] = Arabic إغماء 'swoon, faint, unconsciousness, coma'; cf. par. 15: והשעמום מינים רבים וכולם עם הנשימה ודפיקת העורקים (There are many different kinds of unconsciousness; all are related to breathing and pulsation). Hebrew שעמום is mentioned, as featuring in Rabbinic literature, in the sense of 'melancholy' in EM 1870, and in the sense of 'dullness, idiocy' in JD 1611. Ben Yehuda (BM 7355) refers to it in the sense of a 'mental disease', quoting the passage above. The term features in Zeraḥyah Ḥen's translation of Maimonides, *Medical Aphorisms* 2.16 (ed. and trans. Bos, 1:31) in the sense of '(melancholic) delusion' for Arabic وسواس (cf. NM 1:193).

שער (*Sefer ha-Qanun*, Nathan) = Arabic باب '1. the gate of the liver; 2. the portal vein' (cf. DKT 618–9, 815; FAL 30, no. 569); cf. bk. 1 (fol. 63a): ונתחיל בנתוח העורק הנק׳ השער ונאמר השער[637] הנה תחלה מתחלק קצהו השוקע בחלל הכבד לה׳ חלקים (Let us begin with the anatomy of the vein called 'portal vein' and say first of all that the end of the portal vein which goes deep into the cavity of the liver divides into five branches). In the sense of 'portal vein', Hebrew שער features in BM 7363 in attestations, a.o., from the *Sefer ha-Qanun*; see also SRP 4.

---

636 In addition to שעמום, Judah al-Ḥarizi translates Arabic إغماء as כאב המוח (see entry).

637 Ms השיער emend. ed.: השער.

שפודיי (*Sefer ha-Qanun*, Nathan) = Arabic سفّودي 'shaped liked a spit' (cf. DKT 458–9; cf. bk. 1 (fol. 29a): ושלב מחלק לאורך הראש ישר יאמר לו לבדו חציי וכשיחקר מצד חבורו עם הכלילי אז יאמר לו שפודיי (A suture that divides the head longitudinally [and that is] straight is called 'sagital' when considered on its own, but when it is considered in relation to its connection with the coronal [suture], it is called 'shaped like a spit'). Hebrew שפודיי, adjective coined from the noun שפוד, does not feature in the current dictionaries; for its occurrence in Nathan's translation, cf. RTT 146.

שפוי כובע :שפוי (*Sefer ha-Qanun*, Nathan) I. = Arabic حنجرة 'larynx' (cf. DKT 534–5, 816; FAL 68, no. 1514); cf. bk. 1 (fol. 46b): השפוי כובע אבר שחוסי נברא כלי לקול (The larynx is a cartilaginous organ that was created as an instrument for the voice). Hebrew שפוי כובע features in the current dictionaries in the sense of 'Adam's apple' (BM 7378; EM 1875); 'thyroid cartilage; Adam's apple' (JD 616, s.v. כובע); 'the protruding point where the thyroid cartilage inclines downward, Adam's apple' (LOW LXXXIII). Nathan's faulty translation is the result of reading Arabic حنجرة as خنجري 'xiphoid', which was often used defectively for غضروف خنجري 'xiphoid cartilage' (see next entry). Zeraḥyah Ḥen and Joseph Lorki translate the Arabic حنجرة as גרון. Hebrew שפוי כובע also features for Arabic حنجرة in Nathan's translation of Maimonides, *Medical Aphorisms* 1.47; 3.21, 43; 9.32, 34, 37; 23.12, 24, 76, 77; 25.53, whereas Zeraḥyah has גרון except for one case where he has שפוי כובע; II. = Arabic خنجري 'xiphoid [cartilage]' (cf. DKT 824; FAL 64, no. 1425); cf. bk. 1 (fol. 64b): עד שהגיע אל השפוי כובע ומשאיר מדי עברו שריגים מתפרדים בעצלים אשר בין הצלעות (When they reach the xiphoid cartilage they (i.e., the branches of the vena cava) let out [more] branches that spread out into the intercostal muscles). Joseph Lorki reads the Arabic خنجري as حنجرة and accordingly translates גרון.

שפולי הרגלים :שפול (*Sefer Issur ha-Qevurah le-Galienus*) = Arabic أسفل القدمين 'the soles of the feet'; cf. 144: ותרופת עלות המאמר הרביעי שילקח חלב האתון באשישות רבות אחר יחממוהו בתנור חם ובהקרבו להקפיא יוציאוהו וישימוהו על כל אשישה ליטר דבש ויערבוהו ויטבלוהו החולי וימרחו שפולי רגליו (The illnesses featuring in the fourth section should be treated [as follows]: Take ass milk [that has been poured into] in many flasks, heat them up in a warm oven, take them out of the oven when [the milk] is about to clot, pour into each flask one *raṭl*[638] of honey, beat it into the milk; then completely cover the

638 '*raṭl*': The weight of the raṭl varies according to region and period; in the eleventh and twelfth century its weight in Egypt was 437.5 grams and subsequently 450 grams. See Hinz, *Islamische Maße und Gewichte*, 28–33, esp. 29.

patient with it, and rub (the liquid) on the sole(s) of his feet). Hebrew שפולי הרגלים does not feature in the current dictionaries.

שיפוע: שִׁפּוּעַ (*Sefer ha-Qanun*, Joseph Lorki) = Arabic كبّ 'pronation'; cf. bk. 1 (fol. 15b): וכשיתנענעו אלו ביחד ימתחו החוליא מתיחה עם מעט שיפוע (When these two [muscles of the wrist] act together, they extend the carpus with some pronation). Hebrew שפוע does not feature in this sense in the current dictionaries. For the other translator(s), see entry קבוב.

שְׁפוֹת (*Sefer ha-Shimmush*) = Arabic زبد 'cream, (fresh) butter'[639]; cf. fol. 146b, col. b–147a, col. a: מיץ החלב אמנם כשתוסר שפותו והתחיל להחמיץ הוא טוב לשלשול[640] המתהוה מן המרה הכרכומית עם כחשות הגוף וחולשתו (Buttermilk: When the butter has been removed and it has begun to turn sour it is good for diarrhea[641] originating from yellow bile which comes with meagerness and weakness of the body). Hebrew שפות features as שפות בקר (cf. next entry) in the Bible in 2Sam 17:29. Its meaning is uncertain: cf. BDB 1045: 'perhaps cream'; KB 1620: '… all this means that it designates a foodstuff such as hard cheese or curd cheese made from cow's milk'; cf. the Targum on 2Sam 17:29: וגובנין דחלב (J. Levy, *Chaldäisches Wörterbuch* 1:123[642], s.v. גובנין: 'zusammen geronnene Milch, Milchram, Käse'). Both, Nathan ha-Me'ati and Zeraḥyah Ḥen, translate Arabic زبد, as it features in Maimonides, *Medical Aphorisms* 6.86, as קצף (foam),[643] and in 23.107 as חמאה (curled milk, butter).[644]

שפות בקר (*Sefer ha-Shimmush*) = Arabic زبد 'cream, (fresh) butter'; cf. fol. 139b, col. a: ודחית נזקם למי שירגילם בהכרח על דרך מזון ויזיקוהו לשתות אחריהם מן השמנים הלחים או מן החמאה או מן שפות הבקר או מן החלב תכף שנחלב (If someone eats them (i.e., myrtle berries) as food out of necessity and suffers harm, he can undo their harm by taking fresh oils or cream or fresh butter or fresh milk after their consumption). Cf. entry שפות.

שפלות הקול: שפלות (*Sefer Ṣedat ha-Derakhim*) = Arabic بحوحة الصوت (Greek βράγχος, cf. UW 169) 'hoarseness', cf. introduction, fol. 3a: השער הד' בשפלות הקול הוא בחוח אלצות (Chapter four: On hoarseness, i.e., [Arabic] *buḥūḥ al-ṣaut*). Hebrew שפלות הקול does not feature in the current dictionaries. Cf. NM 3:28, s.v. אפיסת הקול.

---

639 Cf. FL 2:221: 'spuma, cremor lactis, tum butyrum recens' (froth, cream of milk, fresh butter); DAS 6:308: 'frische Butter' (fresh butter).

640 לשלשול המתהוה מן המרה הכרכומית: للخلقة الصفراوية الحارة a.

641 'diarrhea originating from yellow bile': 'hot yellow bile' a.

642 J. Levy, *Chaldäisches Wörterbuch*, 2 pts. in 1 vol. (Repr. Köln 1959).

643 Cf. English translation: 'A foamy stool indicates one of two things' (trans. Bos, 2:19).

644 Cf. English translation: 'Among the names of [different] types of milk are the following: if milk is churned and its butter (*zubd*) removed, the rest is called 'buttermilk'' (trans. Bos, 5:69).

השפיע (שפע) (*Sefer ha-Qanun*, Joseph Lorki) = Arabic أكبّ 'to produce pronation' (cf. DKT 825, s.v. كبّ); cf. bk. 1 (fol. 15b): ואמנם המשפיעים אותו זוג מונח מחוץ (The pronators [of the forearm] are a pair [of muscles] placed on the outer side [of the forearm]). Hebrew השפיע does not feature in this sense in the current dictionaries. For the other translator(s), see entry קיבב (קבב).

שוקד (שקד) (*Sefer ha-Shimmush*) = Arabic لازم 'inherent' (cf. WKAS 2.1:575: 'permanent, inherent quality'; cf. fol. 135b, col. b: ומסגולותיו השוקדת אותם שהם מולידים קיטורים מחשיכים וחלומות רעים (One of its (i.e., of leek) inherent properties is that it produces dark vapours and cause bad dreams). Hebrew שקד features in the sense of 'to last' in BM 7417–8 in an attestation from Abraham Ibn Ezra, *Ḥai Ben Meqiẓ*, and from Nathan's *Sefer ha-Qanun*; see also NM 2:89.

שרין: השריין הורידי (*Sefer ha-Qanun*, Nathan) = Arabic الشريان الوريدي 'venous artery, pulmonary vein' (cf. DKT 604–5, 820; FAL 138, no. 2988); cf. bk. 1 (fol. 60b): ולכן נקרא השריין הורידי (For this reason it is called 'venous artery (pulmonary vein)'). Hebrew השריין הורידי is not attested in the current dictionaries. For Hebrew שרין, a loan word from Arabic شريان, see BM 7465. Ben Yehuda explains the term שרין as עורק (vein). Zeraḥyah Ḥen translates the Arabic الشريان الوريدي as הגיד הורידי (see entry), and Joseph Lorki as הגיד הדופק הורידי (see entry).

השריינים הנרדמים (*Sefer ha-Qanun*, Nathan) = Arabic الشرايين السباتيين 'the [two] carotid arteries' (cf. DKT 608–9, 820; FAL 138, no. 2987); cf. bk. 1 (fol. 61b): וכל אחד משני השריינים הנרדמים מתחלקים אצל כלותו אל המפרקת לשני חלקים (Each of the two carotid arteries, when they reach the neck divides into two branches). Hebrew השריינים הנרדמים is a combined term, שריין, Plur. שריינים, is a loan word from Arabic شريان (see previous entry), and נרדם, Plur. נרדמים, is a loan translation from the Arabic سباتيين. Zeraḥyah Ḥen translates the Arabic الشرايين السباتيين as שני הדופקים הנקראים בערבי סבאתין, and Joseph Lorki as הגידים הדופקים הנקראים סוביתין.

שרייני (*Pirqei Arnauṭ de Vilanova*) = Latin 'arterialis' (arterial); cf. 4.21 (54): אם הדם השרייני יכאיב ויעקוץ אבר מן האיברים כמו העין, לא יספיק בהרקתו הקזת השריין אך יצטרך לחתכו[645] יועיל, ביחוד אל הנזלים הנושנים (If the arterial blood causes a sharp pain in an organ, such as the eye, it is not sufficient to apply venesection but one should cut right through the artery [and tie it off], it will be useful especially for chronic defluctions). Hebrew שרייני, adjective coined from שרין (cf. previous entry), does not feature in the current dictionaries.

שורף (שרף): See entry **סם**.

---

645 ed. Ferre-Feliu להתכו :(Ms Munich, Bayerische Staatsbibliothek 297, fol. 19b =) לחתכו.

שְׂרָף (*Sefer ha-Shimmush*) = Arabic حسو 'broth'[646]; cf. fol. 124a, col. b: שרף קמח החטה הוא ממין שרף הגריסין בהולידו הסתומים והלחה הלבנה (Broth prepared from wheat flour is of the same kind as the broth from grits as it causes obstructions and phlegm). Hebrew שרף features in Rabbinic literature in the sense of 'acrid substance, esp. vegetable sap made thick by inspissation; resin, gum' (JD 1633; BM 7625–6). Ben Yehuda brings some attestations for the term in the sense of 'gum' from medieval literature as well. In his glossary to the *Sefer ha-Qanun*, Nathan ha-Me'ati defines חסו as חסו הוא שם לחביץ קדרה כלומר איזה קמח או פתיתות מבושל בקדרה (This is the name for a type of soup (ḤBYṢ QDRH); i.e., flour or breadcrumbs boiled in a pot) (cf. NM 2:114, 139 (Ḥet 17)). The same Hebrew transcription חסו is used by Nathan ha-Me'ati and Zeraḥyah Ḥen in their translation of Maimonides, *Medical Aphorisms* 17.21. Arabic حسو also features as حسو الشعير 'barley broth' in Maimonides, *Regimen of Health* 2.6, and is translated by Ibn Tibbon as מי שעורים, and by the anonymous translator as שתיתת השעורים. The same Arabic term features as حساء الشعير in Maimonides, *Medical Aphorisms* 8.26 and is rendered as חסו מן השעורים by Nathan ha-Me'ati, and as השורבו מהשעורים by Zeraḥyah Ḥen.

שרש: שרש האזנים (*Sefer ha-Shimmush*) = Arabic أصل الأذن 'parotid gland' (cf. UW 507); cf. fol. 126b, col. a: והמערב קמח הפול עם קמח התלתן ומחבש בהם יתיכו הנפח אשר יקרה בשרשי האזנים ומה שיקרה מן הכהות מתחת העין (If one mixes meal of broad beans with that of fenugreek and applies it as a plaster, it cures tumours of the parotid glands and livid spots beneath the eyes). Hebrew שרש האזנים does not feature in the current dictionaries.

שרש הלשון (*Hanhagat ha-Beri'ut le-Abu 'Ali Ben Zuhr*) = Arabic لهاة 'uvula' (cf. Honofredi: 'uvula'); cf. ch. 8 (variant reading): והרחקת אכילת העצמים הדקים כמו עצם העוף והפרדיץ והצפרים והתרנגולים ואכילת הדגים הקוציים, זולת עצמי השיות והתישים הסריסים כאשר יותך מהם לעיסותם ממה שירכך הקנה והאוילה וירכך הושט וישלשל המעברות ויעזור לירידת המאכל בקערורית האצטומכא (One should avoid the consumption of fine bones such as those of birds, partridges, small birds (sparrows?), chickens and of spiny fish except for the bones of (young) sheep, and castrated billy-goats; when these are chewed so that they become soft it is something that mollifies the trachea, uvula and esophagus, cleanses the passages and helps the food to descend to the concave part

646 Cf. NA 607: 'light, smooth, and thin soup made with water, flour, or fine bread crumbs, and fat … In fact, it may apply to any thin and light soups, which can be sipped'; cf. L 572, s.v. حساء: 'A well-known kind of food; soup; i.e., what is supped or sipped; thin cooked food, that is supped or sipped, made of flour and water and oil or grease, and sometimes sweetened: also called حَسُوٌّ and حَسِيَّةٌ and حَسًا and حَسْو.'

(bottom) of the stomach). Hebrew שרש הלשון features in BM 7475 in an attestation from Isaac Tovim, *Sefer ha-Difteriah*. It also features in EM 1898 as a medieval term without any reference, and is explained by Even Shoshan as הקצה האחורי של הלשון המחבר את הלשון אל דפן הלוע.

שתוק (*Sefer Ṣedat ha-Derakhim*) = Arabic سكتة 'apoplexy, stroke'; cf. bk. 1, ch. 22: והכפיה קרוב מן השתוק כי מקום החולי בשניהם אחד והליחה המולידה אותם קרה לחה אבל כי השתוק יהיה בהעדר הכח אשר ילך אל העצבים כלם והכפיה תהיה בתנועה מצטערת (Epilepsy is closely related to apoplexy for in both cases the illness occurs in the same spot. The humour that causes them is cold [and] moist. However, apoplexy results from the lack of power that goes to all the nerves and epilepsy occurs with convulsions). Hebrew שתוק features, a.o., in BM 7495 in an attestation from Nathan ha-Me'ati's translation of Maimonides, *Medical Aphorisms* 6.1 (cf. NM 2:194). It also features in EM 1902 in an attestation from Maimonides, *Moreh Nevukhim*. Both, Ben Yehuda and Even Shoshan, translate the term as 'paralysis'.

השתין במטה :שתן (*Sefer Ṣedat ha-Derakhim*) = Arabic بال في الفراش 'to wet the bed' (enuresis); cf. introduction (fol. 3b): השער הי"ט ברפואת מי שישתין במטה (Chapter nineteen: On bed-wetting). Hebrew השתין במטה does not feature in the current dictionaries.

תבשיל האספרגוס :תבשיל (*Sefer ha-Shimmush*) = Arabic الهليونية 'the asparagus dish'; for its composition, cf. PK 475: '*Hilyauniyya*: Boil meat and asparagus, then put both upon the other and break eggs over it and sprinkle it with pepper and dry coriander and put it on the fire until done'; cf. fol. 145b, col. b–46a, col. a: ותבשיל הלפת טוב לכליות וכיס מקוה <המים> ואינו מזיק לבעל ההדרקון כנזק תבשיל הנפוס והוא טוב לבעל הקרירות ובלתי טוב לבעלי החמימות ולא בעתים החמים ותבשיל האספרגוס כמוהו (The turnip dish is good for the intestines and urinary bladder and not as harmful for colic patients as the carrot dish; it is good for those with a [cold temperament] and bad for those with a [hot temperament] and when it is hot; the asparagus dish is the same (has the same effect as the [turnip dish]). Hebrew תבשיל האספרגוס does not feature in the current dictionaries.

תבשיל בסר הכרם (*Sefer ha-Shimmush*) = Arabic الحسرمية 'a stew soured with juice of unripe grapes' (NA 607). For some recipes, cf. ISW 163–4 (ch. 62) (Arabic text); NA 289–90 (English trans.); cf. fol. 146a, col. a: תבשיל בסר הכרם והרמונים והתפוחים והדומה להם ואשר יכנס בהם חומץ כלם ראוים לבעלי החמימות ולבעלי הקרבים[647] החמים ובארצות החמות (An unripe grapes stew, a

647 הקרבים: الأُكباد a.

pomegranate stew, and an apple stew and similar [stews] and those prepared with vinegar are all of them good for people with a [hot temperament], or [a burning sensation in] the intestines[648] or [who live] in hot countries). Hebrew תבשיל בסר הכרם does not feature in the current dictionaries.

תבשיל זירבאג': See entry 'זירבאג'.

התבשיל החמוץ (*Sefer ha-Shimmush*) = Arabic المخلّل 'the sour dish' (also called (السكباج) (cf. D 1:389: 'Au Maghrib المخلّل était le nom ordinaire du سكباج, mets aigre, fait de viande avec du vinaigre, de la coriandre, du sel et de l'huile'; cf. NA 617, s.v. *sikbāja*: 'sour stew cooked mainly with beef, but other meats may be incorporated, too. The souring agent used is vinegar. Physicians recommend it for people with hor tempers. It is the dish to have in hot countries and during the summer').[649] For recipes, see ISW 132–7 (ch. 49) (Arabic text); NA 248–55 (English trans.); cf. fol. 145a, col. b: התבשיל החמוץ הנקרא סכבאג' אצל אנשי המזרח והוא בשר וחומץ ותבלין ומי בצל והוא קר (The sour dish which is called *sikbāğ* amongst the people in the East consists of meat, vinegar, spices, and juice from onions and is [a] cold [dish]). Hebrew התבשיל החמוץ does not feature in the current dictionaries.

תבשיל הכרוב (*Sefer ha-Shimmush*) = Arabic الكرنبية 'the cabbage dish'; cf. NA 610: 'cabbage stew, cooked with meat, spices and herbs'; for a recipe see ISW 146 (ch. 53) (Arabic text); NA 265–6 (English trans.); cf. fol. 146a, col. a: תבשיל הכרוב ותבשיל התרובתור מטעמים ערבים מדרכם להוליד תחלאי המרה השחורה וכל שכן תבשיל התרובתור ומסגולת תבשיל הכרוב לשלשל הבטן ולהקל צאת הרוחות ולעזור על רוב שתית היין ולמעט השכרות (The cabbage and cauliflower[650] dishes are palatable dishes that are such that they cause black bile illnesses, especially the cauliflower dish; the cabbage dish has the specific property to empty the bowels, to ease the exit of winds and to help against drinking too much wine and to lessen intoxication). Hebrew תבשיל הכרוב does not feature in the current dictionaries.

תבשיל הלפת (*Sefer ha-Shimmush*) = Arabic اللفتية 'the turnip dish'; i.e., a dish consisting of rice, turnip, and meat (cf. Ibn Ǧazla, *Minhāǧ al-bayān*, Ms. London, British Library, Add. 5934, fol. 185b–186a, s.v. لفتية); cf. fol. 145b, col. b–146a, col. a: תבשיל הלפת הוא מטעם מנפח רב המזון מוסיף בתאות המשגל (The

---

648 'intestines': 'liver' a.

649 Note that al-Zahrāwī, *Kitāb al-taṣrīf*, fol. 574 (trans. Shem Tov, *Sefer ha-Shimmush*, fol. 145b, col. b), distinguishes between both dishes and remarks that '[the dish called] *sikbāğ* in our place (where we live) is prepared from raisin juice, vinegar, spices and is close to [the dish called] *muhallal*, but is slightly less cooling, less harmful for the nerves and for people with a cold temperament because of the raisins'.

650 'cauliflower': For the Hebrew term, i.e., תרובתור and its Arabic equivalent قنبيط, cf. SHS 1:531 (Tav 5).

turnip dish is a food that produces winds [and] that is very nutritious and that increases the sexual lust). Hebrew תבשיל הלפת does not feature in the current dictionaries.

תבשיל הנפוס (*Sefer ha-Shimmush*)[651] = Arabic الجزرية 'the carrot dish'; for its composition, cf. PK 471: '*Jazariyya*: Boil meat with a little water. Put carrots, garlic cloves and peeled onions in it, then put crushed garlic in it. Some people put spinach with it also: some make it without spinach. Walnuts and parsley are put in'; cf. fol. 145b, col. b–146a, col. a: ותבשיל הלפת טוב לכליות וכיס מקוה <המים> ואינו מזיק לבעל ההדרקון כנזק תבשיל הנפוס (The turnip dish is good for the intestines and urinary bladder and not as harmful for colic patients as the carrot dish). Hebrew תבשיל הנפוס does not feature in the current dictionaries.

תבשיל הרמונים (*Sefer ha-Shimmush*) = Arabic الرمانية 'pomegranate stew cooked mostly with chicken' (NA 614). For some recipes, cf. ISW 155–6 (ch. 58) (Arabic text); NA 279–80 (English trans.); AB 45; RR 168–71, 176–8; PD 315–6; PK 472; cf. fol. 146a, col. a: תבשיל בסר הכרם והרמונים והתפוחים והדומה להם ואשר יכנס בהם חומץ כלם ראוים לבעלי החמימות ולבעלי הקרבים[652] החמים ובארצות החמות (An unripe grapes stew, a pomegranate stew, and an apple stew and similar [stews] and those prepared with vinegar are all of them good for people with a [hot temperament], or [a burning sensation in] the intestines[653] or [who live] in hot countries). Hebrew תבשיל הרמונים does not feature in the current dictionaries.

תבשיל התפוחים (*Sefer ha-Shimmush*) = Arabic التفاحية 'apple stew'. For some recipes, cf. AB 44; PD 311, 352; PK 471; cf. fol. 146a, col. a: תבשיל בסר הכרם והרמונים והתפוחים והדומה להם ואשר יכנס בהם חומץ כלם ראוים לבעלי החמימות ולבעלי הקרבים[654] החמים ובארצות החמות. Hebrew תבשיל התפוחים does not feature in the current dictionaries.

תולעים גדולים :תולעת (*Sefer ha-Shimmush*) = Arabic دود 'round worms' (*Ascaris lumbricoides* L., *Ascarididae*; cf. MIG 406); cf. fol. 140b, col. b: וכשיבושל ביין וישתה ממנו תשע אונקי׳ והוא חם יועיל מן הכאב אשר יקרה מן המותרות העבות ויוציא התולעים הגדולים והקטנים מן הבטן (And if it (i.e., olive oil) is boiled with wine and a dose of nine ounces is administered while it is hot, it is good for pain caused by thick superfluities and it expels round worms and tapeworms from the stomach). Hebrew תולעים גדולים does not feature in the current

651 For Hebrew נפוס in the sense of 'carrot', instead of the regular 'radish', or 'rape', cf. SHS 1:344–5 (Nun 17).

652 הקרבים: الأكباد a.

653 'intestines': 'liver' a.

654 הקרבים: الأكباد a.

dictionaries. The same Hebrew term is used by Moses Ibn Tibbon and Zeraḥyah Ḥen to render the Arabic synonym حيّات 'round worms', featuring in Hippocrates' *Aphorisms* 3.26 (cf. NM 3:239).

תולעים קטנים (*Sefer ha-Shimmush*)[655] = Arabic حبّ القرع 'tape-worms' (esp., *Taenia solium* L., and *T. saginata* Goeze, *Taeniidae*; cf. MIG 406); cf. fol. 140b, col. b: וכשיבושל ביין וישתה ממנו תשע אונקי' והוא חם יועיל מן הכאב אשר יקרה מן המותרות העבות ויוציא התולעים הגדולים והקטנים מן הבטן. Hebrew תולעים קטנים does not feature in the current dictionaries. In his translation of Maimonides, *Medical Aphorisms* 22.9 (cf. NM 2:91), Zeraḥyah Ḥen renders Arabic حبّ القرع as תולעים הקטנים הדומים לזרע הדלעת (cf. NM 2:91).

תוספת I. (*Sefer ha-Qanun*, Zeraḥyah) = Arabic نتوء 'prominence [of the head]'; cf. bk. 1 (fol. 17a): ואמנם צורות הראש שאינם טבעיים הם שלשה האחד מהם שיחסר מהם התוספת המקדים (There are three non-natural shapes of the head, one [form] is that where the frontal prominence is missing). Hebrew תוספת does not feature as an anatomical term in the current dictionaries. For the other translator(s), see entry בליטה; II. **Plur. תוספות** (*Sefer ha-Qanun*, Nathan) = Arabic زائدة, Plur. زوائد 'processes (apophyses) of a bone' (Greek ἀπόφυσις, Plur. ἀποφυσέις; cf. LSG 227); cf. bk. 1 (fol. 32a): החוליא הוא עצם באמצעיתו יש נקב יעבור בו החוט ויש לחוליא ארבעה תוספות ימין ושמאל (The vertebra is a bone that has a hole in the middle through which the spinal cord passes and it has four processes (apophyses) at the right and at the left side). In the sense of 'process (apophysis) of a bone', the Hebrew term is a non-attested semantic borrowing from the Arabic زائدة. Zeraḥyah Ḥen renders the Arabic زوائد as תוספות as well. In his translation of Maimonides, *Medical Aphorisms* 24.54, Zeraḥyah uses תוספות for Arabic زوائد in the sense of the 'lobes [of the liver]' (cf. NM 1:194); in his translation of Maimonides, *Medical Aphorisms* 15.21, Nathan uses תוספות for the same Arabic term in the sence of 'excrescenses' (cf. NM 2:91).

התוספות הדומות לחצים (*Sefer ha-Qanun*, Zeraḥyah)[656] = Arabic الزوائد السهمية 'the arrow-like processes' (i.e., the styloid processes) (cf. DKT 540–1, 819; FAL 171, no. 3671); cf. bk. 1 (fol. 25b): ואמנם מושקלי המניעים הלשון הם תשעה מושקלי שנים ברחב באים מן התוספות[657] הדומות לחצים ויתדבקו בשני צדדים (There are nine muscles which move the tongue. Two transverse [muscles] come from the 'arrow-like' (styloid) processes and are inserted into the two sides [of the tongue]). Hebrew התוספת הדומה לחץ, Plur. התוספות הדומות לחצים,

655 In addition to תולעים קטנים, Shem Tov renders Arabic حبّ القرع as גרגרי הדלועים (see entry).

656 For an Arabic and Hebrew synonym, see entry התוספות הדומות למחטים.

657 Ms התוספת emend. ed.: התוספות.

does not feature in the current dictionaries. For the other translator(s), see entry התוספות החצייות.

התוספות הדומות למחטים (*Sefer ha-Qanun*, Zeraḥyah)[658] = Arabic الزوائد الابرية 'the needle-like processes' (i.e., the styloid processes) (cf. DKT 528–9, 818; FAL 171, no. 3674); cf. bk. 1 (fol. 24b): אמנם מושקולי של הפעירה וירידת הלחי יצמחו חוטיה מן התוספות הדומות למחטים (The fibers of the muscle which opens the mouth and lowers the jaw originate from the 'needle-like' (styloid) processes). Hebrew התוספת הדומה למחט, Plur. התוספות הדומות למחטים, does not feature in the current dictionaries. For the other translator(s), see entry התוספות המחטייות.

התוספות הדומות לפיות השדים (*Sefer ha-Qanun*, Zeraḥyah) = Arabic الزوائد الشبيهة بحلمتي الثدى 'nipple-like processes' (cf. DKT 582–3, 819[659]); cf. bk. 1 (fol. 30a): מן המוח צומחים שבעה זוגות מעצבים הזוג הראשון התחלתו מעומק הבתים שבמקדים של מוח אצל מקום שעוברים שתי התוספות הדומות לפיות השדים אשר בהם יריח האדם (Seven pairs of [cranial] nerves originate from the brain. The first pair originates deep in the frontal ventricles of the brain, near the two nipple-like processes through which human beings can smell (olfactory bulbs)). In the sense of 'nipple-like process', Hebrew התוספת הדומה לפי השד, Plur. התוספות הדומות לפיות השדים, does not feature in the current dictionaries. For the other translator(s), see entry התוספות הדומות לשתי טומות.

התוספות הדומות לשתי פטומות (*Sefer ha-Qanun*, Nathan) = Arabic الزوائد الشبيهة بحلمتي الثدى 'nipple-like processes' (cf. DKT 582–3, 819); cf. bk. 1 (fol. 56a): הנה יצמח מן המוח מן העצביים <שבעה> זוגות הזוג הראשון התחלתו מעומֹק שני החדרים המוקדמים מן המוח אצל שכונת שתי התוספות הדומות לשתי פטומות אשר בהם הריח[660]. Hebrew התוספת הדומה לפטומת, Plur. התוספות הדומות לשתי פטומות, does not feature in the current dictionaries. Zeraḥyah Ḥen translates the Arabic الزوائد الشبيهة بحلمتي الثدى as התוספות הדומות לפיות השדים (see entry), and Joseph Lorki as התוספות הדומים בשני ראשי<ם> השדים (see entry).

התוספות הדומים בשני ראשי השדים (*Sefer ha-Qanun*, Joseph Lorki) = Arabic الزوائد الشبيهة بحلمتي الثدى 'nipple-like processes' (cf. DKT 582–3, 819); cf. bk. 1 (fol. 17a): כבר יצמחו מהמוח ז׳ זוגות מה עצלים הזוג הראשון התחלתם מבפנים החדרים המוקדמים מהמוח אצל השתי תוספות הדומים בשני ראשי<ם> השדים ובהם יהיה הרוח. Hebrew התוספת הדומה בראש השד, Plur. התוספות הדומים בשני ראשי השדים,

658 For an Arabic and Hebrew synonym, see entry התוספות הדומות לחצים.

659 According to FAL 171, no. 3673, the Arabic term refers to '1. the condiloid processes [of the mandible]; 2. the mastoid processes'.

660 Ms[1] :הריח.

does not feature in the current dictionaries. For the other translator(s), see entry התוספות הדומות לשתי פטומות.

התוספות החצייות (*Sefer ha-Qanun*, Nathan)[661] = Arabic الزوائد السهمية 'the arrow-like processes' (i.e., the styloid processes) (cf. DKT 540–1, 819; FAL 171, no. 3671); cf. bk. 1 (fol. 47b): העצלים המניעים הלשון הם עצלים תשעה שנים רחבים באים מהתוספות[662] החיציות ומתחברים בצדדיו (There are nine muscles which move the tongue. Two transverse [muscles] come from the 'arrow-like' (styloid) processes and are inserted into the sides of the tongue). Hebrew התוספת החצית, Plur. התוספות החצייות, does not feature in the current dictionaries. Zerahyah Ḥen translates Arabic الزوائد السهمية as התוספות הדומות לחצים (see entry), and Joseph Lorki as התוספות שהם כמו החץ (see entry).

התוספות המחטייות (*Sefer ha-Qanun*, Nathan)[663] = Arabic الزوائد الابرية 'the 'needle-like processes' (i.e., the styloid processes) (cf. DKT 528–9, 818; FAL 171 (no. 3674)); cf. bk. 1 (fol. 45a): ואמנם עצלי הפעירה וירידת הלחי יצמחו פתיליהם מן התוספות המחטייות (The fibers of the muscle which opens the mouth and lowers the jaw originate from the 'needle-like' (styloid) processes). Hebrew התוספת המחטית, Plur. התוספות המחטייות, does not feature in the current dictionaries. Zeraḥyah Ḥen translates the Arabic الزوائد الابرية as התוספות הדומות למחטים (see entry), and Joseph Lorki as התוספות.

התוספות שהם כמו החץ (*Sefer ha-Qanun*, Joseph Lorki)[664] = Arabic الزوائد السهمية 'the arrow-like processes' (i.e., the styloid processes) (cf. DKT 540–1, 819; FAL 171, no. 3671); cf. bk. 1 (fol. 15a): ואמנם העצלים המניעים הלשון הם תשעה עצלים שנים מתרחבים יבואו מהתוספות שהם כמו החץ ונדבקים בשני צדדיו (There are nine muscles which move the tongue. Two transverse [muscles] come from the 'arrow-like' (styloid) processes and are inserted into the two sides of the tongue). Hebrew התוספת שהיא כמו החץ, Plur. התוספות שהם כמו החץ, does not feature in the current dictionaries. For the other translator(s), see entry התוספות החיציות.

תושבת (*Hanhagat ha-Beri'ut le-Abu 'Ali Ben Zuhr*) 'anus'; cf. ch. 15: והאורז מבושל עם החלב החלוב יזון אותם ויחזקם גם כן עד שהוא יועיל מרפיון הרחם ויפתח פיות העורקים אשר בבטן התושבת (Rice boiled with milk feeds the [internal parts of the body] and also strengthens them to a degree that it is beneficial for laxity of the uterus and opens the veins that are inside the anus); see also ch. 19, where Honofredi has 'anus': הטוב שבדברי' לתושבת ושמירת בריאותה הישיבה על כסא עור החיות (The best thing to preserve the health of the anus is to sit on a

661 For an Arabic and Hebrew synonym, see entry התוספות המחטייות.
662 Ms מהתוספת emend. ed.: מהתוספות.
663 For an Arabic and Hebrew synonym, see entry התוספות החצייות.
664 For an Arabic and Hebrew synonym, see entry התוספות המחטייות.

chair made from the hide of an animal). Hebrew תושבת does not feature in this sense in the current dictionaries. It features in medieval scientific-philosophical literature in the sense of 'basis, groundline' (BM 7708; EM 1925; KTP 4:187–8). In the sense of 'anus', it also features in Shem Tov Ben Isaac's glossary to the *Sefer ha-Shimmush* (cf. SHS 1:534 (Tav 12)).

תחתית: תחתית העין (*Sefer ha-Qanun*, Nathan)[665] = Arabic مقلة 'eyeball' (cf. DKT 829; FAL 96, no. 2127); cf. bk. 1 (fol. 56b): והזוג[666] השני מזוגות העצבים המוחיים צמיחתו אחורי צמיחת הזוג הראשון ונוטה ממנו אל הצד החיצוני ויצא מן הנקב אשר בנקרה הכולל על אלמקלה הוא תחתית העין (The second pair of encephalic nerves arises behind the first pair, turns outward and exits through the hole [in the wall of] the cavity which surrounds the *muqla* (Arabic); i.e., eyeball). Hebrew תחתית העין is not attested in the current dictionaries. Zeraḥyah Ḥen translates the Arabic مقلة as עין,[667] and Joseph Lorki as בת העין.

תיק (*Sefer ha-Qanun*, Nathan) = Arabic جُنَّة 'a thing with which a person is veiled, concealed, hidden, covered, or protected; an arm or armour with which one protects oneself,' (cf. L 463); cf. bk 1 (fol. 28b): כלל עצמות קדרת המוח הנה הם תיקי המוח למחסה ולמסתור מן הפגעים (All the bones of the skull serve as a protection of the brain, to protect it against injuries). Hebrew תיק (from Greek θήκη; cf. HM 230) features in Rabbinic literature in the sense of 'casing, sheath' (cf. JD 1665). Zeraḥyah Ḥen renders the Arabic جُنَّة as מגנה (coined from מגן (shield)).

תירוש: תירוש מבושל (*Sefer ha-Shimmush*) I. = Arabic طلاء 'wine of grape juice cooked down to one third of its original amount. Prepared this way, it is a kind of rubb 'concentrated juice', used dilated with water' (cf. NA 556); cf. fol. 131a, col. b: התירוש המבושל הנקרא בלשונם אל טלא ושאר מיני המבושלים הוא יותר חם ויותר יבש ויותר עב מן היין שהוא בלתי מבושל (Wine of grape juice that was cooked down called *al-ṭilā'* in their language (i.e., Arabic) is, in addition to other drinks that are cooked, hotter, drier and thicker than uncooked wine). Hebrew תירוש מבושל does not feature in this specific sense in the current dictionaries. The term תירוש features in BDB 440 in the sense of 'must, fresh or new wine'; in JD 1666 as 'juice, must, wine', and in BM 7740 as 'grape-juice'; II. = Arabic عقيد العنب 'inspissated must' (cf. MIG 566); cf. fol. 142a, col. a: ושתייתם בתירוש מבושל לוטשת החלט החלוק מן הכליות (If one takes them (i.e., pine seeds) with inspissated must it cleanses the viscous humour from the intestines). The same Arabic term is translated by Moses Ibn Tibbon as יין שנתבשל עד שנתעבה in his translation of Ibn al-Jazzār's *Zād al-musāfir* 13.6 (cf.

665 In addition to תחתית העין, Nathan translates Arabic مقلة as כלל העין (see entry).

666 Ms והזוגות emend. ed.: והזוג.

667 In addition to עין, Zeraḥyah translates Arabic مقلة as בת עין (see entry).

IJZ 37, 146). Nathan ha-Me'ati renders the Arabic term as תירוש ענבים קרוש, תירוש ענבים, and תירוש ענבים קרוש בבשול in his translation of Maimonides, *Medical Aphorisms* 8.35; 9.112; 21.61; 22.32; 25.49, and Zeraḥyah Ḥen (ibid.) as יין, תירוש, מירכב הענבים and יין הענבים.

תכלית (*Sefer Ṣedat ha-Derakhim*) = Arabic منتهى 'peak, climax, culmination'; cf. bk. 1, ch. 18 (fol. 26b): ואולם הערבוב המתחדש בתכלית הקדחות החמות יהיה כשיעלה אל המוח עשן נושך חם וכאשר סרה הקדחת ינוח אותו הערבוב והשגעון (But the [mental] confusion (delirium) that occurs during the peak of hot fevers, happens when a hot biting fume arises to the brain. When the fever abates, the [mental] confusion (delirium) and raving will ease). Hebrew תכלית does not feature in this sense in the current dictionaries. Subsequently, Zeraḥyah Ḥen uses תכלית in the same sense in his translation of Maimonides, *Medical Aphorisms* 9.81 (cf. NM 2:92).

תמונה: תמונת הפנים (*Sefer Ṣedat ha-Derakhim*) = Arabic سحنة 'complexion'; cf. bk. 1; ch. 18 (fol. 26a): ויקרה לחולה עם עלות החולי וקרוב חזקתו מקרים מפחידים כמו צמא חזק ונגוב פה ושעירות לשון ושחרותה וסער ודפיקת לב ושלא[668] יראה ועלוף ושינוי תמונת הפנים מן הענין הטבעי אל ענין יוצא מהטבע (And when the illness becomes severe and burning hot, the patient suffers from frightening afflictions such as severe thirst, dryness of the mouth, roughness and blackness of the tongue, distress, cardialgia, fatigue,[669] fainting, change from a natural complexion into an unnatural complexion). Hebrew תמונת הפנים does not feature in the current dictionaries. In his translation of Hippocrates' *Aphorisms* 2.34, Ibn Tibbon renders the same Arabic term as תוכן הגוף (cf. NM 3:204).

תמרי (*Sefer ha-Shimmush*) = Arabic تمري 'date-'[670]; cf. fol 141b, col. b: והמרבה מאכילת השקדים הרטובים החדשים ראוי לקחת עליהם ממרקחת התמרי או ממרקחת החבושים המשלשל (And if someone eats a large quantity of fresh almonds, he should take the date electuary or the quince stomachic after their consumption). Hebrew תמרי, adjective coined from תמר, does not feature in the current dictionaries.

תנועה: תנועה מצטערת (*Sefer Ṣedat ha-Derakhim*) = Arabic حركة مضطربة 'convulsion'; cf. bk. 22, ch.1: והכפיה קרוב מן השתוק כי מקום החולי בשניהם אחד והליחה המולידה אותם קרה לחה אבל כי השתוק יהיה בהעדר הכח אשר ילך אל העצבים כלם והכפיה תהיה בתנועה מצטערת (Epilepsy is closely related to apoplexy for in both cases the illness occurs in the same spot. The humour that causes them is cold [and] moist. However, apoplexy results from the lack of power that

668 a والإعياء :(وعمى) שלא יראה.

669 'fatigue': Trans. after the Arabic.

670 Cf. entry מרקחת התמרי.

goes to all the nerves and epilepsy occurs with convulsions). Hebrew תנועה מצטערת does not feature in the currrent dictionaries.

תנועי: העצבים התנועיים (*Sefer ha-Qanun*, Nathan) = Arabic الأعصاب الحركية 'motor nerves'; cf. bk. 1 (fol. 56a): ואמנם <העצבים> התנועיים הנה מגיעים אל המכוון (Motor nerves assume the role they have been assigned ...). Hebrew תנועי features in BM 7821 and EM 1952 as a modern term only. Zeraḥyah Ḥen translates the Arabic الأعصاب الحركية as עצבי התנועה; the same term features in Joseph Lorki.

תעלה: תעלות העורקים (*Sefer ha-Qanun*, Nathan) = Arabic جدول العروق, Plur. جداول العروق '1. intestinal canal; 2. mesentery' (cf. DKT 815; FAL 62, no. 1369); cf. bk. 1 (fol 62b): ואחר יתפרק מן השריין הזה הגדול שני שריינים מתפרדים בתעלות העורקים אשר סביב המעי הישר (From this large artery [other] arteries detach themselves which spread along the mesentery which surrounds the rectum). Hebrew תעלת העורקים, Plur. תעלות העורקים, does not feature in the current dictionaries. The term תעלות on its own features in the *Sefer Asaph ha-Rofe* in the sense 'vessels, veins' (cf. MM 142). Joseph Lorki translates Arabic جداول العروق as צנורות הגידים (see entry).

תפיחה (*Sefer ha-Shimmush*) = Arabic تَرَبُّل 'swelling'; cf. fol. 129b, col. b: המים הקובצים מועילים משלשול המעים ומתפיחת הגוף (Astringent water is good for diarrhoea and for swelling of the body ...). Hebrew תפיחה features in the sense of 'swelling' in BM 7851 in attestations subsequent to Shem Tov Ben Isaac, namely from Nathan ha-Me'ati's translations of Maimonides, *Medical Aphorisms* 23.51, and of Ibn Sīnā's *K. al-Qānūn*.

תרדמה (*Sefer Ṣedat ha-Derakhim*) = Arabic سبات (= Greek καταφορά; cf. UW 335: 'Tiefschlaf, Koma'; LSG 920: 'lethargic attack') 'torpor, lethargy'; cf. bk. 1, ch. 16 (fol. 23a): התרדמה היא הנטיה אל השינה עם סתימת העינים ויהיה זה על אחד משני פנים אם שנשקע החולה בשינה עד שיקשה להקיצו ואם שתהיה שנתו קלה (A torpor is the tendency to sleep with closed eyes, and this can be the case in one of two ways, either that the patient sinks in a sleep [so deep] that it is difficult to wake him up or that his sleep is light). Hebrew תרדמה features in the Bible in the sense of 'deep sleep' (BDB 922), in Rabbinic literature as 'torpor, trance' (JD 1696), and in medieval medical literature it is attested in BM 7902 as תרדמת האברים, and is explained by Ben Yehuda as התכווצות השרירים באברי הגוף (contraction of the muscles in the limbs); however, cf. next entry and NM 2:93–4 for תרדמת האברים in the sense of 'numbness'. In his translation of Hippocrates' *Aphorisms* 5.25, Ibn Tibbon uses תרדמה for Arabic خدر 'numbness' (cf. NM 3:247). Subsequent to Ibn Tibbon, Nathan ha-Me'ati uses the same Hebrew term for Arabic سبات in his translation of Maimonides, *Medical Aphorisms* 23.58 (cf. NM 2:93–4), and in his translation of aphorisms 9.38, he uses שינה תרדמית for Arabic نوم سباتي (lethargic sleep). Zeraḥyah Ḥen (ibid.) renders the same Arabic term as שינת תרדמה, and in his translation of Hippocrates' *Aphorisms* 3.16, he uses תרדמה to render Arabic سكات 'apoplexy' (cf. NM 3:247).

תרדמת האיברים (*Sefer Ṣedat ha-Derakhim*)[671] = Arabic خدر 'numbness [of the limbs]' (Greek νάρκη; cf. UW 431); cf. bk. 25, ch. 1 (fol. 39b): ואולם תרדמת האיברים הנה היא מקרה גם כן מתערב במה שבין הטבע ובין החולי (Numbness of the limbs is also an affliction that is a combination of something natural and something accidental). Hebrew תרדמת האיברים features in BM 7902 as התכוצות השרירים באברי הגוף, and is explained by Ben Yehuda as 'contraction of the muscles in the limbs' (cf. previous entry). Subsequent to Ibn Tibbon, the term features in Nathan ha-Me'ati's translation of Maimonides, *Medical Aphorisms* 22.43 (cf. NM 2:94), and in the *Hanhagat ha-Beri'ut le-Abu 'Ali Ben Zuhr* (cf. Honofredi: 'obdormitatio membrorum' (recension 1); 'stupor sive dormitatio membrorum'; cf. ch. 28: תרדמת האברים יורה על הפלג' וראוי כאשר יתחדש לדקדק ההנהגה וירגיל בסמים החמים הנזכרי' בשער הפלג (Numbness of the limbs indicates hemiplegia. When that happens one should refine one's diet and use hot remedies that are mentioned in the chapter on hemiplegia).

תרובתור[672] (*Sefer ha-Shimmush*) = Arabic قنّبيط 'cauliflower' (a cultivated form of *Brassica oleracea* var. *botrytis* L.[673]); cf. DT 2:162 (337, n. 6); MMS 184 (91–2); cf. fol. 134b, col. b–135a, col. a: התרובתור יותר עב ויותר מתאחר להתעכל באסטומ' מן הכרוב (TRWBTWR is thicker and slower to digest in the stomach than cabbage). Hebrew תרובתור features in Rabbinic literature and is identified by Feliks (FM 160) as 'garden cabbage' (*Brassica oleraceae capitata*) and by Jastrow (JD 1696) as a 'kind of cabbage'. Maimonides (MK 1:168) states that תורבתור is a kind of wild cabbage with thin stalks. For the identification of قنّبيط as תרובתור, cf. *Sefer ha-Arukh* (KA 8:273–4): תרבתר: מין של כרוב הוא ונקרא בל' ישמעאל אלקרנביט ומתגדל ועושה זרעונין והוא קבוץ ואין העלין נפרדין (TRBTWR: a kind of cabbage, called in Arabic 'LQRNBYṬ; it grows and produces seed (buds), it is compact and its leaves do not separate); cf. LF 1:485–487. According to Ibn Ğanāḥ, *qunnabīṭ* is *kurunb ša'mī* (lit., 'Syrian cabbage'); cf. MIG 489.

תריסי: See entry **צְנִי**.

---

671 The term תרדמת האיברים already features for Latin 'dormitatio membrorum' (numbness) in Do'eg ha-Edomi's translation of the *Viaticum*, bk. 1, ch. 25 (cf. NM 5, forthcoming).

672 For variant spellings of this term, even with initial *kaf*: כר(ו)בתור, cf. FL 1:485.

673 Ibn Māsawayh and al-Ṭabarī (cf. IBA 2:318) maintained that the 'heart' (*ğummār*) of *qunnabīṭ* is white, wherefore green varieties of *Brassica oleracea* L., such as broccoli, cannot be meant here.

תרעלה (*Sefer ha-Shimmush*) = Arabic سدر 'vertigo' (Greek ἴλιγγος, σκοτοδινία, cf. UW 308–9, 619); cf. fol. 135b, col. b: ואמר הכנדי כשישתה מסחיטת הכוסבר משקל ארבע אונקיאו' יורגש ריחו בגוף כלו ויחדש נחרת הגרון ותרעלה או שבוש הדעת עד שוב שותהו כשכור מנבל פיו (Al-Kindī said that if one drinks four ounces of coriander juice, one will notice its smell in one's whole body; it will cause hoarseness, vertigo, and mental confusion to a degree that the one who drinks it will be like a drunk talking obscenely). Hebrew תרעלה does not feature in the current dictionaries. Hebrew תרעלה features in the Bible only in the following combinations: 1) יין תרעלה 'wine of staggering' (cf. Ps 60:5), 2) קבעת התרעלה 'cup, goblet of staggering' (cf. Is 51:17) and 3) כוס תרעלה 'cup of staggering' (cf. Is 51:22) (KB 1794; BM 7917–8). Both, the Hebrew and Arabic term, feature in Shem Tov Ben Isaac's Glossary as well; cf. SHS 1:533 (Tav 9).

תרקוה (*Sefer ha-Qanun*, Nathan ha-Me'ati) = Arabic ترقوة 'collar bone' (clavicle); cf. DKT 815; FAL 150, no. 3226; cf. bk. 1 (fol. 36b): פרק ששה עשר בנתוח התרקוה. התרקוה העצם המונח[674] על כל אחד משני צדי עליוני החזה (Chapter sixteen. On the anatomy of the collar bone. The collar bone is a bone that lies on each side of the higher part of the sternum). Hebrew תרקוה is a loan word from the Arabic ترقوة. Masie (MD 166) remarks that the term features in the *Sefer Asaph ha-Rofe*. Muntner (MM 142) refers to Hebrew תרקבובית in the sense of 'claviculae', featuring in the *Sefer Asaph ha-Rofe*.[675] For the occurrence of תרקוה in the *Sefer ha-Qanun*, see SRP 20 (107). Joseph Lorki renders Arabic ترقوة as שכם (see entry).

---

674 Ms המוח emend. ed.: המונח.

675 Muntner's term תרקבובית is possibly a corruption of תרקוביות, as it features in Ms. Munich, Bayerische Staatsbibliothek, Cod. hebr. 231, fol. 3r. I thank Emunah Levy for this reference.

Bibliography

Adams, F. (trans.), *The Seven Books of Paulus Aegineta* (London 1846).

Adeli Sardo, P. (trans.), *Avicenna: The Canon of Medicine*, vol. 3: *Special Pathologies* (Chicago 2014).

al-Hassan, A. Y., and Hill, D. R., *Islamic Technology: An Illustrated History* (Cambridge 1986).

al-Khouri, M. (ed.), *Abu Marwān Ibn Zuhr: Kitāb al-taisīr fīl-mudawāt wal-tadbīr* (Damascus 1983).

Allgaier-Honal, R. (ed.), *Jehuda ben Jakob: Hanhagat ha-Beri'ut* (*Traktat zur Gesundheitslehre*) (Hamburg 2013).

Bacher, W., *Ein Hebräisches-Persisches Wörterbuch aus dem vierzehnten Jahrhundert*, = XXIII. Jahresbericht der Landes-Rabbinerschule (Budapest 1900).

Bakhtiar, L. (trans.), *Avicenna: The Canon of Medicine* (*al-Qānūn fī 'l-ṭibb*): *The Law of Natural Healing*, vol. 5: *Pharmacopeia* (Chicago 2014).

Béguin, D., 'Un exemple d'exploitation de la base Esculape: Une liste des noms des maladies', in *Nommer la maladie: Recherches sur le lexique gréco-latin de la pathologie*, ed. by A. Debru and G. Sabbah (Saint-Étienne 1998), 172–200.

Bos, G., 'Baladhur (Marking-nut): A Popular Medieval Drug for Strengthening Memory', *Bulletin of the School of Oriental and African Studies* 59.2 (1996): 229–36.

Bos, 'Isaac Todros on Facial Paresis: Edition of the Hebrew Text with Introduction, English Translation and Glossary', *Korot* 20 (2009–10): 181–203.

Bos, 'R. Moshe Narboni, Philosopher and Physician. A Critical Analysis of *Sefer Orah Hayyim*', *Medieval Encounters* 2.1 (1995): 219–51.

Bos, 'The Creation and Innovation of Medieval Hebrew Medical Terminology: Shem Tov Ben Isaac, Sefer ha-Shimmush', in *Islamic Thought in the Middle Ages: Studies in Text, Transmission and Translation, in Honour of Hans Daiber*, ed. by A. Akasoy and W. Raven (Leiden 2008), 197–202.

Bos, 'The Literature of Hebrew Medical Synonyms: Romance and Latin Terms and their Identification', *Aleph* 5 (2005): 169–211.

Bos, 'Two Notes on A Complete Dictionary of Ancient and Modern Hebrew', in *Ha-Lashon* (forthcoming).

Bos (ed. and trans.), *Ibn al-Jazzar On Sexual Diseases: A Critical Edition, English Translation and Introduction of Zad al-musafir wa-qut al-hadir* (*Provisions for the Traveller and the Nourishment of the Settled*), *bk. 6* (London 1997).

Bos (ed. and trans.), *Maimonides: On Asthma*, vol. 1 (Provo, UT 2002).

Bos (ed. and trans.), *Maimonides: On Coitus* (forthcoming).

Bos (ed. and trans.), *Maimonides: On Hemorrhoids* (Provo, UT 2012).

Bos (ed. and trans.), *Maimonides: Medical Aphorisms*, 5 vols. (Provo, UT 2004–17).

Bos, G., and Mensching, G., 'Arabic-Romance Medico-Botanical Synonym Lists in Hebrew Manuscripts from the Iberian Peninsula and Italy (Vatican Library, Fourteenth–Fifteenth Century)', *Aleph* 15.1 (2015): 9–61.

Bouamrane, F. (trans.), *Le traité médical 'Kitab al-taysir' par Ibn Zuhr de Séville* (Paris 2010).

Davidson, I. (ed.), *Joseph Ben Meir Zabara: Sepher Shaashuim* (New York 1914).

Demaitre, L., *Medieval Medicine. The Art of Healing from Head to Toe* (Santa Barbara, CA 2013).

Dietrich, A., *Medicinalia Arabica: Studien über arabische medizinische Handschriften in türkischen und syrischen Bibliotheken*, = Abhandlungen der Akademie der Wissenschaften in Göttingen, Philologisch-Historische Klasse, vol. 3.66 (Göttingen 1966).

Dols, M. W., *Majnūn: The Madman in Medieval Islamic Society*, ed. by D. E. Immisch (Oxford 1992).

Dubler, C. E. (ed.), *La 'Materia Medica' de Dioscórides*. 6 vols. (Tetuan-Barcelona 1952–9).

Dugat, G., 'Études sur le *Traité de Médecine* d'Abou Djafar Ahmad, intitulé: *Zad al-Moçafir*, La Provision du Voyageur', *Journal Asiatique* 1 (1853), repr. in *Beiträge zur Geschichte der arabisch-Islamischen Medizin*. Aufsätze, vol. 1 (1819–69), ed. by F. Sezgin, in collab. with M. Amawi, D. Bischoff, E. Neubauer, (Frankfurt 1987), 169–233 (290–353).

Elgrably-Berzin, G., *Avicenna in Medieval Hebrew Translation: Ṭodros Ṭodrosi's Translation of Ibn Sīnā's K. al-Najāt on Psychology and Metaphysics* (Leiden 2015).

Ferre, L., 'Avicena Hebraico: La Traducción del *Canon* de Medicina', *MEAH* 52 (2003): 163–82.

Freudenthal, G., 'The Father of the Latin-into-Hebrew Translations: "Doeg the Edomite", the Twelfth Century Repentant Convert', in *Latin-into-Hebrew: Texts and Studies*, ed. by R. Fontaine and G. Freudenthal, vol. 1 (Leiden 2013), 105–21.

Freudenthal, G., and Zonta, M., 'Avicenna among Medieval Jews: The Reception of Avicenna's Philosophical, Scientific and Medical Writings in Jewish Cultures, East and West', *Arabic Sciences and Philosophy* 22 (2012): 271–87.

García González, A. (ed.), *Alphita* (Florence 2007).

Gaster, M. (ed.), *Studies and Texts in Folklore, Magic, Mediaeval Romance, Hebrew Apocrypha and Samaritan Archaeology*, 3 vols. (New York 1971).

Grant, M. (trans.), *Galen: On Food and Diet* (London 2000).

Hameed, A. (trans.), *Avicenna: Tract on Cardiac Drugs and Essays on Arab Cardiotherapy* (*Risālah al-adwiyah al-qalbīyah*) (Karachi 1983).

Hinz, W., *Islamische Maße und Gewichte: Umgerechnet ins metrische System*, = Handbuch der Orientalistik, vol. 1, suppl. 1.1 (Leiden 1970).

Kahl, O. (ed.), *Sābūr Ibn Sahl: Dispensatorium parvum* (*al-Aqrābādhīn al-ṣaghīr* (Leiden 1994).

Kahl, *Sābūr ibn Sahl's Dispensatory in the Recension of the 'Aḍudī Hospital* (Leiden 2009).

Kahl (ed.), *Sābūr Ibn Sahl: The Small Dispensatory: Translated from the Arabic together with a Study and Glossary* (Leiden 2003).

Krauss, S., 'Ha-shemot 'ashkenaz u-sefarad', in *Tarbiz* 3 (1931–2): 423–35.

Kühn, K. G., *Claudii Galeni Opera Omnia*, 20 vols. (repr. Hildesheim 1967).

Leclerc, L. (trans.), *Ibn al-Bayṭār: Traité des simples*, 3 vols. (Paris 1877–83).

Leibowitz, J. O., and Marcus, S. (eds.), *Sefer Hanisyonot. The Book of Medical Experiences attributed to Ibn Ezra* (Jerusalem 1984).

Levy, J., *Chaldäisches Wörterbuch*, 2 pts. in 1 vol. (repr. Cologne 1959).

Lieberman, S., *Tosefta kifshutah*, vol. 3: *Sefer Mo'ed* (New York 1992).

Margoliouth, G., *Catalogue of the Hebrew and Samaritan Manuscripts in the British Museum*, 4 vols. (London 1899–1935).

Maxson Stillman, J., *The Story of Alchemy and Early Chemistry* (New York 1960).

McVaugh, M., and Ferre, L. (eds.), *The Tabula Antidotarii of Armengaud Blaise and its Hebrew Translation*, = Transactions of the American Philosophical Society, vol. 90.6 (Philadephia 2000).

Mirkin, M. A. (ed.), *Midrash Rabbah*, 11 vols. (Tel Aviv 1968–74).

Muntner, S. (ed.), *Saladino di Ascoli: Compendium Aromatariorum. The Book of the Pharmacists. Based on a Hebrew Ms. of the early XV. Century* (Tel Aviv 1953).

Neubauer, A., *Catalogue of the Hebrew Manuscripts in the Bodleian Library* (Oxford 1886, repr. 1994), and *Supplement of Addenda and Corrigenda*, comp. under the direction of M. Beit-Arié and ed. by R. A. May (Oxford 1994).

Neubauer, A., and Renan, E., *Les Écrivains Français du XIVe Siècle* (Paris 1893, repr. 1969).

Paniagua, J. A., Ferre, L., and Feliu, E. (eds.), *Arnaldi de Villanova Opera Medica Omnia*, vol. 6.1 (Barcelona 1990).

Preuss, J., *Biblical and Talmudic Medicine*, trans. and ed. by F. Rosner (New York 1978).

Richler, B., *Hebrew Manuscripts in the Vatican Library: Catalogue*, comp. by the staff of the Institute of Microfilmed Hebrew Manuscripts, Jewish National and University Library, Jerusalem; Palaeographical and Codicological Descriptions by M. Beit-Arié (Jerusalem 2008).

Richler, 'Manuscripts of Avicenna's *Kanon* in Hebrew Translation: A Revised and Up-to-date List,' *Korot* 8.1–2 (1981): 145–68.

Sezgin, F. (ed.), *A Presentation to Would-Be-Authors On Medicine: Al Taṣrīf li-man 'ajiza 'an al-Ta'līf by Abū'l-Qāsim al-Zahrāwī, Khalaf ibn 'Abbās (d. ca. 1010 AD)*, 2 vols. (Frankfurt 1986).

Sezgin (ed.), *Provisions for the Traveller and Sustenance for the Resident: Zād al-musāfir wa-qūt al-ḥāḍir by Ibn al-Jazzār, Abū Ja'far Aḥmad ibn Ibrāhīm ibn Abī Khālid (d. 979 AD)*, 2 vols., repr. from the Izmir manuscript, in collab. with M. Amawi and E. Neubauer, = Publications of the Institute for the History of Arabic-Islamic Science, Series C: Facsimile Editions, vols. 59.1–2 (Frankfurt 1996).

Siddiqi, M. Z. (ed.), *ʿAlī b. Rabban al-Ṭabarī: Firdaws al-ḥikma* (Berlin 1928).

Siggel, A. (ed.), *Das Buch der Gifte des Ǧābir ibn Ḥayyān: Arabischer Text in Faksimile (HS. Taymūr, Ṭibb 393, Kairo)* (Wiesbaden 1958).

Spencer, W. G. (ed. and trans.), *Celsus: De medicina* (Cambridge 1977).

Steinschneider, M., *Catalogus Codicum Hebraeorum Bibliothecae Academiae Lugduno-Batavae* (Leiden 1858).

Steinschneider, *Die hebräischen Handschriften der K. Hof—und Staatsbibliothek in München*, 2nd rev. enl. ed. (Munich 1895).

Steinschneider, *Die hebräischen Übersetzungen des Mittelalters und die Juden als Dolmetscher* (Berlin 1893, repr. 1956).

Stroumsa, S., *Maimonides in His World: Portrait of a Mediterrean Thinker* (Princeton 2009.

Tallmadge May, M. (trans.), *Galen: On the Usefulness of the Parts of the Body*, 2 vols. (Ithaca 1968).

Tamani, G., *Il Canon medicinae di Avicenna nella tradizione ebraica: Le miniature del manoscritto 2197 della Biblioteca Universitaria di Bologna* (Padova 1988).

Ullmann, M., *Die Medizin im Islam* (Leiden 1970).

van der Heide, A., *Hebrew Manuscripts of Leiden University Library* (Leiden 1977).

Wallis, F., *Medieval Medicine: A Reader* (Toronto 2010).

Weiss, J. G., *Middot u-Mishkalot shel Torah* (Jerusalem 1985).

Westberg, F. (trans.), 'Ibrâhîm's-ibn-Jaʿḳûb's Reiseberight [für Reisebericht] über die Slawenlande aus dem Jahre 965', in *Mémoires de l'Académie Impériale des Sciences de St.-Pétersbourg*, ser. 8, *Classe historico-philologique*, vol. 3.4 (St. Petersburg 1898), repr. in *Studies on Ibrāhīm ibn Yaʿqūb (2nd Half 10th Century) and on His Account of Eastern Europe*, ed. by F. Sezgin et al., = PIHAIS: Islamic Geography, vol. 159 (Frankfurt 1994).

Zotenberg, H., *Catalogues des Manuscrits hébreux et samaritains de la Bibliothèque Impériale* (Paris 1866).

Corrections and Additions to NM 1–3

NM 1:23–4, s.v. התחכחות, correct התחכחות as: התחככות; also index, 202.

NM 1:60–1, s.v. מצנפות, correct as מצנפת, Plur. מצנפות; ‘bandage’, correct as: ‘bandages’.

NM 1:77–8, s.v. אִסָּר or אֱסָר: correct ‘tendon’ (= trans. Spink-Lewis) as ‘nerve’ (עצב) (Arab. عصبة).

NM 1:85, s.v. דליות: correct Arab. دوالى as Arab. دالية, Plur. دوالٍ.

NM 1:85–6, s.v. דרדני: correct Arab. لثّة as لثة.

NM 1:86, s.v. הברה, correct ‘borborygmi’ as ‘intestinal rumbling’ (borborygmus), and delete the reference to UW 239, as the Greek ἐμπνευμάτωσις seems to be rendered as أرواح and قرقرة.

NM 1:90–1, s.v. חבל הזרוע: חֶבֶל: correct Arab. حبل لذراع as حبل الذراع.

NM 1:92, s.v. חיק העין: חיק: correct ליהורי as ליהודי.

NM 1:93, s.v. תחת החלציים: חלצים: correct: תחת החלציים: חלץ; ibid.: ‘hypochondria’; correct: ‘hypochondrium’.

NM 1:120, s.v. תער הגלבים, correct: (fol. 203b; SL 6–8) as: (fol. 203b; SL 17, 6–8).

NM 1:129–30, s.v. אספוגות: correct והאספוגות האבר as ואספוגות האבר.

NM 1:143, s.v. הזיר (זור): correct: הֲזָרָה.

NM 1:144, s.v. זַכּוּת: Add: Arab. ذكاء.

NM 1:151, s.v. חֶנֶק: correct ודומה as ודומהו.

NM 1:155–6, s.v. ירידת המים בעין: ירידה: The term features in BM 2968 in an attestation from the *Sefer ha-Qanun*.

NM 1:168, s.v. נמשך זו אחר זו: משך correct as: נמשך זה אחר זה: משך.

NM 2:35, s.v. גִּעוּשׁ: correct ותשתקק as ותשתוקק.

NM 2:37, s.v. דפוס: correct הצטרך as תצטרך.

NM 2:39–40, s.v. הנחה: correct: הנחָה חמה: הנחה.

NM 2:44–5, s.v. חולים חדים: חד: ‘acute diseases’: add: cf. 7.11.

NM 2:49, s.v. חפף: correct Pi‘el חיפף as Pu‘al חופף.

NM 2:55, n. 72: correct الرمض as الرمص.

NM 2:60, s.v. מכחול: The quotation from Nathan ha-Me’ati also features in BM 2990, while the term itself is defined by Ben Yehuda as something with which a medicine is dripped into the ear and the like (see also entry מכחול).

NM 3:6, n. 33: add: ‘For the translation by Hillel, I consulted Ms Berlin, Staatsbibliothek, Or. Qu. 517’.

NM 3:25, s.v. אַמָּה: ‘nerve’; added after the Arabic عصبة.

NM 3:34, s.v. בלבול השכל: בלבול: correct ‘north [winds]’ as ‘north winds’.

NM 3:51, s.v. דן (דון) (Hillel; fol. 24b) = Latin ‘indicare’; read: Latin ‘iudicare’.

NM 3:53–4, s.v. דֶּפֶק 'tetanus'; Actually the regular Hebrew term for 'tetanus' featuring in the *Sefer Agur* is not דפק but דפק הגידים as in the following entry.

NM 3:55, entry דרך השתן: correct כל מי שבדרך השתן יולדו as כל מי שבדרך השתן הנה יולדו.

NM 3:142, s.v. מראות: מַרְאָה: correct as: מַרְאֶה, Plur. מראות.

NM 3:165–6, s.v. נתן הרפואה: correct the Ibn Tibbon quote as: אמר אבקראט: ראוי שתנתן הרפואה למעוברת כאשר יהיו הליחות מתעוררות אחר שיעבור על הולד ארבעה חדשים עד שיעברו עליו שבעה חדשים ויכניס עצמו בזה מעט ואולם המעט מזה והיותר הנה ראוי שישמור ממנו.

NM 3:172, s.v. עִוּוּת: correct Arab. مغص 'colic' as 'colic' (Latin 'torsio').

NM 3:181–2, s.v. עצר: עוֹצֵר: correct ליראו as לירא.

Index

Greek

Arabic

Latin

Romance (Occitan)